CLINICAL SOCIAL WORK SUPERVISION
Second Edition
Carlton Munson, DSW

SOME ADVANCE REVIEWS

"Provides a comprehensive and insightful examination of social work supervision. An historical and ethical context anchors the subject. The author's discussion of supervisory styles and practitioners' practices of these styles is particularly noteworthy."

Alex Gitterman, EdD, MSW
Professor of Social Work
Columbia University

"Provides an expanded, even more definitive treatment of current dimensions of supervision than the highly regarded *An Introduction to Social Work Supervision*. This book presents a careful and thoughtful analysis of the many facets of clinical supervision. . . . Timely and significant, this book is essential reading for practicing supervisors and those who wish to become supervisors."

Margaret R. Rodway, PhD
Professor, Faculty of Social Work
The University of Calgary

"A must for all clinical social workers because social work education gives scant attention to supervision during MSW education; skilled supervision will pick up on unresolved personal problems of young social workers and provide appropriate referrals. Dr. Munson provides the information necessary for the science part of the science/art equation in supervision. I strongly recommend it to new and experienced practitioners."

Donald R. Bardill, PhD
Dean and Professor, School of Social Work
Florida State University

NOTES FOR PROFESSIONAL LIBRARIANS AND LIBRARY USERS

This is an original book title published by The Haworth Press, Inc. Unless otherwise noted in specific chapters with attribution, materials in this book have not been previously published elsewhere in any format or language.

CONSERVATION AND PRESERVATION NOTES

The paper used in this publication meets the minimum requirements of American National Standard for Information Sciences–Permanence of Paper for Printed Material, ANSI Z39.48-1984.

Clinical Social Work
Supervision
Second Edition

HAWORTH Social Work Practice
Carlton E. Munson, DSW, Senior Editor

New, Recent, and Forthcoming Titles:

Management and Information Systems in Human Services: Implications for the Distribution of Authority and Decision Making by Richard K. Caputo

The Creative Practitioner: Creative Theory and Method for the Helping Services by Bernard Gelfand

Social Work Theory and Practice with the Terminally Ill by Joan K. Parry

Social Work in Health Settings: Practice in Context by Toba Schwaber Kerson and Associates

Gerontological Social Work Supervision by Ann Burack-Weiss and Frances Coyle Brennan

Group Work: Skills and Strategies for Effective Interventions by Sondra Brandler and Camille P. Roman

If a Partner Has AIDS: Guide to Clinical Intervention for Relationships in Crisis by R. Dennis Shelby

Social Work Practice: A Systems Approach by Benyamin Chetkow-Yanoov

Elements of the Helping Process: A Guide for Clinicians by Raymond Fox

Clinical Social Work Supervision, Second Edition by Carlton E. Munson

Intervention Research: Design and Development for the Human Services edited by Jack Rothman and Edwin J. Thomas

Forensic Social Work: Legal Aspects of Professional Practice by Robert L. Barker and Douglas M. Branson

Now Dare Everything: Tales of HIV-Related Psychotherapy by Steven Dansky

Clinical Social Work
Supervision
Second Edition

Carlton E. Munson, DSW

The Haworth Press
New York • London • Norwood (Australia)

For additional information about the contents of this book, video and audio tape supplements, and supervision seminars contact:

Dr. Carlton Munson
Washington Area Supervision Institute
218 Mealey Parkway
Hagerstown, Maryland 21742

Telephone: (310) 733-3714

The Haworth Press, Inc., 10 Alice Street, Binghamton, NY 13904-1580

Library of Congress Cataloging-in-Publication Data

Munson, Carlton E.
    Clinical social work supervision / Carlton E. Munson. — 2nd ed.
      p. cm.
    Rev. ed. of: An introduction to clinical social work supervision. 1983.
    Includes bibliographical references and index.
    ISBN 1-56024-284-1 (alk. paper) — 1-56024-285-X (pbk: alk. paper).
    1. Social workers — Supervision of. I. Munson, Carlton E. Introduction to clinical social work supervision. II. Title.
    [DNLM: 1. Social Work — organization & administration. 2. Social Work, Psychiatric — organization & administration. HV 41 M969c]
HV40.54.M86   1992
361.3′2′0683 — dc20
DNLM/DLC
for Library of Congress
                                                     92-1462
                                                     CIP

To my wife, Joan Smith Munson

ABOUT THE AUTHOR

Carlton Munson, DSW, is Professor of Social Work and Doctoral Program Director at the School of Social Work, University of Maryland at Baltimore. He has served as a consultant to numerous educational programs, hospitals, long-term care facilities, and criminal justice programs and has conducted a number of workshops and seminars on clinic supervision throughout the United States and abroad. Dr. Munson has published over sixty articles in professional journals and is the author of several books including *Social Work Education and Practice* (JoVon Books), *Social Work Supervision* (The Free Press), *Family of Origin Applications in Clinical Supervision* (The Haworth Press), and *Social Work with Families* (The Free Press). Dr. Munson maintains a public clinical practice near Washington, DC and directs the Washington Area Supervision Institute. An editorial board member for a variety of professional journals, he has been Editor of *The Clinical Supervisor* since its inception in 1983 and is Senior Editor, Social Work Practice, for The Haworth Press.

CONTENTS

Preface   **xv**

Chapter 1: Introduction   **1**

Introduction to the Book   2
Background Research Studies   4
Style of Reading   5
Activity and Practice Differentiation   7
Clinical Practice and Clinical Supervision Defined   8
Function of Supervision   11
Supervision Perspectives   13
What Good Supervisors Do   15
Supervisory Thought Process   16
Cost of Supervision   17
Style   18
Need for Supervision   19
Supervisor Preparation   25
Characteristics of Supervisees   26
Beginning Professionals   27
Organizations   28
Needs of Supervisees   29
Clinical Assessment and Diagnosis   32
Beginning Guidelines   34
Characteristics of Supervisors   35
On Becoming a Clinical Supervisor   35
Authority   36
Avoiding Supervision as Treatment   36
Support for Supervisors   37
Unanticipated Consequences   37

Supervisee Bill of Rights   39
Suggested Readings   43

Chapter 2: History of Supervision   **45**

Practice Knowledge   46
Early History   47
The Freudian Influence   51
Mary Richmond   53
The 1920s   54
The 1930s   56
The 1940s   58
The 1950s   59
The 1960s   63
The 1970s   65
The 1980s   69
The 1990s   70
Supervision Issues   76
Conclusion   77
Suggested Readings   78

Chapter 3: Values and Ethics   **81**

Introduction   82
Values   83
Values and Knowledge   85
Ethics   88
Ethics Knowledge   90
Extent of Ethics Violations   92
Advancing Ethics Knowledge   93
Suggested Readings   93

Chapter 4: Supervisor Styles   **95**

Introduction   96
Observing Styles   97
Style as a Resource   98
Style as a Concept   99
Applying Style   103
Supervisor Styles   105
Style and Theoretical Orientation   114
Suggested Readings   115

Chapter 5: Practitioners' Reactions to Supervisor Styles 117

Introduction 118
Supervisee Expectations 118
Interactional Reactions 120
Conclusion 128
Suggested Readings 129

Chapter 6: Technique in Supervision 131

Introduction 132
Educational Assessment 132
Case Material 135
Case Presentations 137
Level of Knowing and Technique 138
Continuity 139
Treatment Patterns 140
Mechanics of Technique 140
Overcoming Difficulty 141
Technical Difficulty 143
Questioning Technique 144
Contracting as a Technique 145
Reading as Technique 146
Latent Supervision 148
Supervisor Resistance 149
Guidelines 150
Suggested Readings 151

Chapter 7: The Role of Authority and Structure 153

Introduction 154
Organizations and Authority 155
Authority and Supervision 156
Interaction and Authority 159
Authority and Structure 161
Style and Authority 163
Age and Authority 165
Autonomy 165
Group Supervision 169
Conclusion 173
Suggested Readings 173

Chapter 8: Use of Theory 175

Introduction 176
Theory in Supervision 176
Confusion About Theory 177
Teaching Theory 181
Theory and Practice Connection 183
Elements of Theory 184
Functions of Theory 188
Components of Theory 190
Theoretical Speculation 192
Timing 193
Theory and Technique 193
Theory Abandonment 194
Creativity and Theory 197
Theory Application 197
Theory and Supervision Interaction 198
Guidelines for Applying Theory to Clinical Material 200
Conclusion 201
Suggested Readings 201

Chapter 9: Evaluation of Practice 203

Introduction 204
Evaluation of Learning 205
Simplicity 206
Practice Errors 208
Follow-Up and Evaluation 210
Criticism of Clinical Material 210
Reactions to Criticism 212
Evaluation and Self-Assessment 214
Research and Practice 215
Note Taking 217
Record Keeping 218
Administrative Evaluation 221
Practice Research and Supervision 222
Suggested Readings 225

Chapter 10: Stress Reactions   **229**

Introduction   230
Research on Stress Among Social Workers   230
Students and Stress   232
Supervision and Stress   233
Supervisor Stress   234
Role of Support   235
General Principles   236
Contributing Factors   243
Dealing with Stress   244
The Supervisor's Role   246
Unanswered Questions   247
Supervisor Training   250
Despair and Isolation   250
The Beginning Professional   253
Suggested Readings   255

Chapter 11: Administrative Activities   **257**

Introduction   258
Record Keeping   258
Legal Issues   261
Duty to Warn   262
Violence and Safety   264
Credentials and Examinations   267
Dealing with the Administrator   269
Administrator Styles   270
Suggested Readings   280

Chapter 12: Audiovisual and Action Techniques   **283**

Television (Videotape)   284
Knowledge Gap   284
Taping the Therapy to Be Supervised   287
Audiotaping   291
Audio/Video Separation   292
Role Play   292
Role Play Procedures   293
Live Supervision   299

Intrusion of Privacy   301
Ranking of Techniques   301
Suggested Readings   302

Chapter 13: Supervision in Different Settings   **305**

Different Settings   306
Medical Settings   306
Geriatrics and Gerontology Settings   310
Criminal Justice Settings   317
Rural Practice Settings   324
Suggested Readings   331

Chapter 14: Supervision in Unique Situations   **333**

Introduction   334
Practitioners Who Are in Therapy   334
Family Therapy Supervision   335
Family of Origin Material in Supervision   342
Cotherapist Activity   349
Consultation   356
Gender and Supervision   362
Ergonomics   375
Suggested Readings   376

Chapter 15: Art and Science in Social Work Practice   **379**

Introduction   380
Traditions   381
Art Terminology Confusion   383
Artistic Elements and Scientifically Based Practice   383
Elements of Art   385
Art as Defense   390
Patterns and Art   391
Science   392
Social Work and Artistic Qualities   395
Book Conclusion   397
Suggested Readings   400

References   **401**

Appendix 1: Assessment Scale for Becoming a Clinical
  Supervisor   423

Appendix 2: Educational Assessment Scale   425

Appendix 3: Credentialing, Accrediting, and Service
  Organizations in Social Work   429

Appendix 4: Code of Ethics of the National Association
  of Social Workers   433

Appendix 5: Knowledge Survey for the NASW Code
  of Ethics   445

Appendix 6: Practitioner Self-Assessment Form   449

Appendix 7: Short Form Stress Scale   453

Appendix 8: Supervision Questionnaire   457

Appendix 9: Long Form Stress Questionnaire   467

Index   473

List of Visuals

Visual 1.1. Correlation of Supervisee Satisfaction and Level
of Interaction with the Supervisor   30

Visual 1.2. Correlation of Supervisor Satisfaction with Supervisory
Role and Level of Interaction with Supervisees   31

Visual 4.1. Conceptualization of Main and Substyles   104

Visual 5.1. Matrix of Supervision Styles and Supervisee Reactions   130

Visual 7.1. Models of Supervisory Intervention   166

Visual 9.1. Practitioner's Perception of Sessions   207

Visual 9.2. Practitioner Perception of a Session   207

Visual 10.1. Coping, Strategies, Practice Demands, and Stress   251

Visual 11.1. Typical Clinical Forms   259

Visual 11.2. Diagram of Typical Treatment Process   260

Visual 11.3. Administrator Styles   271

Visual 14.1. Combinations of Interactions for Treatment Situations   336

Visual 14.2. SEES System for Analyzing Family Therapy
Interactional Sequences   343

Visual 15.1. Elements of Practice Style   398

Preface

I have been writing this book for the past 24 years. It has evolved through much reading, note taking, journal article and professional paper writing, course teaching and taking, and workshop conducting and attending. It was put aside twice — to write a dissertation on supervision and to edit a book on supervision. Over the past year I have returned to the notes, the libraries, and my desk to complete the second edition of this book. During the 24 years, social work practice and supervision have changed substantially. Every page, line, and word of this book has been reviewed for relevance to modern practice. This has resulted in numerous alterations, deletions, and additions that I hope make this book as clinically up to date as possible. The title of the book has been updated. "An Introduction" has been dropped because it was felt when the manuscript was completed that the coverage was more than an introduction to the topic of supervision. This book is a comprehensive treatment of clinical social work supervision.

In 1983 the first edition of this book appeared. From the day it appeared, I began collecting information for the second edition. There have been major revisions with much new material that relates to the enormous changes in practice that have occurred over the last decade. The changes emerged from my own practice and the comments and suggestions made by practicing supervisors who have attended workshops and seminars I have conducted. I owe a tremendous debt to the many people who have attended these workshops and seminars and so clearly articulated strengths and weaknesses of the first edition of the book. The information they provided was invaluable in revising the book.

My own learning and reflection about the profession have been sharpened by the effort that went into writing the first edition of this book and rewriting for the second edition. Above all, I think I have become a better supervisor and practitioner as a by-product of this arduous task. My hope is that others can benefit from reading this book, as I feel I have from writing it.

Any task that covers so many years involves literally hundreds of people who have contributed to the final product. My own teachers, students, and colleagues have nurtured the creative thought process. My wife, Joan, to whom this book is dedicated, deserves more credit than I can express. I hope I can somehow make up to her all the lost days of sharing and that those days can be recaptured. I appreciate the initial reviews of the manuscript by Al Roberts and Max Siporin, and owe much to Bill Cohen who has had faith in this and other projects we have worked on. Also, I appreciate the thorough editorial assistance of Trudy Raschkind Steinfeld on the first edition of the book. I want to thank my many classroom students at Fordham University and the field instruction students from University of Maryland School of Social Work I have supervised over the last five years. I have learned so very much from my classroom students and my field instruction students.

When writing a book, an author gets so caught up in the process that the rightness and necessity of certain things begin to seem self-evident, and it is hard for an author to understand why the rest of the world does not see what he sees. I have come to think that the writer is the one who does not see. In one's devotion to a topic, one may fail to consider many of the other models, other methods, and other approaches that exist. One may be blinded by one's focus. I am glad that this book is now completed so that I can begin to see again.

> Teaching is even more difficult than learning . . . because what teaching calls for is this: to let learn. The real teacher . . . lets nothing else be learned than learning.
>
> Martin Heidegger
> *What Is Called Thinking?*

Chapter 1

Introduction

This chapter is an overview of supervision. Background conceptions, a definition of clinical supervision, and the function of supervision are covered. The interactional framework that serves as background for subsequent chapters is summarized. Current issues and conditions that give rise to the need for supervision are delineated. Characteristics of supervisees and supervisors are summarized along with factors that need to be considered when becoming a clinical supervisor.

INTRODUCTION TO THE BOOK

If this book delineated all the things the supervisor must know and do in order to be effective, helpful, and appreciated, after reading it most of us would ask: Why would anyone want to become a supervisor? The answer to this question is complex, but to save time and space, it can be answered with: Because we want to be effective, helpful, and appreciated. Otherwise, we would have chosen some other, less humane, endeavor as a career.

Few supervisors have the luxury of devoting all their time to their supervisory roles, so they must be highly organized and efficient to be successful, helpful, and appreciated. Some people find that supervision is more demanding than they expected, and they return to practice activities full time. Others resign themselves to limited effectiveness, proceed through trial and error, become cynical and disillusioned, and pass this attitude on to their supervisees. Some struggle to do a good job and work harder and harder until they eventually succumb to distress. In all three of these situations, the knowledge and skills of good people are not passed on to the next generation of practitioners. Our profession cannot afford such losses.

This book is designed to help the profession avoid the loss of transmission of this knowledge and skill and to facilitate the passage of practice wisdom from one professional generation to the next. I hope that the practices and guidelines presented here will make the supervisory job easier without sacrificing substance and quality. Too often we have failed and abandoned our supervisory responsibility because we lacked adequate coping mechanisms. It was simply less demanding or more rewarding to devote oneself to other endeavors.

We are fortunate to live in an era and work in a professional generation that still allows us to trace our own supervisory heritage directly to such people as Mary Richmond, Jane Addams, Bertha Reynolds, Porter Lee, Mary Conyngton, Lucille Austin, Ida Cannon, Frances Scherz, Yonata Feldman, Fred Berl, Dorothy Hutchinson, Jessie Taft, Virginia Robinson, and Sigmund and Anna Freud. I have interviewed, talked with, and read the published and unpublished works of many colleagues who studied under and were supervised by these great contributors to our own knowledge, skill, and practice. I have been supervised and taught by people with such connections to our heritage, and feel a part of a legacy that sustains **my commitment to the profession of social work.**

Through my supervisory work, my teaching, and through this book, I hope to make my contribution to passing on this legacy and to promote the possibility of others' doing the same. Too many of our students and supervisees think social work began some time around 1960. If our profession is to endure, we must transmit more of an understanding of and appreciation for our history to those who come after us.

I decided to write this book because there has never been one devoted exclusively to clinical social work supervision. That no such book has been written in the past is difficult to understand, given that casework has been the foundation of the profession since the beginning and that clinical treatment has in the past decade reemerged as the major practice area. Social work treatment has remained the major area of specialization among graduate students. Social workers are the largest professional group delivering psychotherapy services in the United States, and the National Association of Social Workers (NASW) has reported that social workers are the largest single professional group offering treatment services in mental health centers and the numbers continue to increase. From 1987 to 1990, the percentage of social workers practicing in mental health increased from 28 to 31 percent of NASW membership. Since approximately 50 percent of trained social workers join NASW (129,092 members), the total number of social workers practicing in metal health is substantial. Nine percent of the NASW membership report that they are doing full-time supervision. NASW research data regarding functional activity indicates that approximately 30 percent of the members are performing functions that would involve some supervision (National Association of Social Workers, 1991:5). So, a significant percentage of social work professionals are engaged in clinical practice and supervision of clinical work. The few books that have been written on supervision have a much more general approach to the topic than is helpful to the supervisor in such clinical settings and situations.

At a broader level, social work education has increasingly placed emphasis on generic skills, even though specialization in agencies has expanded greatly. This basic incongruity has led many agencies and organizations to place renewed emphasis on supervision as a means of overcoming this gap between educational focus and practice demands. Supervisors attempting to help new practitioners develop their skills have very few guidelines to use. What I have attempted to do in this book is to provide some very practical guidelines to assist the supervisor of clinical practitioners.

Most books on supervision to date have focused on what to learn and how to learn regarding clinical work through supervision. This book covers the essential aspect of supervision, but another component has been added by placing this material in the framework of the supervision process itself. What has to be learned about and done in practice is presented in the context of how the supervisor acts—what the supervisor says, hears, and writes. Organizationally, supervisors receive limited training, feedback, and support group help for what they do. This book is for and about supervisors.

BACKGROUND RESEARCH STUDIES

Throughout the book I make reference to research studies I have done on supervision. Some of these studies have been reported in the literature, and they are cited and referenced in the text. Other studies I refer to are so recent that they have not yet appeared in the literature. Rather than repeat the details of these studies in the text each time they are referred to, I have listed the studies here.

- A survey of 34 graduate students, representing a 10 percent random sample of students in one school of social work. The students completed questionnaires regarding their clinical activity and their supervisory activity (Study A).
- An intensive content analysis of the supervisory experience of three graduate social work students. Weekly one-hour research interviews were done over a nine-month period in which supervision activity was systematically analyzed based on the students' perceptions (Study B).
- A study of 26 field instructors selected at random from all the field instructors at one graduate school of social work. Each participant was administered an interview schedule that took an hour to complete. The supervisors were surveyed regarding their style of supervision, theoretical orientation, and philosophy of supervision and practice. In addition, demographic data were gathered (Study C).
- A survey of 183 workers and supervisors in a department of public welfare regarding their experiences in and attitudes toward supervision. The questionnaire also included a series of questions regarding the amount of stress the participants had experienced (Study D).
- A survey of 82 graduate students in a school of social work regarding the degree of stress they experienced in connection with classroom and field components of their educational program (Study E).

- A survey of 40 clinical social work practitioners regarding their therapy work with respect to type of therapy performed, theoretical orientation, cotherapy activity, and conflict with colleagues (Study F).
- A survey study conducted through interviews with 30 practitioners regarding the styles of administration of supervisors and administrators. This study resulted in six administrative types that have been used with over 300 practitioners to test the accuracy of the classifications (Study G).
- A content analysis study of video tape sessions of master therapist. The tapes of Ackerman, Bowen, Framo, Minuchin, Papp, Rubentstein, Satir, and Whitaker were analyzed for common techniques and themes. This resulted in the development of the SEES classification system (Style, Enabling, Encountering, and Shifting dysfunction) of intervention sequences (Study H).
- A survey of 50 social workers' knowledge of the National Association of Social Workers Code of Ethics through administration of a 50-item instrument (Study I).

In addition to these formal studies I have used case examples and comments made by supervisors and supervisees in connection with teaching, consultation, and training I have done in various settings. Throughout the book I have attempted to blend empirical research findings with practical observations to form sound, logical, reasonable suggestions and recommendations for supervisors. Questionnaires used in some of this research can be found in the appendixes.

STYLE OF READING

Although many suggestions and guidelines are offered for use in supervision, I refrain from providing any suggestions on how to read this book to avoid hampering creative use of it. The only suggestion is to follow the advice of Virginia Woolf (1932; 1960):

> The only advice, indeed, that one person can give another about reading is to take no advice, to follow your own instincts, to use your own reason, to come to your own conclusions. (p. 281)

Given Woolf's suggestion, I offer only one recommendation as you begin. **Avoid getting defensive about some of your own practices in light of the new and different guidelines I suggest, because the moment you become** defensive, learning ceases. Again, Woolf advocates a point of view I recommend to the reader:

> Do not dictate to your author; try to become him. If you hang back, and reserve and criticize at first, you are preventing yourself from getting the fullest possible value from what you read. But if you open your mind as widely as possible, then signs and hints of almost imperceptible fineness, from the twist and turn of the sentences, will bring you into the presence of a human being unlike any other. (p. 282)

Abstract discussion in this text has been minimized and only used to lay the foundation for the practical guidelines that are offered. The book is designed as a text for learning good supervisory practices through formal academic course work, but it can also serve as a resource for the practicing supervisor. The theoretical material and practice principles are interlaced with case material to illustrate major points.

Each chapter concludes with a list of suggested readings including brief summary statements about the usefulness of each citation. These suggested readings were drawn on for much of the material in each chapter, and can be used to supplement that particular chapter. I hope that these lists will be a valuable, quick reference tool for the busy educator and supervisor who do not have large blocks of time available to engage in many hours of extensive library research.

The concept of style is used a great deal in this book because it has been my experience that it is one of those simple, but powerful, terms that can be used to organize large amounts of helpful information. Style is defined and then used to identify the major styles of supervision. Very little has been written elsewhere about style as a concept. I have discovered the usefulness of this concept only in the past several years, and continue to develop its use in my supervisory practice. The ideas about style used here are tentative.

In this book the terms practitioner, worker, and therapist are used interchangeably. All of these terms are used to refer to those actively engaged in short-term and long-term contact with clients for the purpose of some type of intervention to resolve problems in functioning. Also, in the same vein, the terms client and patient are used interchangeably.

Edgar Allen Poe believed that to make an impression, any literary work must be able to be read in one sitting. I have tried to keep this rule of brevity in mind while writing this book. At the same time, each chapter is constructed as a reference source so that the supervisor and/or supervisee can come back to it many times until the suggestions and guidelines become a natural part of the supervisory process.

ACTIVITY AND PRACTICE DIFFERENTIATION

The practice of clinical social work is difficult to achieve. Often, *activity* masquerades as practice. Immanuel Kant distinguished *practice* by noting that it is the "pursuit of a purpose which is thought of as application of certain general principles of procedure," and "there needs to be a connecting and mediating link between theory and practice'; but at the same time, practice cannot be directly deduced from theory. Practice is disciplined conduct that rules out certain random activity. The Kantian conception of the relation between theory and practice that stresses rational, enlightened, practical conduct based on theory (Holzner & Marx, 1979:36) is of paramount importance to the supervisor. The supervisor's chief function is to minimize activity and maximize practice. Much of the interaction between supervisor and practitioner is related to transforming activity into practice. Inexperienced as well as experienced practitioners engage in activity that must be translated into practice if treatment is to be effective. At times all practitioners need minor and major help in giving meaning, purpose, and discipline to what we do in relation to clients, and this is the function of supervision.

Too often with adult learners in social work, supervisors have taken Heidegger's concept of "to let learn," cited above, to mean let the student alone. This is not what they need; in fact, it can be detrimental. Knowles (1970) has argued that when adults are given responsibility for their own learning, their initial reaction is usually shock and disorganization, and this reaction has been confirmed in a research study of andragogical methods (based on learning applied with self-directed, experienced, and problem-centered adults) used to train a group of social workers (Gelfand et al., 1975). When learners are asked to be more responsible for their own learning, the supervisor becomes more important rather than less important. What is critical is the way in which the supervisor relates to the supervisee. The guidelines in the following chapters are focused on relating to supervisees as adult learners without abandoning them.

CLINICAL PRACTICE AND CLINICAL SUPERVISION DEFINED

The term clinical social work is used because that is the most descriptive, in current phraseology, of what a certain group of social work practitioners perform. In the past clinical social work has been referred to as casework, social casework, psychiatric social work, social treatment, psychotherapy, and probably many other things. The desire here is to keep terminology from becoming a barrier to advancing our knowledge and understanding of supervision. It has been argued that the term "clinical social work" in the past decade has "become a euphemism for 'social casework,' treatment — oriented 'social group work,' 'social treatment,' 'psychiatric social work' and 'direct practice'" (Minahan, 1980:171). At the same time efforts are being made to conceptualize a definition of clinical social work consistent with our heritage of evolving a coherent knowledge base and practice domains (see Goldstein, E. G., 1980; Simon, B. K., 1977).

The term clinical social work is relatively new (Ewalt, 1980:23). It still lacks specificity and has given rise to divergent definitions, as manifested in the proceedings of a national conference on clinical social work held in Denver, Colorado in 1980 (Ewalt, 1980). In all of the definitions that have been offered, a common idea is that it involves work with individuals, families, and groups. The comprehensive term "clinical social work" appears to be designed to unite the diversity of practice that exists. There seems to be a view that clinical social work encompasses psychotherapy, but goes beyond this form of practice. There has been a tendency in the practice literature, and especially in the supervision literature, to use a very broad definition of clinical practice based more on setting than on tasks. Some of the supervision literature mixes clinical psychotherapy and case management oriented supervision (Kadushin, 1991). Practice literature indicates that agencies are making distinctions between case management practice and clinical practice. For example, practice in child welfare has been characterized as:

> . . . public child welfare is now believed to be that of a conduit to private-for-profit or not-for-profit agencies that provide direct services rather than provider of direct services itself. Referred to as "case management," public child welfare practice now involves **referring clients** to appropriate external service providers, monitoring them, and maintaining liaison with external service providers. (Samantrai, 1991:359)

This observation is most likely associated with the reported increase of social workers in private practice from 10.9 percent in 1982 to 16.1 percent in 1990 (National Association of Social Workers, 1991). Such changes will require more precision in our definition of what constitutes clinical social work practice.

The definition of clinical social work has been evolving over the last two decades. This evolution has resulted in refinement of the definition, but also has led to some diversity that has resulted in multiple definitions that are used by different organizations which has resulted in some confusion (Kenemore, 1991: 83-93). For example, The National Registry of Health Care Providers in Clinical Social Work was guided by the following statement:

> Clinical social work practice includes provision of mental health services for the diagnosis, treatment and prevention of mental and emotional disorders in individuals, families and groups. Clinical Social Work Practice is based on knowledge and theory of psychosocial development, behavior, psychopathology, unconscious motivation, interpersonal relationships and environmental stress. Treatment interventions include, but are not limited to, individual, marital, family and group psychotherapy. (National Institute for Clinical Social Work Advancement, 1987)

The National Association of Social Workers uses a slightly different definition:

> Clinical Social Work shares with all other social work practice the goal of enhancement and maintenance of psychosocial functioning of individuals, families, and small groups. Clinical social work practice is the professional application of social work theory and methods to the treatment and prevention of psychosocial dysfunction, disability, or impairment, including emotional and mental disorders. It is based on knowledge of one or more theories of human development with a psychosocial context.
>
> The perspective of person-in-situation is central to clinical social work practice. Clinical social work includes interventions directed to interpersonal interactions, intrapsychic dynamics, and life-support and management issues. Clinical social work services consist of assessment, diagnosis and treatment, including psychotherapy and counseling, client-centered advocacy, consultation and evaluation. The process of clinical social work is undertaken within the objec-

tives of social work and the principles and values contained in the NASW Code of Ethics. (National Association of Social Workers, 1987)

The American Board of Examiners in Clinical Social Work, a group formed to certify advanced practice, uses a different definition:

> Clinical social work practice is the professional application of social work theory and methods to the treatment and prevention of psychosocial dysfunction, disability or impairment, including emotional and mental disorders. It is based on knowledge and theory of psychosocial development, behavior, psychopathology, unconscious motivation, interpersonal relationships, environmental stress, social systems, and cultural diversity with particular attention to person-in-environment. It shares with all social work practice the goal of enhancement and maintenance of psychosocial functioning of individuals, families and small groups. (American Board of Examiners in Clinical Social Work, 1989:7)

For the purposes of this book, clinical social work practice is defined as:

> *organized efforts by graduates of accredited schools of social work to assist people to overcome physical, financial, social, or psychological disruptions in functioning through individual, group, or family intervention methods.*

The definition of clinical supervision in social work must naturally parallel the definition of clinical practice. With the above definition in mind the following definition of clinical supervision in social work is used by the author:

> *Clinical supervision is an interactional process in which a supervisor has been assigned or designated to assist in and direct the practice of supervisees in the areas of teaching, administration, and helping. The supervisees are graduates of accredited schools of social work who are engaged in practice that assists people to overcome physical, financial, social, or psychological disruptions in functioning through individual, group, or family intervention methods efforts.*

Supervisory assistance is not necessarily limited to these areas, but they are the main ones that traditionally have been associated with supervision in social work. The key words in this definition that distinguish supervision from consultation are *assigned*, *designated*, and *direct*. A supervisor has been assigned or designated by an agency, organization, or statute to supervise another's practice, and the supervisee is expected to be accountable to the supervisor. The supervisor is a person who has some official sanction to direct and guide the supervisee's practice.

Consultation, on the other hand, has no such official sanction. The practitioner is free to decide whether to seek consultation, and is free to decide whether to implement the advice and recommendations of a consultant. This is an important distinction because, in recent times, there has been a tendency to use the two terms interchangeably. The trend toward referring to supervision as consultation to minimize the authority involved in supervision has been problematic for some supervisors and supervisees. (This difficulty is discussed in Chapter 7 in the section "Authority and Supervision.")

FUNCTION OF SUPERVISION

Just as the scientific method can be applied to any problem or question, supervision can be applied to any clinical problem or question. Supervision can be superimposed on any theory or technique used in practice. Although we do not have precise rules to guide us in supervision, as is the case with the scientific method, it is possible to identify some basic, general rules that can be useful in approaching practice situations and problems. A major purpose of this book is to identify those basic rules. The principles and guidelines presented in the following chapters can be applied by any supervisor, regardless of his or her theoretical orientation or the theoretical orientation of the supervisees.

Treatment often requires that the client and practitioner have faith in the process of treatment without much empirical evidence to justify this faith. Because of this, supervision becomes important as it serves as the arena in which data are accumulated, documented, evaluated, and made known as a measure of the success or failure of the treatment. Supervision is the only check and balance on the alliance of faith and action of treatment. The investment of faith is as important to the practitioner as it is to the client, and supervision is where faith is sustained and reinforced for the practitioner. The client must rely on himself or herself and the practitioner for perpetuation of therapeutic faith. For this reason the supervisor is important to the practitioner as well as the client, although the client rarely knows it. This makes rules in supervision crucial. In some respects supervision is research on specific clinical practice that is abstract and defies concrete interpretation.

If we enter supervision viewing it as the place where supervisors give answers, check up on the practitioner's work, and find solutions for the clinician, we will have started off on the wrong foot and will stumble. Supervision should be a mutual sharing of questions, concerns, observations, speculations, and selection of alternative techniques to apply in practice. I call this process the *congruence of perceptions in supervision*. Practitioners should, and want to, participate in supervision rather than be recipients of it. Such mutual understanding requires mutual trust. If mutual trust is missing, then the supervisory relationship is bound to falter and eventually fail.

All of the material in this text is based on the assumption that the supervisor and supervisee trust each other. If there is any doubt about trust, most of the guidelines provided in the following pages will be of little use. Supervision cannot proceed in a climate of mistrust. Where mistrust exists the supervisory process becomes a stand-off, a struggle for survival. Supervision must be viewed as a safe place to share and struggle with concerns, weaknesses, failures, and gaps in skill. The supervisor must work to establish a trusting climate and be diligent to avoid using the information learned in the supervisory process against the supervisee. One must avoid the suspicious philosophy expressed by one supervisor in an initial session with a supervisee: "Different people bring different agendas to supervision." Fortunately, in this situation, the supervisee gave the right answer when she said, "My agenda is to learn."

There is nothing magical, mystical, or arcane about good supervision. There are five basic propositions that serve as the foundation of effective supervision, and they serve as the basis of the material covered in this book. To be effective, supervision must be:

1. *Structured.* There should be a formal structure for the supervision that is made clear to the supervisee. Structure refers to the formats for conducting supervision such as individual supervision, group supervision or a combination of these formats.

2. *Regular.* Regardless of the structure used the supervision should be conducted on a regular basis. It is easy for a busy supervisor to fail to formalize the regularity of supervision and as a result supervision often gets put off.

3. *Consistent.* The supervisor should work to ensure that the style and approach used with the supervisee is consistent. There should be a logical connection between the style and pattern of decision making so the supervisee can anticipate what the expectations are from a situation. The supervisee who has to wonder and guess how the supervisor will react to each situation will be limited in their ability to grow and learn through supervision.

4. *Case oriented.* Supervision, to be effective and efficient, should be case oriented at all times. All other matters are extraneous or secondary. Administrative issues, personal matters, and learning should all be connected to case material when discussed. This material does not have to involve only specific cases, but can also be related to general case discussion. The objective is to keep the supervision focused. Any supervision discussion should be able to be related to the practitioner's cases. If it cannot be related to cases it most likely means the supervision has lost sight of its primary focus.

5. *Evaluated.* The supervision itself should be evaluated. It is the responsibility of supervisors to periodically solicit formal and informal feedback about the supervision practice they are conducting.

SUPERVISION PERSPECTIVES

There are several perspectives from which one can discuss supervision. The most prominent ones are listed here.

1. *Personality perspective.* This perspective involves the characteristics and traits that the participants bring to the supervisory situation and how these influence the practice activity and the supervisory relationship.

2. *Situational perspective.* This approach relates to the specific situations and problems that the participants encounter as part of the supervision process. The focus is on the situations and problems and how to deal with them.

3. *Organizational perspective.* In this model the emphasis is placed on the function of the organization and how the supervision serves to effectively implement the organizational goals and objectives.

4. *Interactional perspective.* This approach, which is the predominant model used in this book, focuses on the interaction between the supervisor

and the supervisee. The emphasis is on how the participants interact and how interaction is varied to fit the specific content of the supervision.

Each of these perspectives is quite complicated. They can produce similar as well as different outcomes. It is common for participants to intermingle the various perspectives. This book is based on an interactional approach to supervision and the styles that emerge from interaction. Organizational, personality, and situational content are included in this perspective, but are analyzed as interactional processes. The content is considered in the context of the interaction. The notion underpinning this book is that the process of supervisory interaction is as important as the content of supervision. Claude Levi-Strauss has succinctly described this view:

> We have tried to introduce into the social sciences the fundamental idea that we are looking at things which are extremely complicated and difficult, sometimes even impossible to describe because of their complexity. Yet if instead of looking at the things themselves we look at the relations which prevail between them, then we will discover that these relationships are altogether more simple and less numerous than the things themselves, and that they can give us a firmer base for investigation. (1978:30)

Following Levi-Strauss' view, the focus in this book is more on the relationship between participants in supervision rather than on supervision as a concept.

Heidegger pointed out that becoming a teacher is much more difficult than becoming a famous professor. The supervisor's job is more difficult than that of the professor because, as Heidegger further argued, teaching is more difficult than learning since the teacher must know how *to let learn*. We have repeatedly failed to recognize the importance of the supervisor as a teacher. Rather than being viewed as a difficult task, letting a person learn has been perceived in much modern social work as a simple process of letting the supervisee alone.

When the supervisor is ill prepared for the role of teacher, there is a tendency to shift the emphasis to interaction about administrative functions, which can create more social and professional distance in the process. This shift in focus illustrates the interactional nature of supervision.

WHAT GOOD SUPERVISORS DO

An important question is: What do supervisors do? A more difficult question is: What do good supervisors do? or, What should supervisors do? The answer to the first two questions is that the five basic actions of the supervisor are:

1. *Reading.* It is essential that the supervisor keep up with the literature and be prepared to guide the supervisee to appropriate literature. There has been an explosion of practice research and vast expansion of practice specializations. Supervisors must devise a method to systematically keep up with the literature if they are to be effective with and helpful to supervisees.

2. *Writing.* The supervisor is required to do various forms of writing in addition to charts and records that are a part of practice. This can vary from setting to setting, but preparing reports, drafting grant proposals and writing articles for publication or presentation are common writing activities. Supervisors need to develop a system to manage all the writing tasks they must do. The supervisor can be an effective role model by recommending works they have written to the supervisee. Engaging in joint writing efforts with the supervisee can also be rewarding for both participants.

3. *Watching.* Supervisors need to be keen observers, using the same observational skills that are necessary for good clinical practice. The supervisor must continually be alert to the performance of supervisees. Not all observations need to become the focus of the supervision, but supervisors should be aware of more than what their supervisees present to them. The supervisor that relies completely on input from the supervisee for judgements and decision making is at a disadvantage.

4. *Talking.* Most supervision activity is accomplished through discussion. The supervisor must possess skill at talking about material with supervisees. This is also the same skill that is needed to be an effective clinician, but the discussion and the techniques used to promote participation need to be altered from the manner in which they are used in the practice situation. Supervisees become uncomfortable and frustrated when the supervisor treats them like clients.

5. *Listening.* This is a crucial skill that the supervisor must possess. It is the same listening skill that is essential to good clinical work. The difference is that, at times, the supervisor will need to be more active in supervision than in the clinical situation. Supervisees sometimes complain that

supervisors are good listeners, but they do not provide enough direct information to assist the supervisee. The supervisor who "just listens" will be of limited help to the supervisee.

Any action of the supervisor fits one of these five categories. This book deals with answering the question: What should supervisors do in these five areas to be effective? It is based on research about the actions of people who have been identified as good supervisors. Each chapter in some way deals with what to read, what and how to write, what and how to watch, what to say and how to say it, and how to listen.

SUPERVISORY THOUGHT PROCESS

Teaching in supervision involves an interactional process, but this must be based on a concomitant thought process. This thought process incorporates the following five components, which can provide a comprehensive approach to most supervisory practice situations.

1. *Perception.* This involves selection of stimuli in the environment, including both the obvious and the not so obvious. There will be areas in which the supervisor perceives that the practitioner needs improvement. This need may or may not be perceived by the worker. The need must be agreed on before learning is pursued.

2. *Imagination.* This relates to creating ideas that were not known to the creator previously, regardless of whether the ideas are known to or in the surrounding environment. The supervisor must be able to translate for the practitioner accumulated knowledge and experience from the collective practice wisdom and practice literature to apply in unique practice situations. The supervisor can avoid problems by resisting the tendency to assume that generally accepted practice procedures will always be available to the practitioner in a common or uncommon practice situation. Knowledge of practice procedures must be confirmed or made known through the process of supervision.

3. *Analysis and Redefinition.* This process requires separating elements of a complex whole and reorganizing them into a new whole, creating a different form of understanding from what appears to be a known situation. This is the heart of supervisory interaction. Difficult cases can result in the practitioner's creating a complex orientation and comprehension of the case that is inaccurate diagnostically or in terms of treatment. In order for the practitioner to develop a new focus that will take him or her in a new direction with a case, the supervisor needs to guide the practitioner

through an analysis to produce a new comprehension of the dynamics of the case.

4. *Pattern Recognition.* The repeated elements of any situation form a pattern that permits consistent recognition and understanding. As the supervisor engages in several case analyses with the practitioner, repeated patterns of client problems, client interaction, and worker interaction will become apparent and should be highlighted. This can occur over a series of cases or in a single case. If the worker is to learn to practice independently, recognition of these patterns of problems, interaction, and communication must become part of his or her observational and interventive skills.

5. *Prediction.* One can project outcomes or behaviors from known situations to unknown situations. This is the ultimate goal of independent practice based on learning in supervision. For learning in supervision to be successful, the practitioner must develop skill at achieving this transfer of learning. Once the supervisor has worked through the four previous elements with the practitioner, the supervisor must provide opportunities for the practitioner to apply what has been learned from previous cases to new cases.

These elements have been explained separately, but they become integrated in the supervision process to formulate a complex network of thinking and interaction that can be identified when the supervisory process is observed. One important factor that has become apparent from attempting to observe these elements in supervision interaction is that, for the learning to be successful, the elements should occur in the order that has been listed. None of the elements can be effectively applied unless the previous elements have been applied and understood. These five elements serve as the general principles of learning that are a basis for all the other facets of learning covered in this book.

COST OF SUPERVISION

Time and expense are rarely mentioned in connection with supervision. If more attention were devoted to them, more supervisors and practitioners would be conscious of the importance of making effective use of supervisory time. Depending upon the training, experience, and salary of the supervisor and supervisee, each hour of individual supervision can cost between $60 and $95. Over a typical professional year of weekly sessions, the cost can range from $3,000 to $6,000. If supervision involved more awareness of supervision cost, time would undoubtedly be used more effectively and efficiently. Tardiness, cancelled sessions, small talk, lack of content planning, and rambling clinical speculation on the part of either the supervisor or supervisee are costly and unjustifiable. Every question, every interpretation, every comment should be clinically relevant and related to a treatment or learning goal. Another objective of this book is to offer some guidelines that aid in more effective use of supervision time.

In business and management, the recent emphasis has focused on decreasing costs by eliminating supervision rather than increasing productivity through supervision. This has been the pattern in social work over the past three decades. Cost in administering treatment can be decreased by structuring supervision in a manner that *decreases* the need for it. We should not eliminate supervision in social work, but we can make it more cost effective.

The management field does have some conceptual ways of aiding us in this area. In management, supervision is being related to *what to do* and *how to do it*, while in professional social work, we have assumed that professionals generally know these things. In most cases, supervision has been obliquely focused on checking whether or not you are doing it, and in some instances, supervision has been all but eliminated. We need to devote more attention to the "what" and "how" of doing treatment.

As financial demands for decreased administrative costs become more important in social work education and practice, supervision gets harder to justify. Ironically, we need more rather than less supervision — more genuine supervision that is structured and specific to learning. This will not mean an overall increase in the amount of supervision since, in many settings, it is already being provided, but not on a sound basis. What is needed is more effectiveness and efficiency within the existing time frame of supervisory practices and structures.

STYLE

Some attention has been devoted to *style* in clinical practice, but limited attention has been devoted to styles of supervision. The concept of style emerged as a natural and useful tool to organize the interactional perspective used in this book. There is a difference between structure of supervision and style. Style relates to the pattern of interaction that is fostered directly or indirectly by the supervisor. A major thesis of this book, based on my research, is that the supervisor's style gives rise to the style that the practitioner adopts in supervision.

There is no theory of supervision, and no attempt will be made to create one in this book. Our knowledge and research are not sufficient to permit development of a substantial theory at this point. Instead, the attempt has been to create a paradigm of supervision based on interactional styles. (A paradigm is a set of concepts, descriptive categories, and a common language that allows researchers to work in a given area using consistent guiding principles. [See Lachman et al., 1979:1-34]) Others are doing research within the paradigm; additional research and other paradigms will surely follow. Only with continued research efforts can supervision be utilized to contribute to quality treatment. (See Chapter 4 for a detailed discussion of style.)

NEED FOR SUPERVISION

A relevant question in the clinical practice of social work is: Why do we need supervision? This question is of importance because of the increased emphasis on the autonomy of the practitioner in the past two decades in a profession that historically has placed heavy emphasis on close supervision. The idea of consultation replaced the idea of supervision as the autonomous model of professionalism was developing. The focus on autonomy has emerged more as a supportive indicator that we are truly professionals than as a reflection of the self-directed practitioner. There are indications in the characteristics of new BSW and MSW graduates that support this view.

Several general professional trends that support the need for clinical supervision can be identified. These trends are: the resurgence of clinical practice, the social work dominance inmental illness treatment, the theory explosion, changes in professional standards, limited supervision training, practitioner stress and burnout prevention, unethical practice, complex external controls on practice structure, complicated documentation, sophisticated outcome measures, and new highly specialized practice areas. These developments are beyond what social work education can effectively teach within the existing curriculum and time constraints. New graduates need assistance to integrate the many practice demands that are marginally covered in educational programs. It is a mistake to assume that the recent graduate is totally prepared to be a practitioner. This book in part is designed to guide the supervisor in efforts to enhance and refine the functioning of the recent graduate.

Resurgence of Clinical Practice

Since the retreat of clinical practice during the 1960s under the pressure of several social reform movements, a large-scale resurgence of clinical practice has transformed what were called casework and group work into a more specialized and generic classification of psychotherapy. Social workers functioning in this area do individual, group, and family therapy. By the 1970s statistics revealed that social workers were the largest single group providing psychotherapy; more than 29,000 social workers perform this service, compared with 26,000 psychiatrists, 18,000 psychologists, 12,000 nurses, and 10,000 other practitioners (Sobel, 1980). By 1990 this figure had grown to 60 percent. Although social workers deliver the majority of psychotherapy services, there has been scant mention of this shift in the social work literature. Even though the trend has been emerging for two decades, few schools have adapted to this change in practice function, and few schools prepare students exclusively for this form of practice. The profession and the schools will need to adapt to the dramatic changes in practice activity or risk being co-opted by other disciplines.

Clinical Social Work in Mental Health

The trend of social workers as the predominant group offering mental health services and psychotherapy will most likely continue, since the definition of mental illness has expanded over the decades as mental illness has become better understood and as mental health treatment has become more accepted. As the number of psychiatrists remains constant, other professionals move into doing psychotherapy, and most of these are social workers. The number of psychiatrists is declining, leaving to the social worker much of the modern talking therapy for mild neurotic behavior, communication problems, and situational stress. With the decline in the number of new practitioners, psychiatric practice is focusing more on the severe mental illnesses (e.g., schizophrenia and manic depressive illness), and psychiatric research is focusing more on the biological aspects of mental disorders. Increasingly, social workers will be treating situational and psychological dysfunctioning, and psychiatrists will be treating biological disorders. This trend is a return to a pattern of service delivery of three to five decades ago.

At the same time that this is occurring the schools and the professional literature have de-emphasized the teaching and practice of supervision. **This in part has been the result of developing the concept of the social worker as a full-fledged professional.** The view that a genuine professional must be independent and autonomous was believed to be necessary to professional status. Supervision and professionalism were seen as antithetical. There is a trend to a more balanced approach, and this book is an effort to help fill the gap in the supervision practice that has evolved over last 30 years.

Theory Explosion

As these functional and structural changes have taken place, there has been a simultaneous increase in emphasis on practice theory to the point of confusion. There are now over 130 different theories of practice competing for utilization. Social work practice theory is in a period of diversified unrest. Some trends can be vaguely identified. Systems theory appears to have reached the apex of its contribution to practice knowledge, and along with it Gestalt therapy and the ecosystems approach are reaching their theoretical limits. There is a resurgence of psychoanalytic theory in the broadest sense from an interactional perspective. There have been fascinating developments in communication theory, and empirical research on linguistics-based theories is producing intriguing results and insights.

Social work in general seems to be fostering a plateau of theoretical dormancy, and in some respects we are returning to an earlier era of developing methodologies such as individual, group, and family treatment rather than developing theories of intervention based on behavioral patterns. Clearly, the era of "do your own thing" is over. Self-help and do-it-yourself approaches, which began with Karen Horney and bloomed in different arrangements during the 1960s and 1970s, are losing favor. Supervisors need to keep abreast of these developments if they are to aid supervisees in their theoretical and conceptual learning. (See Chapter 8 for a more detailed discussion of theory in practice and supervision.)

Changes in Professional Standards

The responsibility for setting standards for entry into the profession has passed from the schools to the profession through licensing. The number of comprehensive examinations in schools has decreased as the number of states that have passed licensing laws has increased. There is great variation in the requirements of supervision for licensing.

Learning and standards are being separated as licensing laws for social work are increasing. Over 40 states now have laws regulating social work practice. Most of these laws require an examination for certification. Some do not have any requirements for supervision. The examinations are not associated with supervisory requirements, so there is no connection between learning, the examination, and supervision. Some examinations contain questions about supervision, but they have limited relationship to the supervision process and practice activity.

There is reason to believe that educational testing services have more experience than the social work schools in measuring competence today. However, the question remains whether examinations are sufficient to measure competence. In earlier times social work relied more on supervision to monitor competence of practitioners. This was accomplished through discussion of cases, theories, techniques, evaluation, and administrative matters. The profession now depends more on the licensing examinations to evaluate competence. With the decreased emphasis on verbal exchange to promote competence, the professional seems to have lost something. We must ask ourselves: What can be accomplished and what is accomplished through such examinations? What are their limitations? Adler has pointed out that, "if the aim were to discover the student's familiarity with a specific branch of knowledge, one way to do that might be to test the individual's ability to use correctly a particular discipline's technical terms" (1981:16). This might be all we can expect to accomplish with licensing examinations. We cannot expect written tests to deal with supervisee's fears, anxieties, doubts, learning to recognize patterns of behavior, developing a philosophy of practice, identifying a basic effective style, and numerous other interactional factors. We need to renew our discussion of such areas in supervision if we expect our supervisees to become truly well-rounded practitioners.

Continuing Education

Continuing education is taking on increased significance, as it is now required by many professional organizations and licensing boards to maintain professional standards and status. However, some professionals consider these programs to be of limited value in promoting competence, to be of little importance or effectiveness, and in some instances, actually to be detrimental since there is minimal monitoring of what is learned, consistency of learning, and degree of application in practice. Supervisors have a responsibility to monitor continuing education courses attended by supervisees, and to evaluate how they contribute to learning about social work practice.

Continuing education programs are the chief source of learning for practitioners. They serve a valuable function in preparing for specialized practice areas. Continuing education is abstract learning since it usually is conducted outside the actual practice setting. Continuing education learning should be supplemented by structured application in the treatment setting and supervision is the natural arena for this to occur. Continuing education should be viewed as a supplement to supervision instead of a substitute for it.

Supervision Training

With increased pressure on schools to expand content in a number of areas including minority concerns, women's' issues, feminist practice, oppression, human biology, human behavior in the social environment, research, and policy, there has been a decrease in courses devoted to practice content and supervision. For clinical majors, 10 to 12 percent of the courses taken as part of a BSW or MSW program are exclusively devoted to practice subjects. A two-year graduate curriculum is limited in its content. Committed students who recognize the limits of their practice knowledge are increasingly seeking third-year fellowship programs upon graduation, but there are few such programs. Given these conditions, supervision of the beginning practitioner will become increasingly important as a way of giving the social worker a unified view of practice and orienting him or her to the breadth of the profession.

That the schools are providing limited training to prepare workers for autonomous clinical practice is illustrated by the findings of a research project, in which students undergoing a two-year graduate education averaged 15-20 cases and conducted 120-150 interviews, including an average of 120 individual sessions, 20 group sessions, and 13 family interviews (Munson, 1981a). This is hardly a basis upon which to base an autonomous practice.

The Council on Social Work Education's revised Curriculum Policy Statement, implemented in July 1983, does not mention supervision as a concept or require any curriculum offerings in the area of supervision. In a survey, it was found that only 13 percent of graduate schools of social work required a course in supervision (Munson, see Study C). At the same time, schools are placing emphasis on specialization (e.g., health, aging, mental health, rural practice). Cooper has argued that universities are not interested in developing clinical training programs, and are incapable of adequate training for clinical practice because of disharmony between the schools and the field (Mishne, 1980:29-30). As long as academicians and practitioners are so polarized, little hope can be held that there will be any basic agreement about requirements for supervision of students and practitioners.

Supervision has made limited adjustment to changes in motivation of **students entering graduate schools of social work.** In one study, 53 percent of students indicated that they had undergone therapy themselves. A majority of these students indicated that they had entered graduate school because of a desire to emulate their own therapist (Munson, see Study A). This desire to accomplish a personal fantasy — rather than a strong, altruistic commitment to help others through social work — is consistent with Yankelovich's observation that "in our preoccupation with self-fulfillment we have also grown recklessly unrealistic in our demands on our institutions" (1981:5).

As the emphasis on the role of supervision has decreased, we have failed to recognize both this change in motivation of practitioners and their tendency to draw on their experiences with their own therapist as the model for their own practice techniques.

Stress

In this era of decreased emphasis on supervision, we have witnessed an increase in concern about burnout among practitioners. Although there is some question about the amount and degree of burnout (Streepy, 1981), it is ironic that the increased concern has occurred at a time when supervision is being de-emphasized since good supervision has been held to be effective in preventing burnout. If burnout actually is accelerating, it possibly can be traced to the decline in emphasis on supervision. If this is the case, renewed requirements for supervision could be of value in combating burnout. Burnout, in many instances, is associated with lack of coping mechanisms. When practitioners cannot cope with practice demands, they need to turn for help to a trustworthy source. The supervisor should be and is the most appropriate resource for dealing with such difficulties. Without supervision as a resource, practitioners will struggle on their own, turn to colleagues, or as mentioned before, in some cases draw on experiences from their therapy. Rarely do these measures aid the worker, and in some instances they can make the burnout worse.

In supervision, as in any endeavor, anxiety, fear, frustration, and failure are the result of inadequate coping mechanisms. As was pointed out at the beginning of this chapter, graduates are being provided fewer coping strategies for practice and for supervision even though practice demands are becoming more difficult. This could be the source of distress (Streepy, 1981) and disillusionment (Reiter, 1980) among practitioners and supervisors. Coping strategies are specific techniques to use in response to difficult situations, and are discussed in detail in later chapters.

Research on stress in the workplace has repeatedly demonstrated that effective supervision is a powerful antidote to stress. For this reason alone **we should consider reviving and expanding supervision in agencies.** Administrators rarely associate stress prevention and supervision. More attention needs to be given to this function of supervision as excess stress, or "burnout" as it is commonly labelled, increasingly becomes a problem for practitioners and supervisors. (Chapter 10 provides a thorough discussion of stress and supervision as a way to minimize the negative effects of stress.)

Ethics in Practice

Unethical practices seem to be on the rise in society in general and among mental health practitioners specifically. There is increasing evidence of sexual activity between practitioners and clients (NASW, 1982). Given the intensity of the therapeutic relationship and the lack of preparation in psychotherapy training programs to deal with sexual content (Edelwich & Brodsky, 1982), it is understandable that ethical problems are surfacing in this area. Supervision is an important arena for dealing with sexual content in practice and for helping the practitioner to develop appropriate and ethical ways of handling such material (Edelwich & Brodsky, 1982:135-138). With the increase in the number of private practitioners, more practice is removed from monitoring by others. The unethical practices are an elusive problem, but exposure of practice through good supervision is the best safeguard we have against such problems. Some agencies have reinstituted supervision as a means of ensuring that abuse of the client/practitioner relationship is minimized.

SUPERVISOR PREPARATION

In spite of these trends and the indication that they are giving rise to more complexity in supervision and practice, formal learning about supervision and how to do it has been declining in the social work profession. In one survey, over 60 percent of the supervisors had no formal academic training in supervision. The majority of the supervisors reported that they learned to do supervision through an agency training program (20 percent) or through on-the-job training (28 percent) (Munson, see Study A). There is limited information about the quality or quantity of learning in such programs. The survey revealed that only 13 percent of the graduate schools required a course in supervision as part of the MSW curriculum. Twenty-eight percent did not have a course in supervision, and 58 percent offered a supervision course as an elective (Munson, see Study C).

These statistics reveal that, although most states that license and certify practitioners require a period of supervision, there is little assurance the supervision will be of high quality or uniform from state to state or agency to agency because we lack consistent universal standards. There is no national association of supervisors, and only recently has a journal been developed that is devoted to supervision (*The Clinical Supervisor*).

Most supervisors tend to supervise in reaction to the way they were supervised. When asked how they developed their style of and attitude toward supervision, supervisors cite about equally the emulation of admired qualities and the avoidance of negative aspects of their own past supervisors (Munson, see Study C).

CHARACTERISTICS OF SUPERVISEES

In order to understand the needs of supervisees it is important that the supervisor have knowledge of the characteristics of supervisees. Each supervisee is unique, but it is helpful for supervisors to know general characteristics of supervisees as a group. This is especially important for new supervisors.

There is a 70 percent likelihood that the supervisee will be female (Kadushin, 1974:289; Munson, 1975:96). Supervisees on the average are 34 years old, making them generally ten years younger than their supervisors. There is a 60 percent chance that they are married, and on the average they have two children. The majority (43 percent) hold MSW degrees, while one-third (36 percent) hold BA degrees, and only 6 percent hold BSW degrees. The remaining 15 percent hold various degrees in related areas.

There is a slightly better than 50 percent chance that the supervisee is employed in a public agency; the remainder work in private agencies. The workers are generally employed in family and children's services (40 percent), health and mental health settings (30 percent), and social service (public welfare) agencies (29 percent). The supervisee will most likely have six years' social work experience, and half of that experience will have been in the agency where he or she is currently employed. The majority (54 percent) of supervisees report being supervised in the traditional, one-to-one, individual model of supervision, while 17 percent report undergoing group supervision, and 29 percent experience the independent model of supervision in which they function autonomously and use supervision only occasionally. Over 60 percent of the supervisees report being satisfied with their supervisory experience. These are general characteristics of social work supervisees. They are summarized here to give the reader an idea of what the profession looks like generally and to give the supervisor something to compare with his or her individual situation. Each supervisee is unique, and should be recognized as such.

BEGINNING PROFESSIONALS

With these general observations in mind, we can turn to consideration of the nature and characteristics of beginning professionals who come to you for supervision. These neophytes will have wide variation in amount and type of clinical practice, techniques, theories, and supervision they have experienced. Some will have strong foundations in a theory or theories and will have experienced good, sound supervision in which specific clinical material has been explored and appropriate strategies and techniques of intervention have been applied.

Many more supervisees will come to you who have experienced poor, limited supervision in agencies that are under the practice gun and shoot from the hip theoretically and practically. Such supervisees have been left with partially learned theory and techniques. Many of them have surveyed several theories and have mastered none, or have developed a repertoire of fragmented and unrelated techniques that lack a coherent pattern. In many agencies, theories and concepts are used only as code words, which results in their misinterpretation and misapplication. Products of such settings make such statements as "I am a Gestalt therapist" or "I am a systems person" or "I use paradoxing" or "I do TA." Such descriptions reveal little about what the practitioners know or can and cannot do.

For these reasons, the supervisor must do a thorough educational diagnosis as he or she begins supervision. In the past, educational diagnosis was equated with a personality assessment of the practitioner. This is too narrow for today's practice demands. An educational diagnosis measures what the person knows and has experienced. The more relevant questions that go into an educational diagnosis are: What do supervisees know? What do they know about theory? What kind of practice settings have they worked in? What kind of and how many cases have they treated? How many in-depth cases have they had? What kind of outcomes have they produced in the cases they have treated? What do they know about diagnosis and assessment? What do they see as their practice strengths and weaknesses? What is their style of practice? What kind of and how much supervision have they experienced? What do they hope to accomplish from supervision? (Appendix 2 contains a form for doing an educational assessment.)

Many students enter graduate education today because of a personal problem they have experienced. Because of contact with a therapist they want to emulate, they have developed the desire to help others. This connection between being the helped and being the helper is perpetuated in schools through therapeutically oriented supervision. In cases in which this model is used, the student and beginning practitioner show a tendency to model themselves after their therapist rather than their supervisor. This can result in deficient practice style because the worker adopts as a general practice style the techniques that were utilized with him or her. These may not be appropriate to a variety of cases with diverse problems. Where the therapeutic model of supervision does not work for the supervisee, there is a tendency on the part of the supervisors to be leery of such practices in supervision.

Depending on their student supervisory experience, beginning practitioners are either eager for self-analysis in supervision or will resist it strongly. Research has demonstrated that the supervisor needs to encourage a healthy balance with respect to the amount of self-analysis, because some students seek self-analysis to avoid dealing with other important components of their practice, and others avoid self-analysis to the detriment of their own growth and development as practitioners (Munson, see Study B). Self-analysis should always be encouraged by the supervisor in the context of how it will make the practitioner more effective in a specific case. Individual or group supervision focused only on the worker's personal dynamics in order to help him or her to learn abstractly about practice is usually inappropriate. Supervisors who focus primarily on supervisees' personal dynamics have been characterized as poor supervisors and poor therapists (Haley, 1976:187).

ORGANIZATIONS

Some have argued that under new demands of practice, clinical learning must be integrated with organizational theory (see Cottle & Whitten, 1980:3-19). This seems to be a generalization that confuses certain issues for practitioners. Organizations do have an impact on clinical practice, but this varies with the practice setting. The experiences of hospital patients differ from those of private outpatients in a group practice. Where there is an overemphasis on the organization in supervision, organization can become the scapegoat for avoiding clinical issues or justifying clinical failures. Organizational issues in supervision are relevant to the extent that they impede the progress of the treatment. Supervisees should be given full credit for any organizational obstacles they can identify. The supervision should be focused on the question: Given the organizational obstacles, what can be done to overcome them to the benefit of the client?

NEEDS OF SUPERVISEES

An extensive review by Hansen and Warner (1971) of research on counselor practicum supervision answers some questions about the impact of supervision and reinforces some old doubts. The survey revealed that supervisors rely predominantly on teaching through questioning as the interactional structure. Although supervisors do not like to rely on teaching of specific techniques, this is what supervisees perceive themselves as needing, especially in the early stages. Also, technique-oriented supervision produces more effective learning than supervision that has a therapeutic orientation. This finding has implications for supervisor styles that are discussed later.

Supportive supervision was found to produce more effective learning than nonsupportive or negative supervision. In the nonsupportive model, supervisees showed a significant tendency to shift the focus of the supervision interaction from the clients to themselves. This finding has implications for supervisees' reactions (discussed in Chapter 5). Also, supervisee learning is significantly greater when the supervisor's theoretical orientation is taken into account.

Social workers show a tendency to prefer characteristics in supervisors different from those in the disciplines of psychiatry and psychology. Respondents in a study of psychiatry and psychology supervisees ranked interest in supervision and experience as a therapist as the preferred characteristics, whereas social workers ranked genuineness and ability to provide feedback as the preferred characteristics (Nelson, 1978:548). Social workers tend to look for more specific characteristics in supervisors than do workers in other disciplines. The importance of feedback in supervision was highlighted and refined in a study by Thigpen (1979), who found that a group of supervisees in mental health settings preferred client-focused feedback and that supervisees did not regard highly feedback focused on themselves.

Although these research studies indicate that supervisees can change on the basis of specific components of supervision, we still know very little about the specific reason for change, and we do not know what supervisors can do to make supervisees more effective with their clients. One of the problems has been lack of adequate research methodology in studies of supervision. Many variables remain uncontrolled. The need for more in-depth and extensive research on supervision cannot be overemphasized.

Research has begun to expose some of the inconsistencies that need to be addressed. In a controlled study of graduate social work students, Joel Fisher (1975) found that students who had received specific instruction in core practice conditions had higher levels of learning and performance and higher evaluative ratings by their field instructors than two control groups that had received less specific instruction. An unexpected finding in all three groups was that field instructors' evaluations of students' empathy, warmth, and genuineness were inversely correlated with academic grades.

A more disturbing finding came from two studies. In a study of 65 supervisees in various settings (Munson, 1975), supervisees perceived their level of accomplishment and various types of supervisory satisfaction to be highly correlated with the amount of interaction they had with the supervisor (see Visual 1.1). Another study, involving 26 field instructors of graduate social work students (Munson, see Study C), found no correlation between the amount of instructor interaction with supervisees and the instructors' own satisfaction with helping the supervisees grow professionally, sharing knowledge with them, and discussing administrative matters. The only variable that produced a significant correlation with interaction was their sense of obligation to direct the work of the supervisee (see Visual 1.2). These findings show that the factors that produce high levels of satisfaction and meet the needs of supervisees produce little

VISUAL 1.1. Correlation of Supervisee Satisfaction
and Level of Interaction with the Supervisor

Satisfaction Variable	Level of Interaction* (Correlation Coefficient)
Job Satisfaction	.63
Helping Satisfaction	.84
Teaching Satisfaction	.81
Control Satisfaction	.78
Administrative Satisfaction	.84
General Satisfaction	.83
Sense of Accomplishment	.50

Correlation Coefficients are Kendall Tau. All coefficients were significant at the .05 level or better.

*Level of Interaction scale based on frequency of contact, approachability of supervisor, supervisor encouragement of discussion, ability of supervisor to put supervisee at ease, clarity of supervisor communication, and degree of congruence in supervisor and supervisee communication. All of these components are based on the supervisees' perception.

Source: Munson 1975:288.

VISUAL 1.2. Correlation of Supervisor Satisfaction with Supervisory Role
and Level of Interaction with Supervisees

Satisfaction Variables	Level of Interaction*
Helping supervisees grow professionally	.01
Sharing knowledge with supervisees	.14
Discussion of administrative matters	.07
Sense of obligation to direct and guide supervisees	.35

Correlation Coefficients are Kendall Tau. The only variable that was significantly correlated with level of interaction was sense of obligation to direct and to guide supervisees (p = < .04).

*Level of Interaction scale based on frequency of contact, approachability of supervisor, and supervisor encouragement of discussion ability of supervisor.

Source: Munson, Study C.

satisfaction for the supervisors. Although most studies reveal that supervisees are satisfied with their supervisory experiences, the findings of this study raise the question: At what price to the supervisor are these supervisee satisfactions being achieved? We do not know the extent to which the supervisory role has negative impact on the supervisor. These findings could help to explain why some supervisors neglect and emotionally and physically withdraw from their supervisory responsibilities.

In many settings workers express what I call *diminished perceptions* regarding their supervisors when the supervisees experience supervisor withdrawal. When asked about the supervisor's performance, the worker will list numerous dissatisfactions; but when asked to rate the adequacy of the supervisor, the worker will indicate fairly high levels of satisfaction. When questioned about this inconsistency, supervisees will explain that they know they are not getting what they should from supervision, but accept it because they understand that their supervisors are busy and overworked and because they do not wish to burden them further. The supervisee adopts perceptions of supervision that lead to a diminished expectation of the supervisor. It is at this point that the supervisory process has broken down and fragmentation of learning sets in.

It is common to hear supervisees justify supervisor withdrawal and aloofness on the basis that more supervisory contact just creates anxiety in the supervisee out of the fear of emotional dependence on the supervisor.

It appears that in reality supervisee anxiety grows out of lack of mechanisms to cope with problems encountered in practice. The social worker who has difficulty tolerating clients who get upset, combative, and aggressive is like the medical student who cannot stand the sight of blood. Although medical students may be shocked at their first sight of blood, they learn and are taught to deal with it. Too often we fail to teach student clinicians to deal with highly emotional reactions of clients. As a result, these clinicians continue to be upset by these occurrences and conduct their treatment in a way that aims at preventing them, even if it is essential for the client to have reactions of this nature. In both situations these reactions negatively affect the treatment. Providing sound, helpful supervision through a trained, qualified, committed supervisor on a regular basis is the best antidote for practitioner anxiety about clinical activity.

In a series of surveys (Munson, see Study A), the following major categories of learning needs were the ones most identified by graduating MSW's as they began their professional careers:

- exposure to specialized cases
- criticism of work
- exposure to different practice approaches
- more exposure to theory
- cotherapy experience
- exposure to the work of others
- more direct supervision
- developing more self-awareness
- feedback on work
- support and encouragement
- training in group therapy
- help improving diagnostic skills.

It is clear from these responses that new supervisees generally recognize a need for help in developing their skills, applying theory, fostering self-awareness, being exposed to different practice modalities, and getting support as they struggle to develop self-confidence.

CLINICAL ASSESSMENT AND DIAGNOSIS

It is important for the beginning practitioner to learn to avoid attempting treatment before doing a basic diagnostic assessment. There is a difference between a diagnostic assessment and a diagnosis. A diagnostic assessment is a process of gathering various forms of information, and permits planning sound treatment intervention; a diagnosis is a limited process of applying a label or diagnostic category to the client based on identifying symptoms and behaviors. Students and beginning practitioners frequently feel that they are under a great deal of pressure to apply treatment strategies and interventions. (The pressure may be imagined or real.) This results in interventions being made without an adequate information base to support them, which can lead the treatment astray. It is true that we must always make intervention without sufficient information upon which to base our treatment. However, beginning practitioners show a tendency to act without weighing the amount of information that serves as the basis for the intervention. The practitioner must be helped to understand that there is nothing wrong with asking questions until the client's problems are comprehended in the context of the therapy and the client's situation.

Educators, writers, and supervisors unwittingly contribute to this rapidity of treatment by minimizing the importance of the diagnostic phase and emphasizing that treatment begins as soon as the first interview starts. Although this is true, it is confusing to the practitioner because we lack clarity about both the distinction between and the interrelatedness of the diagnostic and treatment phases. Beginning professionals feel a need to produce results for their clients and supervisors, which makes them vulnerable to questioning or engaging in weakly supported interventions. They are caught in a supervisory double bind of sorts: they are fearful of hesitating to intervene soon enough, but are open to concerns about the basis for hastily planned interventions. The supervisor must be sensitive to this and help the learner balance the two realms. The supervisor has a responsibility to ensure that assessment and treatment are accomplished in a sound, thorough, and sequential manner.

This balancing act is important because prolonged diagnostic activity can be a barrier to intervening and learning about intervention. This is the basis of what I call *persistent diagnosis*. Just as Parkinson (1957:2) has observed that "work expands so as to fill the time available for its completion," so does diagnosis expand in direct relation to the time available for its completion. The supervisor has a responsibility to aid the beginning practitioner in adequately planning and preparing a diagnostic assessment as well as giving it some form of closure, and in initiating treatment. When this process is clear, the client can also be reassured that the worker is proceeding in an orderly fashion.

In achieving an assessment/treatment balance the supervisor must recognize that the beginning practitioner shows a tendency to need to be in control and a tendency to be overactive in the treatment. The supervisor can guard against this by encouraging the neophyte practitioner to explore interactionally, rather than to explain when the client asks questions about the quality, type, or purpose of the treatment, the program, or the agency.

BEGINNING GUIDELINES

Research conducted with supervisees (Munson, see Study A, Study B, Study E) has revealed a number of factors the new supervisor must be aware of and prepared to deal with. These factors are particularly appropriate to beginning supervisors and beginning practitioners, but they apply in most cases to any supervisory situation:

1. Consider that the supervisee will likely have limited experience at applying theory, concepts, and techniques.
2. The supervisor should be prepared to demonstrate what he or she wants the practitioner to do.
3. The emphasis should be on evaluation of the supervisee's practice as well as some emphasis on evaluation of the supervision process itself.
4. The supervisor should observe the supervisee's practice periodically.
5. The supervisor should make the details of his or her expectations clear.
6. The supervisor should refrain from criticizing the supervisee's educational program or experience.
7. The supervisor should avoid criticizing the profession.
8. The supervisor should refrain from using supervision as a forum to criticize other professions or other agency staff.
9. The supervisor should avoid comparing the supervisee's performance to that of other supervisees or other staff.
10. The supervisor should make sure that the supervisee has enough work.
11. The supervisor should be willing to share his or her knowledge and skills with the supervisee.
12. The supervisor should remember that the supervisee is supposed to be working under the direction of a competent and informed master teacher and professional.

CHARACTERISTICS OF SUPERVISORS

Research has revealed that supervisors are on the average 42 years of age and are usually about 10 years older than their supervisees (Munson, 1975). Supervisors have an average of 15 years of social work experience, and an average of seven years of experience in the agency that currently employs them. Fifty percent of supervisors are female. Slightly more of the supervisors are employed in public agencies (53 percent) than private agencies (47 percent). The overwhelming majority (77 percent) holds the MSW degree. The majority (92 percent) of supervisors have some form of preparation for their supervisory roles, such as university-taught courses, agency training programs, and on-the-job training. One-third of supervisors carry a caseload in addition to their supervisory roles, 21 percent do not carry any cases, and 45 percent periodically carry cases. Of those supervisors who do see cases, one-third report that these cases are seen in private practice and are not connected with the agency in which they perform supervisory roles. (This probably accounts for the small degree to which supervisors share their practice with supervisees; this lack of sharing was reported by supervisees in the same study.) The supervisees reported that in the majority of situations (64 percent) they were satisfied with and valued their supervisory experience.

ON BECOMING A CLINICAL SUPERVISOR

Becoming a supervisor in clinical practice is somewhat different from becoming a supervisor in the more traditional management sense. There are many subtle differences, but the major one occurs in the area of role and function in relation to authority. The traditional supervisor makes a complete shift from being a rank-and-file employee to assuming a new, full-time function as manager. This requires the mastery of a new perspective on work, new basic concepts, new emphasis on function, new sources of job satisfaction, new status, and new relationships with others in the organization (Reeves, 1980:1). The traditional supervisor must adjust to regulating the work rather than doing the work, and must adapt to the authority that goes along with the new role. Frequently the most skilled worker experiences a high degree of difficulty in making the transition to supervisor and focusing on getting the job done through other people.

On becoming a clinical supervisor, the shift in responsibility is often **vague and unclear.** Most clinical supervisors are autonomous, professional practitioners rather than exclusively subordinate employees before they become supervisors, and upon assuming supervisory responsibilities, they often continue to practice. The assumption has long been that to be a good supervisor, you must be an active practitioner. This is undoubtedly a good premise, but it can create dilemmas for the supervisor carrying a dual role, such as the problems of time management and establishing priorities when the demands of practice and supervision conflict.

AUTHORITY

The role of authority is unique for the clinical supervisor. Since the supervisor is accustomed to working as an autonomous professional and since the majority of the supervisees are trained professionals, the nature and extent of the supervisor's authority is vague, unstructured, and limited in sanction. Even with student practitioners, authority is vague because the supervisor is often a remote representative of the educational institution and because trainees are encouraged to prepare to be autonomous practitioners. The authority of the clinical supervisor is indirect. It resides in one's ability as a skilled practitioner as in the sanction provided by the agency and the profession. The doing of the work remains in the hands of the supervisee, and the results are rarely seen by the supervisor. This is true in traditional supervision. However, in clinical supervision learning to do is the focus, and there is always a terminal point in mind; whereas in traditional supervision the regulation of the doing is ongoing even after learning the task has been accomplished. A major problem of the clinical supervisor is determining when the learning is complete and regulation is no longer needed.

AVOIDING SUPERVISION AS TREATMENT

The new supervisor is generally an experienced practitioner, but unfortunately, this is all too often the only basis for assuming the supervisory role. The transition from practitioner to supervisor is an important change that often is lacking in adequate preparation. Usually, all the new supervisor has to draw on is his or her own therapeutic orientation and experiences derived from supervision. This is unfortunate since the beginning supervisor is being asked to assume the most intensive teaching role imaginable.

Educational supervision is much different from teaching a course or presenting lectures to small or large groups. Instead, the clinical supervisor is in an intensive teacher/learner relationship (involving one or several students) that is vaguely defined, lacking in precise guidelines, and consisting of unstructured format. Since most practitioners who become supervisors lack the knowledge or skills of general or specific teaching techniques, they fall back on their treatment skills to get by in supervision. This is especially the case when they encounter difficulty in supervising. This mismatch of needs and performance capability gives rise to many of the problems in supervision. The incongruence is heightened by the increasing belief that doing therapy with the supervisee leads to frustration, resentment, and anger on all parts.

Trust in the supervisor is essential to effective supervision, but there is evidence that using therapeutic strategies as a focus in supervision results in distrust of the supervisor (Munson, see Study A, Study B). Supervisors who engage in this approach are simply attempting to develop skills to cope with the situation. The only problem is that such coping mechanisms rarely work. The function of this book is to provide alternate coping strategies based on sound educational principles.

SUPPORT FOR SUPERVISORS

In traditional supervision, supervisors are supervised. They must account for their own performance as well as that of their subordinates. Rarely do clinical supervisors have to account for their own performance, as practitioners or supervisors. Just as they do not have to account for their performance, there is little recognition of their accomplishments and little support when they encounter problems. Clinical supervisors need some form of support system as well as some accountability. When support is not provided from within the organization or from the profession outside, the supervisor will internalize problems, fail to acknowledge the difficulty, or perhaps seek support through supervisees. None of these alternatives is acceptable or appropriate; when utilized they can lead to additional problems. When supervisors turn to their supervisees for support they are open to manipulation. This does not mean that supervisors should avoid support by supervisees, only that they should not be put in or get in the position of having to depend upon supervisees for it.

UNANTICIPATED CONSEQUENCES

The clinical supervisor will encounter some unexpected consequences of the new role that are accepted in traditional supervision. Practitioners will bring to supervision organizational problems, service gaps, and interpersonal staff problems that the supervisor, eager to provide clinical supervision, failed to anticipate and for which he or she has little tolerance. The differing expectations of the supervisor and the supervisee regarding the functions and purposes of supervision can be a source of frustration and disappointment for both sides.

In traditional supervision promotion to the supervisory position brings concomitant increases in pay benefits, status privileges, and access to higher level members of the organization. For the clinical supervisor assuming the supervisory role often does not result in any of these rewards. Supervision is an added responsibility with few tangible benefits. Supervisory positions in psychotherapy are viewed more as a professional responsibility and an opportunity to make a contribution to the next generation of practitioners.

Although most traditional supervisors receive some form of training or assistance for their new roles, clinical supervisors receive little if any training for their new responsibilities. Most have to rely on their own judgment, experience, reading, and relationships with their own supervisors. There is a long-held assumption that clinical experience can serve as a basis for and be converted easily to supervisory practice. This assumption can lead to problems. Some of the techniques and skills of direct treatment can be used in supervision, but they are insufficient for good comprehensive supervision practice. Weak practitioners rarely make good supervisors, and good practitioners do not necessarily make good supervisors. When clinical skills are relied on to conduct supervision, they can lead to problems because supervisees feel they are being placed unwillingly in therapy rather than being supervised. This is why it is important that supervisors be trained in distinguishing therapy skills and supervisory skills. This book is devoted to identifying and applying the skills that are basic to good supervisory practice, so that some of the problems just mentioned can be avoided or overcome.

Many people enter clinical supervision without much anticipation of the adjustments required, but they should possess or be willing to develop certain characteristics. They should:

- enjoy teaching others
- have patience when others cannot understand
- be able to make indirect suggestions
- be able to plan effectively
- have a positive attitude when expected to answer questions and explain actions
- be able to discuss organizational problems in a constructive way
- be able to tolerate others' making mistakes

- be able to give and take criticism
- enjoy decision making
- be able to work with others in a team approach
- be able to effectively manage paperwork.

Appendix 1 contains a scale that covers these areas, among others, in assessing suitability for clinical supervision. Anyone who is considering becoming a clinical supervisor should complete the scale and discuss it with others before accepting a supervisory position.

In addition, becoming a clinical supervisor involves some general shifts in attitude and functioning that one should be prepared in advance to accept (see Reeves, 1980:1-13). Some of these are:

- assuming more responsibility for managing the work of others and doing less practice
- assuming more responsibility in general
- having more authority
- carrying a broader decision-making role
- having more status
- having a changed relationship with coworkers
- being privy to more "inside" information about the organization, its employees, and its functioning
- having greater job pressures
- manifesting a greater commitment to the functions of the organization.

SUPERVISEE BILL OF RIGHTS

There are many aspects of supervision that are collective wisdom that have not been recorded or mandated by any ethical codes or social work licensure laws. The following "Bill of Rights" for supervisees was developed by the author in an effort to establish a basic foundation of expectations for supervision that could guide both the supervisee and supervisor. This "Bill of Rights" is the basis for all the material in this book. The supervisee "Bill of Rights" states that every clinical social work supervisee has the right to:

1. a supervisor who supervises consistently and at regular intervals;
2. growth-oriented supervision that respects personal privacy;
3. **supervision that is technically sound and theoretically grounded;**
4. be evaluated on criteria that are made clear in advance, and evaluations that are based on actual observation of performance;

5. a supervisor who is adequately skilled in clinical practice and trained in supervision practice.

Expectations of the Supervisor

The "Bill of Rights" based on the five criteria of consistency, growth-orientation, stable requirements, clear evaluative criteria, and a knowledgeable, competent supervisor leads to the requirement for clear explication of expectations of the supervisor and the supervisee. The best way to explicate the basic ideas of a succinct bill of rights is by developing a list of expectations a supervisee should have of a supervisor. In addition to the basic rights, a supervisee can and should have certain expectations of the supervisor.

Supervisees have a right to know what to expect from a supervisor. This is especially true in the case of students. While supervisees rarely inquire about this, supervisors should ask themselves this question as they strive to improve the quality of the supervision they provide. Given the nature and pattern of supervisee complaints about supervisors listed in evaluations and research studies, it would appear that supervisors should spend more time in reflection on how to best meet supervisee expectations.

Knowledge of what to expect of a supervisor is important for the supervisee as well as the supervisor. It is important for the supervisee in order to be an educated consumer and to adequately evaluate the supervision. It is important for the supervisor because the primary method of training for supervision today is self-education.

Supervision is the most important educational experience any clinical practitioner undergoes. Classroom courses and workshops are abstractions that are remotely connected to the realities of practice. Student evaluations of educational programs overwhelmingly indicate that the practice supervision component of the program was the most helpful.

Even though we are quick to acknowledge the importance of supervision, in the past two decades its use as an educational experience has diminished. Schools have minimal supervision time requirements; they increasingly give credit for work experience that has limited educational focus; they have downgraded qualifications to be a supervisor, and have given marginal recognition and support to internship faculty and administrators. Agencies are de-emphasizing supervision because it is costly. Some professional organizations minimize emphasis on supervision because it is viewed as a threat to the professional autonomy.

Some would perhaps argue that incompetent supervision is worse than no supervision at all. It is unfortunate that we have reached the point this is the choice we face. Even though supervision is being used less, there are many practitioners in agencies who must undergo supervision, and of course all students have one or two educational experiences on the path to a professional degree. The de-emphasis of supervision requirements at the agency and professional level has decreased the pool of supervisors qualified to offer student supervision. In the past, schools could draw on the agency and professionally trained supervisors for internship supervision. Presently, schools are required to develop their own training and educational programs for supervisors. Most schools have limited resources to provide the level of training needed. This means that the educational supervisor is left to become self-educated about good supervision practices. It is the self-education process that the expectations below are designed to promote.

In an effort to assist supervisors in this important professional reflection, the following list of expectations is provided. The supervisee has the right to expect that a supervisor:

1. is a master teacher;
2. is able to guide learning by virtue of superior knowledge and skill;
3. is able to transmit knowledge that integrates theory and practice activity;
4. has in-depth knowledge that can be applied to practice with precision;
5. is able to apply research knowledge and methodology to practice;
6. is confident in their knowledge, but open to questioning;
7. is able to accept criticism without becoming defensive;
8. is fair, honest, candid, but supportive and patient;
9. can provide cases that are appropriate, but challenging;
10. is appropriate in appearance, courteous, and clear in communication;
11. is thorough in providing orientation to the agency or setting;
12. is prepared for conferences and avoids wasting precious supervision time;
13. is involved in the agency, the community, and the profession;
14. is knowledgeable about the agency, the community, and the profession;
15. is knowledgeable about the code of ethics and faithfully adheres to its tenets.

It is important the supervisor adopt these criteria as an internal code of self-directing principles because the supervisee normally has limited expectations of supervision. Schools, agencies and the professional organizations offer little or no advance information about supervisee rights.

Since supervision is increasingly conducted in private there is no exposure of the activity. Supervisors do not experience supervision or consultation, so that their work as supervisors is not evaluated.

Expectations of the Supervisee

There are also expectations that the supervisor can have of the supervisee. The supervisee should be on time for conferences; should be prepared with cases to discuss; should be open about difficulties; should be open about stress; and should be open about cases that they have limited ability to work with.

In a study of supervisors (Study C) the major expectations of supervisees that were repeatedly identified were that the supervisees would:

- take that extra step in dealing with difficult cases;
- take responsibility for the job organizational matters;
- manifest a willingness to work hard;
- freely talk about problem cases and situations;
- be honest about how they are feeling;
- show respect for the supervisor;
- demonstrate basic interpersonal skills;
- have a genuine interest in learning;
- be willing to work with supervisor;
- be motivated to learn;
- be able to set goals with assistance;
- be willing to discuss work and their thoughts about work;
- present themselves as professionals;
- be aware of themselves;
- have integrity;
- have a sense of respect for others;
- be a person who will effectively engage clients as well as agency staff members;
- ask questions on an ongoing basis;
- take notes on a timely basis;
- be willing to read up on topics in area of practice;
- be open and curious about learning;
- have an ability to assess his or her own learning needs.

The rights and expectations listed here are general in nature, and supervisors and supervisees can draft their own list of rights and expectations based on the demands of individual or unique settings or situations.

SUGGESTED READINGS

Leopold Caligor. *Clinical Perspectives on the Supervision of Psychoanalysis and Psychotherapy.* New York: Plenum Press, 1984.
Overview of psychotherapy supervision from the psychoanalytic perspective.

Theodore Caplow. *How to Run Any Organization: A Manual of Practical Sociology.* Hinsdale, 111: Dryden Press, 1976.
A practical approach to functioning in any organization. Many helpful suggestions for supervisors. Specific strategies are recommended for beginning supervisors.

Gordon M. Hart. *The Process of Clinical Supervision.* Baltimore: University Park Press, 1982.
Overview of clinical supervision.

Ludmila W. Hoffman. *Old Scapes, New Maps: A Training Program for Psychotherapy Supervisors.* Cambridge, MA: Milusik Press, 1990.
Description of a system for training for psychotherapy supervision.

Stephen Holloway and George Brager. *Supervising in the Human Services: The Politics of Practice.* New York: The Free Press, 1989.
An overview of primarily administrative supervision in public social services.

Alfred Kadushin. *Supervision in Social Work.* New York: Columbia University Press, third edition, 1991.
Overview of basic social work supervision.

Ernest Kramer. *A Beginning Manual for Psychotherapists.* New York: Grune and Stratton, 1978.
A book to help the beginning practitioner become oriented to clinical practice.

Jerry M. Lewis. *To Be a Therapist: The Teaching and Learning.* New York: Brunner/Mazel, 1978.
This book describes the learning of theory, concepts, techniques, and skill from an interdisciplinary model developed in a psychiatric facility. This book is of value in individual supervision as well as in setting up a supervisory training program for a large number of trainees.

Carlton E. Munson (ed.). *Social Work Supervision: Classic Statements and Critical Issues*. New York: The Free Press, 1979.

A collection of 31 articles that serves as an introduction to the history and current practice of social work supervision.

James O. Palmer. *A Primer of Eclectic Psychotherapy*. Monterey, CA: Brooks/Cole, 1980.

A book to help the beginning practitioner become oriented to clinical practice.

Dorothy E. Pettes. *Staff and Student Supervision: A Task-Centered Approach*. Boston: Allen & Unwin, 1979.

Overview for beginning supervisors, especially on the administrative aspects of supervision.

Elton T. Reeves. *So You Want to Be a Supervisor!* New York: AMACOM, 1980.

Practical explanation of management-oriented supervision that can be applied to clinical supervision in some areas.

Whatever may be ahead, it is certain
that the new profession of social work
is now being given the greatest
opportunity which has ever come to it
to aid in the directing of economic and
social change for the welfare of
society. And it does not seem likely
that the social worker will ever lose
this advantage which he has gained.

Esther Lucile Brown
Social Work as a Profession

Chapter 2

History of Supervision

This chapter traces major developments in the history of supervision in the area of clinical practice, from the earliest conceptions of preparation for casework practice to the latest views of clinical practice. There is as much emphasis on the evolution of practice knowledge as on ideas about supervision because the two areas cannot be separated. Several themes have been central to every era of practice and supervision history. These themes are: the art and/or science of practice, treatment versus social reform, and the psychological versus sociological explanation of behavior.

What follows is not a comprehensive or rigorous analysis; social work has a rich and diverse heritage that cannot be completely covered briefly. This chapter is designed to give the practicing supervisor a summary understanding of over 100 years of history.

PRACTICE KNOWLEDGE

The history of supervision cannot be separated from discussion of the history of practice theory. Concern about supervision practices has increased and subsided over time in relation to development of, competition between, and conflict over intervention theories. Theories, and the people who develop them and use them, change over time. What are judged to be problems and the best ways to approach them also change with time (Veroff et al., 1981:9).

The history of social work practice reveals a fairly consistent pattern of inductive reasoning to advance our knowledge and deductive reasoning to measure our effectiveness. The early efforts were focused on defining problems and identifying social ills. Later efforts were focused on searching for theories to explain the problems and to guide our interventions, and on evaluating whether those interventions fit the theory. It is only when we take a sweeping historical look at our knowledge-building efforts that this pattern becomes apparent. Supervision has played an important role in this process over the decades, and almost all of our great theoreticians wrote about supervision as well as practice theory.

The history of social work practice is characterized by two recurring, related themes. The first theme has been the quest for a scientific approach to practice knowledge. In 1884 Josephine Shaw Lowell referred to social work as "our science" (Robinson, 1930:xii), and this characterization has continued to the present. In every era, social work leaders have striven to adhere to the scientific principles of the time. Until recently, supervision has been an important component in the application of the science and the evolution of our knowledge. The second theme has been the shifts in practice orientation. These two themes are naturally related. The purpose of science is the evolution of knowledge. The continual application of scientific principles to a body of knowledge produces dynamic shifts in the way practice is defined and oriented.

This persistent quest to expand our knowledge has brought about many of the changes in our practice that are explored in this chapter. Clearly, not all changes are brought about by the pursuit of knowledge, but it is an important part in our history that often goes unrecognized, and the evolution of our practice has not been totally the reflection of economic or political forces, as some have held.

EARLY HISTORY

It is not known for certain where, when, or how the traditional model of social work supervision originated. It probably was based on the model of consultation and supervision developed in the field of medicine in England, which subsequently became the model for American medicine (Kaslow, 1979:1-24). It is reasonable to assume that the medical model of supervision was adopted by early social workers since they had many close connections with physicians. These connections were personal as well as professional. Some of the early social workers' parents and spouses were physicians. Physicians taught in the earliest social work training programs, a pattern that has continued in some schools to the present. Physicians served on the boards of various early charitable societies and had much influence on how these organizations were structured and operated.

Supervision, as we conceptualize it in clinical practice, began to emerge in the late 1800s within the Charity Organization Societies, in which paid agents became the model for casework practice. These paid agents were supervised within the agency as part of apprenticeship programs. There has been disagreement over the extent of administrative and educational focus of this supervision (Kaslow, 1979:28-34). When the apprenticeship programs became burdensome for the agencies to administer, perhaps because of increased focus on the educational component, leaders of the profession reluctantly agreed to training programs' becoming affiliated with universities. These programs did not become part of the university, but were appendages of them. This led to a modified version of the earlier apprentice programs, and field instruction, as we know it today, evolved from this arrangement.

The form and structure of supervision have remained fairly constant from the late nineteenth century to the present. The supervisor was responsible for a number of supervisees, who were provided supervision through periodic individual conferences. Much later the idea of group supervision was applied on a limited basis. Group supervision has not been widely adopted in clinical settings, although it has been conceptually confused with team approaches in some settings.

Although the structure of supervision has not changed, its content has evolved and shifted over the years. Social work practice has traditionally reflected the attitudes and values of society, and supervision has been the **arena in which practice** strategies and societal patterns are consolidated and integrated.

By 1840 there were over 30 private organizations in New York City alone whose focus was on moral uplift combined with the provision of relief. Society's response to this effort was mixed because there was a fear that organized attempts to decrease poverty would actually contribute to its increase, an attitude that has persisted to the present in segments of the society. In these early efforts, social work was associated more with the assessment of the deserving nature of the individual and determining the extent of poverty than with offering moral uplift. The initial focus was on the individual and the characteristics that contributed to poverty. Later this focus shifted to the family and the effects of poverty on its members.

Institutional Supervision

During this era the concept of supervision was more general than it is today. It dealt more with supervising institutions to ensure that clients or patients were being treated and that the institutions were being run effectively and efficiently. As the role of assessment emerged, the idea of individual case supervision developed. It was gradually recognized that to make a good assessment, to determine who was deserving, and to know what information was important in understanding problems, one needs training and practice under a skilled supervisor. This training function was carried by agencies for several decades before it was gradually taken over by universities and training facilities associated with universities. This process of transferring responsibility for training was slow, occurring over several decades, and raised many conflicts about whether agencies or universities were best prepared to train social workers (see Munson, 1979a: 1-5).

Field instruction as part of educational programs has contributed a great deal to the evolution of supervision in social work. The earliest educational programs were agency-based apprenticeships. Classroom instruction, as we know it, emerged later and was "considered supplemental to rounding out of agency-based learning by doing" (Hollis & Taylor, 1951:230-231).

Assessment

At the turn of the century there was a quest for a theory of explanation of poverty and reaction to disease as medical social work emerged. This focus continued social work's emphasis on assessment. What had begun as work with poor persons served by relief agencies became the identification of the social and emotional elements of illness. It was in the move to develop medical social work that the psychological component was first introduced into the profession. At this stage the emphasis was not on treatment, but was still on assessment and identification of problems. Social work was founded on the basis of assessment, first in the area of relief and then in health. Soon after, the same pattern occurred in the area of psychiatric social work.

The social work profession emerged in direct relation to the quest for assessment in dealing with individualized social services. The assessment function of social work grew from the economic assessment of the Charity Organization Societies, to the physical assessment of hospital social work, to the diagnostic assessment of later work with psychiatrists. Ironically, but understandably, as the profession evolved through these forms of assessment it became narrower in focus. It can be argued that Mary Richmond recognized this trend and that her book, *Social Diagnosis*, was a major attempt to reverse the trend. Within the profession, social assessment in individual cases was connected to the larger societal concern with social reform, and as society's concern with social reform waned after World War I (Weinberger, 1974:83), so did social work's interest in assessment.

Sociology and Social Work

During the decades social work was struggling with assessment, it enjoyed a natural connection with sociology. In 1909, this connection was depicted thus:

> Charitable work has become so closely allied with all forms of social effort that general conditions must be taken into account before one can do good work, even among individuals. This involves some study of the whole situation, or in other words, some attention to sociology. (Conyngton, 1909; 1971:326)

This connection is understandable since, in the broadest sense, social work is a practice within society, while "sociology is not a practice, but an attempt to understand" (Greenberg, 1971:4). When social work lost interest in assessment during the1920s, its relationship with sociology deteriorated rapidly (Munson, 1979e; Siporin, 1980:14). Sociology and social work have since been toiling separately in their "little 'gardens of knowledge'" (Greenberg, 1971:10), but social work has been further divided in its devotion to individual treatment and social reform. This division has distracted it further from developing and refining systems of assessment.

Everett Dirksen once said that political parties do not defeat one another, but defeat themselves. The same is true of professions. The cause-and-function debate has distracted social work since its inception. Mary Richmond perceived this division and its destructive effect on the profession. She saw a place for both levels of functioning within the profession, and advocated cooperative efforts in these areas. What Richmond proposed was only a beginning, but social work had failed to recognize this. We had not organized our social reform efforts around sociologists' succinct conception that "there are three requirements for a given social condition to be regarded as a social problem: (1) It must be social in origin. (2) It must be regarded by society as a problem. (3) It must require some form of social intervention" (Greenberg, 1971:13).

In the literature it has been held that a turning point for the profession was reached when Abraham Flexner addressed the National Conference of Charities and Corrections in 1915 and declared that social work was not a profession. Historians have accorded this speech more significance than it appears to have had at the time. In fact, Flexner's pronouncements were nothing new for social work and hardly came as a surprise.

The theory used during this era was practical and inductive. Psychological and sociological theories of poverty were not highly developed, and efforts to explain poverty on the basis of individual personality were not very successful (Robinson, 1930:10-11). Supervision, during this era of the development of assessment knowledge, was focused on developing skill at identifying and classifying individual problems and needs. Mary Richmond succinctly summarized the role of supervision at this stage of our history:

> What should a supervisor look for in a case record in which the work has reached the stage of evidence gathered but not yet compared or interpreted? . . . Good supervision must include this consideration of wider aspects . . . . Every case worker has noticed how a certain juxtaposition of facts often reappears in record after record, and . . . this recurring juxtaposition indicates a hidden relation of cause and effect . . . . It is here that the "notation of recurrence" . . . becomes a duty of supervisor and case worker . . . . The getting at knowledge that will make the case work of another generation more effective **may be only a by-product of our own case work, but it is an important** by-product. (1917; 1965:351-352)

THE FREUDIAN INFLUENCE

At the time Richmond wrote of this view of supervision, a new era of theory-building was emerging. Freud visited Clark University in the fall of 1909, and along with others gave a series of lectures on his theory. There is disagreement about the influence this visit had on the spread of Freud's ideas in the United States. Press coverage of the lectures was "spotty" and limited (Clark, 1980:259-276). It is apparent that the lectures had very little direct impact on social work. It took many years for Freud's influence on social work to become apparent, and it occurred in a way different from what is commonly believed.

Freud's ideas were promoted in the United States by people who traveled to Europe, were analyzed by Freud, and returned to the United States to work and lead the psychoanalytic movement. After World War I, Freud "had around him a flock of young Americans who came to Europe for training" (Roazen, 1974:378) — persons like Horace Frink and Adolf Meyer. Horace Frink was a brilliant American who was analyzed twice by Freud and selected by him to lead the psychoanalytic movement in the United States. But he was a tragic figure: he suffered from prolonged mental illness and died in a mental hospital. At one time he was treated by Adolf Meyer at Johns Hopkins. That Frink turned to Meyer is testimony to Meyer's reputation as a "famous psychiatrist" (Roazen, 1974:380).

Born and trained in Europe, Meyer migrated to the United States at the age of 26. Meyer was regarded highly by social workers and had much influence on their approach to psychiatric social work. He spoke before the National Conference of Charities and Corrections in 1911, and the Smith College School of Psychiatric Social Work, the New York School of Social Work, and the Pennsylvania School of Social and Health Work in 1918 (Robinson, 1930:28-54). Meyer drew heavily on the ideas of Freud, but he had a much more comprehensive view of functioning. Meyer once remarked, "The main thing . . . is that your point of reference should always be life itself and not the imagined cesspool of the unconscious" (Lief, 1948:vii). Meyer's wife worked closely with him. She became the first volunteer psychiatric social worker and was the model for the first paid psychiatric social worker hired in New York in 1907. At about the same time, Richard C. Cabot in Boston was advocating utilizing social workers to work with psychiatrists (Lief, 1948). This brief example of Meyer's influence on social work illustrates the complex, but subtle, **manner in which Freud's ideas found their way into social work.** Also, Meyer was typical of psychiatrists who influenced the ideas of social workers in that the ideas shared by these psychiatric leaders were often sprinkled with Freudian conceptions, but were much broader and not exclusively focused on Freudian conventions.

The Americans who traveled to Europe to study under Freud and returned to the United States to practice introduced to social work the concept of exploring personal dynamics in supervision as well as the idea of group discussion, which became the forerunner of group supervision. An article in the April 1929 issue of *The Family*, titled "Supervision" and written anonymously by a Family Welfare Society worker, includes a description of a discussion group that paralleled Freud's Wednesday Society (which later became the Vienna Psychoanalytic Society) (Clark, 1980: 213-219):

> Through the stimulus of lectures at the local school of social work, an evening reading group was organized, we discussed novels from the caseworker's point of view, and occasionally we studied books of a professional nature.

During this period the "staff conference" was refined as "a method of supervision" in which a caseworker presented a problem case in the presence of the supervisor and staff from other disciplines, such as psychiatry and "home economics." The case was discussed at length, and treatment recommendations were made (Heston, 1929:46). This method of supervision became the model for introduction of group supervision in social work and the team approach of several decades later.

The introduction of social work into the medical setting was promoted by Richard C. Cabot (Chaiklin, 1978:475). Cabot was advocating the social work role in medical settings in Boston at the same time that the psychiatrist Adolf Meyer and his wife were developing psychiatric social work as a specialty in New York (Lief, 1948:149-152). Cabot presented a broad view of the role of social work in medical settings:

> In our own case work in the social service department of the . . . hospital we are accustomed to sum up our cases in monthly reports from the case records by asking about each case four questions: What is the physical state of this patient? What is the mental state of this patient? What is his physical environment? What is his mental and spiritual environment? The doctor is apt to know a good deal about the first of those four things, the physical state, and a little about the second, the mental, but about the other two almost nothing. The expert social worker comes with those four points in mind to every case. It is of interest to notice that this fourfold knowledge

is not the goal of the social worker merely; it is the goal of every intelligent human being who wants to understand another human being . . . . Social work, as I see it, takes no special point of view; it takes the total human point of view, and that is just what it has to teach doctors who by reason of their training are disposed to take a much narrower point of view. They can safely and profitably continue that narrow outlook only in case they have a social worker at their elbow, as they should have, to help them. Each of us has his proper field, but we should not work separately, for the human beings who are our charges cannot be cut in two. (Cabot, 1915a:220)

MARY RICHMOND

Mary Richmond was familiar with Adolf Meyer and his work. Until the appearance of Richmond's *Social Diagnosis* in 1917, social casework focused exclusively on social forces and the effects of large-scale economic need. The individual was seen in the context of larger social problems. Meeting individual economic need and character building were essential components of service, but there was no doubt in the literature about the societal causes. Historical analysis that attributes paramount importance to Richmond's *Social Diagnosis* as the initial and seminal work on casework practice is, in my opinion, not completely accurate. However, such analysis has caused more recent observers to neglect the evolutionary contribution of this work. Richmond's work is not the initial description of the comprehensive casework process. Seven years earlier, Mary Conyngton published *How to Help: A Manual of Practical Charity* (1909), which was a comprehensive explanation of the nature of social casework from a sociological perspective. Richmond's book was more a synthesis of the psychological and the sociological in the context of the family. This view is epitomized in her observation that "a man really is the company he keeps plus the company that his ancestors kept . . . ." (Richmond, 1965:369).

Freud's visit to Clark University in 1909 had gone largely unnoticed, and he is not mentioned in Richmond's book, although American psychiatrists and psychologists are mentioned. Whether this lack of recognition was deliberate or due to lack of Freudian influence in casework circles will never be completely known. Much later Virginia Robinson argued this was due to lack of Freudian influence (Robinson, 1930). There is reason to believe that Richmond did anticipate the gradual shift to exclusive focus on the individual and psychological determinism, and that her aim in *Social Diagnosis* was in part to offer some balance in this trend.

THE 1920s

Family Focus

In an analysis of trends in textbooks on the family, it was found that attention devoted to social work with families increased dramatically after World War I (Hart & Hart, 1935:vi). Many agency names were changed to reflect this trend (e.g., Associated Charities changed its name to Family Welfare Society in 1922). These two developments reflected two important trends (see Siporin, 1980).

It was during this era that it became apparent that supervisors needed more formal preparation. The failure to prepare supervisors adequately often led to "floundering" by workers, disillusionment of workers, and a frustrating "sink or swim" approach to treatment that caused deep frustration for the worker. The situation was aggravated when workers suffering such self-doubt were promoted to supervisory positions. This situation was highlighted by a rare article, published in 1929 in *The Family*, giving one supervisor's account of these problems (Anonymous, 1929). It was at this time that "field work teaching" as a requirement in schools of social work was begun in family welfare societies and spread rapidly to many other agencies (Brown, 1936:56). Also at this time specific literature devoted to supervision techniques began to emerge. The idea of the staff conference as a method of supervision was devised as a way to be more effectively and efficiently oriented to the new knowledge, and it refocused service orientation (Heston, 1929:46-47).

Social Work as Art

The concept of art was introduced into social work practice and supervision after the concept of science. The idea of art was drawn on at points when science failed to further our understanding (see Chapter 15); it came to social work through our close ties with medicine, and was formalized with the publication of Richard Cabot's *Social Service and the Art of Healing* in 1915.

The concept was solidified in 1924 with the publication of DeSchweinitz's *The Art of Helping People Out of Trouble*. DeSchweinitz considered living an art, and he associated this with the art of helping. Several years later Porter Lee and Marion Kenworthy (a physician) further expanded the idea of social work practice as an art in their book *Mental Hygiene and Social Work*. Subsequently, this concept has been applied loosely by most writers about practice.

The idea of the art of living and the art of practice was used to unite personal growth and practice. DeSchweinitz explained:

> Growth is a product of the years. Man, being but part of the whole, may become impatient, content with what would be incomplete. Nature is comprehensive and eternal.
>
> To have grasped this lesson is to have made a beginning of learning the art of helping . . . . Transcending the vicissitudes of experience is the challenge of the greatest of the arts. (1924: 224-231)

Also, the emphasis on art as opposed to identifying the specifics of practice was observed by Dorothy Hutchinson in an article on supervision:

> The word "technique" as applied to supervision in social case work has a dull and rigid sound. The word "art" is more stimulating, if we can release ourselves from a certain shop-worn feeling in its presence. (1935:44)

During the same period, the participants at the Milford Conference concluded: "A social case worker whose own personality development is not furthered through his contact with his clients is probably not an effective social case worker" (National Association of Social Workers, 1974:31).

It was through this process of the connection among physicians, the concept of art, and social work that the analysis of personality found its way into supervision, rather than directly through the introduction of psychoanalysis into the United States.

The shift in focus to the client during this era led to the emergence of marriage counseling distinct from family treatment by social work and other disciplines. Also, prevention from a psychological perspective grew out of the new orientation. The literature of this period addressed premarital counseling in connection with marriage counseling as a preventive measure. Interestingly, the professional emphasis on prevention in mental health grew out of concern about what was termed "popular counseling," which reached the public at large through newspapers, magazines, books, and radio. Karen Horney was typical of this movement and her book, *Self-Analysis*, was most likely the first self-help book even though she cautioned against people engaging in self-help without the aid of a professional therapist. Such broad-based counseling was viewed as dangerous when offered by "professional lecturers" rather than professional practitioners (Groves, 1940), and paralleled the modern concern over "pop psychology" available through the print and electronic media.

THE 1930s

A Shift in Focus

In the decade prior to the depression a great irony occurred in social work. Relief efforts were pushed into the background when poverty was actually increasing. The depression resulted in the solidification of a dichotomy between public and private agencies that had been emerging for some time. Public agencies focused on relief, and private agencies were free to devote attention almost exclusively to treatment.

There was also a distinction in private agencies that resulted in some offering brief treatment, which has been rediscovered in recent times, and psychiatrically oriented agencies focusing on long-term treatment (Chapin & Queen, 1937; 1972:18-22). Prior to the depression, professional education for social work declined, and with the onset of the depression, the professional schools could not supply enough practitioners to meet the need. This created problems for field instructors, who scurried to meet the demands for workers and raised the issue of generic training versus specialization for schools (Chapin & Queen, 1937; 1972:91-95).

Rank-and-File Movement

A major outcome of the depression was the "rank-and-file" movement, based on power through political and union groups. This led some to argue that this movement within the profession was at the expense of functional knowledge aimed at skillful analysis of service and social betterment (Chapin & Queen, 1937; 1972:97). The rank-and-file movement gave new inspiration to trained caseworkers in private agencies, who had been dissatisfied "with the thinking of the social work establishment," and attracted employees of the public relief agencies, who were primarily untrained professionally (Fisher, J., 1980:93). The disgruntled professional caseworkers were reacting to the triumph in the 1920s of psychiatry and psychoanalysis in practice, with their emphasis on the role of the "individual psyche in human affairs." This division of practitioners was based on what was called "large-order problems" versus "small-order problems," and was epitomized by Mary Richmond's earlier view that "social work was in the retail not the wholesale business" (Fisher, Jacob, 1980:17-18).

The division continued through World War II, as the split centered around large-scale political ideologies that became the essential struggle of the war. These ideologies were replicated in a somewhat different context in the 1960s in the United States during the Vietnam War and several social movements. In both eras these conflicts reached down to the most basic levels of practice and often diverted attention from treatment issues in supervision.

Emerging Treatment Services

Social agencies made a shift to offering treatment services in the 1930s when the growth of public programs during the depression relieved them "of routine financial relief for clients" (Stevenson, G. S., 1940:131). A major change of emphasis occurred in these agencies during the 1930s, causing an increase in demand for psychiatric social workers. The demand caught schools of social work off guard and "confused" about how to train such workers. This confusion has a modern-day equivalent in schools of social work (see Chapter 1). Psychoanalytic theory was used to fill many of the conceptual training gaps because it was readily available and was a "practical theory of interpersonal relationship" that fit the mental hygiene movement emphasis on "the personality needs of the client." There was concern that the renewed emphasis on psychological and personality factors was at the expense of "constitutional factors," but concessions were guardedly granted that such swings of the practice pendulum were necessary to advance knowledge. In this context the primary supervisory evaluative question became: "What is this experience with me (a worker) or this agency doing to the development (mental growth) of this client?" (Stevenson, G. S., 1940:131). This same question could be couched in the psychotherapeutic orientation specifically, and was indicative of the shift away from diagnosis and environmental manipulation in treatment.

Field Instruction

By the 1930s field instruction, which originated in the family welfare societies, was highly developed. The schools utilized several models. Some schools paid the salaries of supervisors of students in agencies, a few schools required faculty members to supervise students, and most schools had cooperative agreements with selected agencies that permitted their paid staff to supervise students (Brown, 1936:57). Field instruction was a significant portion of the educational program. In many programs students were required to undergo a general field placement before entering a more specialized placement. The emphasis in field instruction was upon developing practice skill through integration of "knowledge, philosophy and technique" (Brown, 1936:58).

THE 1940s

Therapeutic Eclecticism

It was in this era that the idea of therapeutic eclecticism emerged to fit the needs of the individual case rather than continuous commitment to one theory or approach that the case would be molded to fit. This trend was considered a major change from the practices in the earlier child guidance clinics, and was depicted as occurring rather rapidly. A survey of clinics reported by Stevenson showed a dramatic shift in practice orientation between 1936 and 1939. The sudden onset of this new focus was recognized by Jessie Taft in 1940, when she observed, "In the Philadelphia area, the past decade has witnessed a realization of psychological insight in terms of actual, day-to-day practice that was not dreamed of in 1930" (Taft, 1940:179). The new focus on the client—and not on the qualifications, emotional maturity, and mastery of psychoanalytic concepts of the worker—introduced a new balance of concern in supervision, and required supervisors who had a broader perspective than had been the case in the past.

Child Guidance

The child guidance movement had begun in the early 1920s, spearheaded by psychiatrists who had travelled to Europe to study with Alfred Adler who had invented the movement. Treatment of children was originated in Europe but developed in the United States (Barton, 1987:112). By the 1940s the field of psychiatry, concerned over childhood responses to war, began a shift in focus from the children to the parents that laid the foundation for the family therapy movement. As Plant quipped in 1944, "Why talk of child guidance—it's the parents who need guidance!" This represented a major shift in theoretical orientation from the intrapsychic psychoanalytic position to an interactional educational one. The concern about children was in part based on statistical trends revealing that delinquency had increased rapidly during the 1920s, had decreased in the 1930s, and that a significant rise had occurred at the beginning of the 1940s (Plant, 1944:1-2). It is interesting that when child-focused treatment was called into question, it was attributed to social work and not psychiatry. The following observation by a psychiatrist illustrates this:

The "lost generation" of the depression is in large measure doing our fighting now. One who remembers the dire prognostications of our social-work group has to pinch himself as he reads today's news. Should we not temper all our theory with a healthy regard for the adaptability of the human being? (Plant, 1944:2)

Lawyers and judges turned on social workers in this theoretical debate from a slightly different perspective. For them the idea of individual treatment was not fair. One judge went so far as to say, "Stripped of all its elaborate wrappings, the doctrine of individual treatment may be expressed by one word—*injustice*" (Perkins, 1944:47). The debate emerged around problems with adolescents because this group fit the transitions that were occurring in the theoretical perspectives. If the extremes of psychology and sociology did not satisfy all the requirements for a good approach to practice, a social psychology had to be shaped that would guide intervention.

The behavioral adaptations of adolescence fit the explanatory requirements for the new theory that was needed. Hawkins described the behavioral adaptations necessary in an article that was a response to the attack on social work by the judiciary:

Each adult who gets along even moderately well must reach and maintain some sort of workable balance between himself as an individual with strong individual needs, impulses and drives, and himself as a member of society which makes various and urgent demands upon him. Moreover, in our society it is during the adolescent years that the psychological problem of achieving such a balance is at its peak, and many of the difficulties of the adolescent can be traced to his conflict over his own individuality and his relation to the community as represented by his parents, other adults, such institutions as school, church, and law and society's customs in general. (Hawkins, 1944:129)

Through the professional conflicts, the new theoretical orientation was being forged in the fires of the debate.

THE 1950s

Psychiatry and Social Work

By the 1950s social work had developed a conceptual basis for its connection to psychiatry generally and psychoanalysis specifically. In commenting on the practice of field instruction during the 1950s, George Gardner, a physician, observed:

> It is comparatively of minor importance to cite that the present day individual supervisor-student method of instruction is but a reactivation of the old physician-medical student apprenticeship system or that it has borrowed heavily from the more modern psychoanalyst-analytic control student approach. The fact remains that this educational device as it relates to students in the field of mental health has been brought to its order of excellence by educators in social work. (Garrett, 1954:iii)

It is not clear whether social workers and psychoanalysts were ever as close theoretically as has been argued over the years. However, there seems to be no close association at present. This is epitomized by an Italian psychoanalyst's statement: "Minuchin has a very shallow theory of family therapy. It's just a theory for social workers really." Selvini-Palazzoli later retracted her statement about Minuchin, but not about social workers (Simon, R., 1982:30).

Resurgence of Social Science Focus

Social work has not enjoyed as positive a relationship with medicine in general as it has with psychiatry. This is epitomized by the fact that in 1951 the president of the American Medical Association mounted a successful campaign to have unsold copies of Charlotte Towle's *Common Human Needs* destroyed and publication dropped by the Federal Security Administration, because he interpreted the use of the word "socialized" to mean "socialistic" (Perlman, 1969:12). The 1950s' reaction against psychoanalysis, expert helpers, and long-term treatment has been attributed to everything from mass transportation and mass media to the decline of religion and a reaction against science. In the eyes of many, the gains of half a century were in jeopardy, and many problems were dumped back on the community (Veroff et al., 1981:3-12). The shift back to the social sciences and away from psychiatry in practice and supervision in modern times was identified by Siporin in 1956. In 1959 Charlotte Towle gave a sweeping account of this and how social work had chosen psychiatry over social science as the source of its theoretical underpinnings at the turn of the century, but in the 1950s she saw social work turning back to social science to conceptualize practice demands (Perlman, 1969:268-277). The "reunion" brought emphasis in practice to the nature of roles and functions. This carried over to supervision and led Towle to perceive the "process" of supervision as consisting of three functions: administration, teaching, and helping (Perlman, 1969:166), a conceptualization that has persisted to the present.

Field Instruction

By the 1950s the field instruction supervisor was viewed as a necessary and important link in the partnership of the classroom and the field. The way in which field instruction applied casework theory and developed technique was clear. Rather than focusing on differentiation, the emphasis was on integration. In her book *Learning Through Supervision*, which described the school/agency relationship in detail, Annette Garrett observed: "Theory without cases is empty; cases without theory are meaningless" (1954:5). There were "functional" and "diagnostic" theoretical orientations in different schools, but each school put much effort into ensuring that classroom and field learning were theoretically compatible. There were close ties between the schools and agencies. By this time most schools of social work had become well-established within the university, and field instruction was considered an essential element of the educational program. Doctoral education for social work expanded during this era, giving educators a more theoretical and scientific orientation to practice, which resulted in further diminution of the agency-practitioner's approach to education. This shift in orientation had been taking place gradually since the turn of the century, when the first schools were being established, and this reorientation was fairly complete by the late 1950s (see Kahn, A., 1973:147-168).

Theory Integration

The Freudian influence continued in the 1950s, and was highlighted by the publication of Gordon Hamilton's text on the psychosocial approach to casework in 1951. Based on Freud's psychology, this approach expanded the ideas to include the social context of behavior, and became the foundation for the formulations of Florence Hollis (1966), which were published over a decade later. Hamilton's work called attention to the growing importance of environmental factors. The renewed attention devoted to social factors was also illustrated by the publication of Helen Harris Perlman's popular casework text in 1957. Perlman drew on ego psychology, learning theory, and role theory from the perspective of the client's environmental or interactional problem. Internal dynamics were important for Perlman only in connection with the client's presenting problems (Strean, 1978:14-15). Perlman's work has had considerable influence on social work practice theory, and serves as a forerunner of the problem-centered and interactionally based practice theories that emerged in the late 1970s.

Professional Status

It is ironic that, at the same time social work came into its own as a profession in the 1950s and 1960s, it diverted much of its concern from theory building and a scientific orientation to concern about the status of the profession. At the time that an organizationally unified profession was in great demand in many settings, the profession was questioning its own validity and continued existence. During this era supervision concerns took a back seat as professionalization was characterized as antithetical to supervision. The truly professional practitioner was viewed as independent, sufficiently if not completely educated, generically trained, and self-regulating with respect to evaluation, monitoring of practice, and being scientifically oriented. Towle, commenting on this trend in 1961, pointed out that the profession's orientation to causes, unhappily, had been lost. She observed that Mary Richmond and Jane Addams were "devoid of professionalism"; that they went beyond it, and "gave to their colleagues and subordinates a vital sense of something to work for, not just something to do in the way of performing a task" (Perlman, 1969:280-281).

Interdependence

Systems theory emerged in the 1950s at the same time that sociologists and psychologists for the first time recognized that interdependence of individuals, governments, and societies was a basic fact. As this notion of interdependence gained ascendency in our society, a reaction set in because we are a nation of individualists. This reaction took the form of all sorts of self-development theories and do-it-yourself strategies and philosophies. It was in this societal context that the vision of the autonomous professional social work practitioner emerged.

Supervisors' Calm Existence

During the 1950s supervisors had a relatively calm existence, compared with previous decades and with decades since. There was a general acceptance of the combined role of psychological and sociological factors as determinants of behavior. It was a relatively conservative period with a stable social structure. There were no massive social upheavals. Social roles were well defined, and clinical practice was focused on clients' becoming adjusted to these fairly clear-cut role expectations. Practice theory was evolving systematically, concisely, and slowly, allowing time for integration of new knowledge.

The theories of the 1950s became the basis for much of the practice for the next two decades and remain as a major influence on practice to this day (Strean, 1978:13), although the methods of casework, group work, and community organization forged during this era have been reconceptualized into generalist/specialist models.

THE 1960s

Change and Unrest

The 1960s saw massive political, social, cultural, and economic upheaval. Social roles were changing, and there was much experimentation with new life-styles. The civil rights movement, the sexual revolution, the technological revolution, and the student movement all combined to bring new opportunities and new problems. Social agencies expanded to address unmet needs in a bold effort to combat poverty, and mental health centers saw clients who were expressing feelings and reporting situational adjustment problems that also required new and bold interventive efforts.

A knowledge explosion in practice theory erupted that had been gradually building since the 1950s. At the same time the unified profession of social work, which had emerged with the founding of the National Association of Social Workers in 1956, became a stabilized professional force in the 1960s. Simultaneously, social casework came under attack from within the profession with more intensity than it had from outside during the early 1940s. During this decade supervisors had great difficulty integrating the vast new knowledge and fostering a commitment to practice at the same time, as the entire philosophical base of clinical practice was under attack. Some supervisors retreated; others persisted and struggled with consolidating the new knowledge and theory. Those who took the challenge seriously made commendable efforts not only to apply psychological and sociological theory to cases but to integrate this theory with social reform efforts.

The integration of the new practice knowledge and resolution of the casework-versus-psychotherapy debate was greatly aided in 1966 with the publication of a casework text by Florence Hollis that cast casework in the context of "a psychosocial therapy." This book integrated the psychological and sociological in a usable manner. At the same time the idea of casework as therapy or psychotherapy gave rise to renewed concern that such a conception of practice would tend to dissolve the knowledge base of social work practice that over the years had led to its being unique among the helping professions (Turner, 1978:1-4). Some would argue that although it has taken 20 years, today this dissolution of the social work practice base has, in fact, taken place.

Conflicting Views

For supervisors the calm of the 1950s seemed far away. The new technology and increased emphasis on research produced conflicting views of what to do and how to do it in order to help clients. The old debate of residual treatment versus social reform intensified greatly, but even within the treatment field new theories and new methods escalated, along with conflicting and competing claims of how to intervene most effectively. It is understandable that supervisors and practitioners alike began to question the efficiency of their own practices. To some extent, the social work profession turned on itself during this decade.

The new life-styles and freedom of expression of the 1960s in part contributed to the de-emphasis of supervision. This was the era of the popular slogan "do your own thing" and its corollary of autonomous practice in social work. There was a feeling that the schools needed only to arm students with enough of the new knowledge so they could go forth and forge it into effective independent practice. Faced with all the stresses that were emerging at the societal level, within the profession, and within agencies, supervisors were also willing to accept this view.

New Opportunities

The experimentation and research orientation of the 1960s produced a number of studies assessing the effects of different supervision. One, conducted at the University of Michigan (Sales & Navarre, 1970), found that individual supervision required more time of the supervisor than group supervision; student performance was equally good in group and individual supervision; the content of supervision was the same in both models; group supervisors were more likely to follow a prearranged agenda than individual supervisors; students were more likely to seek and accept advice in individual supervision; and supervisors were equally satisfied with both models.

Despite all the turmoil, the 1960s opened up exploration of and experimentation with new models and structures of supervision. Dual models of **supervision and consultation, first discussed in the 1950s,** were applied in many agencies. Mixed structures of individual and group supervision were used with much success. New models of field instruction were tried, and the use of "faculty-based" field instructors became common practice in schools of social work. Employed primarily with federal grant money, field instructors were placed in agencies full time to supervise students exclusively, individually and in groups. These field instructors worked side by side with "agency-based" field instructors, who were employees of the agency and supervised students as a part of their other agency duties. Even though the faculty-based model of field instruction was quite successful, it has been greatly curtailed because of decreased funding of social work training by the federal government.

Demand for Practitioners

The 1960s were similar to the 1920s in that the demand for trained practitioners was much greater than the supply that could be provided by schools of social work. This led to reemphasis in the 1960s on generic practice and reinstituting of training programs for BSW graduates to meet the manpower needs. Ultimately, and paradoxically, this led to more specialization among MSW practitioners in the decade of the 1970s, with BSW practitioners providing generic services. Supervision has become more specific in its functions when relating to the specialized nature of MSW practitioners. This orientation to practice has placed new demands on supervisors to be more job specific in their approach.

THE 1970s

Disillusionment

In the 1970s the rapid changes of the 1960s slowly subsided. There was a growing sense of disillusionment when all the promises and hopes of the 1960s were not fulfilled (Yankelovich, 1981). This mentality characterized many of the problems clients presented. The economy began to decline, and for the first time in decades, social workers experienced cutbacks in the number of jobs available.

Technology and Specialization

Technology continued to advance. For example, new and dramatic medical treatments of the 1960s became commonplace in the 1970s. Organ transplants became routine. Drug therapies and radiation treatments became widespread. Such expansion created new but highly specialized jobs for social workers. Medical social work and geriatric social work were faced with new practice demands. The increase in specialization has just now led the profession to reconsider the role of supervision in many settings. The 1960s view of making large amounts of knowledge and theory available to students and then sending them off to practice independently is giving way to the view that practitioners need help more than ever as they attempt to integrate so much knowledge as well as master a complex practice specialization, such as oncology social work or practice on a renal dialysis ward in a hospital.

Supervision for specialized practice is the dominant focus at the present time. There has been some emphasis on the role of practitioners as drawing on a common core of knowledge, at the same time that the importance of individualizing treatment has been recognized (Kahn, A., 1973:99). However, the specifics of this combined approach remain a challenge of integration for the profession and supervisors. It remains unclear how this dichotomy of orientation can be effectively presented in supervision. There is some doubt whether specialized knowledge is being conveyed to practitioners. For example, in a study of a sample of social workers by Pratt (1969) it was found that knowledge of social factors affecting health was marginal.

Field Instruction

In the past several years there has been renewed interest in field instruction. With the renewal of undergraduate social work education and the elimination of faculty-based field instructors, there is increasing interest in the role of the agency-based field instructor (see Wilson, 1981). Also, increased interest in field instruction could be related to concern about the limited specialized knowledge of beginning practitioners. The limitations of beginning practitioners and the growing concern about this were epitomized by a position statement of the Family Service Association of America Directors, formulated in 1972 (Anonymous, 1973:108-110). The directors took the stand that graduate schools of social work were providing "general" training that did not adequately prepare practitioners for work with individuals, families, and small groups. It was their view that theoretical learning was weak, that field instruction did not foster knowledge and skill that promoted a minimum level of practice competence, and that faculty were not adequately qualified to teach effective casework practice. The statement called for more cooperation between schools and agencies to overcome these problems. No clear steps have been taken to deal with this issue, and in many communities, the schools and agencies remain at odds about how best to prepare practitioners. This conflict had been building for over a decade and remains as a major source of conflict a decade later.

Continued Professionalization

In the 1970s the professionalization of social work continued mainly through passage of licensing and certification acts in a number of states. The National Association of Social Workers has supported this legislation and has strengthened its own standards for membership in the Academy of Certified Social Workers. By the end of the decade, over two dozen states had laws regulating social work practice. There is much diversity in state laws with respect to supervision and requirements for various levels of clinical practice, including private practice.

Emergence of Private Practice

The essence of social work practice had remained essentially unchanged for 50 years. In the past decade there have been two major developments that will bring about fundamental changes in all that we do: the development of private practice, and renewed denial that what we do is psychotherapy. Two decades ago Briar and Miller pointed out that the debate over psychotherapy versus casework dealt not with practice method or orientation but with professional identity and legitimation (1971:22). Currently, private practice is increasing on a full-time and part-time basis. Many private practitioners purchase supervision and consultation from practitioners in other disciplines, mainly psychiatrists. This is in part due to insurance company requirements that therapy performed by social workers be under the direction of a physician to qualify for reimbursement. The older consultative, collaborative relationship between physicians and social workers has evolved into a formal, official, supervisory relationship based on bureaucratic sanction.

These developments have caused some social workers to raise concern about internal control of professional activity and the orientation of private practitioners to the social work profession. Others have expressed the view that the profession needs to be more active in setting standards for private practitioners. For example, some MSWs begin private practice immediately upon graduation, and the question has been raised whether such practitioners possess the knowledge, skills, and experience to offer competent private psychotherapy. Major issues in the years ahead will be how best to supervise private practitioners and what the content of such supervision should be.

Social work has historically had high expectations for supervision without being rigid in its application. In some respects we could be on the verge of an era in which the application is rigid but the expectations not very high. Licensing, certification, vendorship, third-party payments, and various bureaucratic mandates could lead to changes in structure and content, and could bring about control of supervision that is external to the profession.

Focus on Relationship

Gradually, the shift in practice and supervision has been to the relationship the practitioner has with the client. Research has supported the idea that, regardless of the theoretical orientation of the practitioner, the outcome of the treatment depends on the relationship the practitioner has with the client (Stein, 1961:94-127). In recent times research reveals that supervisors have placed paramount importance upon interpersonal skills of relating as opposed to theoretical knowledge, research knowledge, practice wisdom, and ability to relate to the community (see Brennan, 1976). The idea of relationship found its way into supervision through practice knowledge and was reified into practice by supervisors who drew on their practice knowledge when they became supervisors. As Hutchinson put it in 1935:

> In the actual day-by-day process of supervision probably the greatest and most important factor for us is the kind of relationship we create between our workers and ourselves. We have heard a good deal about the worker-client relationship . . . . The relationship between supervisor and worker has perhaps shown the same trend. (Munson, 1979a:36)

Systems Theory

In the 1970s the idea of systems theory became widespread in social work education and practice. This seems to have been a direct by-product of the obsession with science during the 1950s. It is interesting to note that in the social work interpretation of systems theory by Hearn (Turner, 1979:333-359), he traces systems theory to the 1940s and 1950s, and does not mention Parsons, although Parson's work first appeared in 1937 and his second book, published 14 years later, was titled *The Social System*. The approach to systems that social work adopted came from biology, chemistry, and physics via psychology (Turner, 1979:333). It is interesting that we adopted this limited approach to systems when Parsons' more comprehensive theory wasavailable to us. Perhaps the historical split between social work and sociology was greater than we thought, or it could have been due to the cause-and-function split in the profession. Regardless, systems theory was adopted in a more general way from psychology, and in a more specific way from the family therapy field in more recent years (Bowen, 1978).

Family Therapy Movement

The family therapy movement has contributed significantly to social work practice and supervision in recent years. Although there is no coherent theory of family therapy, the movement has generated much information about the specifics of systems functioning, assessment, application of techniques, and interactional patterns in treatment, and has developed new approaches to supervision.

THE 1980s

Theory Stagnation

The 1980s have produced more advances in specialized practice. The knowledge explosion that has been occurring for three decades has produced many new specializations and subspecializations in the established areas of practice. This has produced some confusion for the evolution of theory of practice. Theory in social work has been historically generic and education programs have followed the same model. The response of the 1980s has been to emphasize *functioning* rather than *knowing*. This decade produced much information about how to perform in specific settings and no new comprehensive theories of intervention have emerged. This trend had been occurring for several decades, but appears to have reached its peak in the 1980s.

During the 1980s social work expanded its use of systems theory, primarily because it fit nicely within the comprehensive orientation of social work. There is some evidence from research that in clinical settings clients have negative responses to the use of systems orientations to treat their problems (Howe, 1989). There is a range of theories that have emerged over the years and social work most likely will engage in more outcome measurement research that analyzes effectiveness of differing approaches.

It remains to be seen if there will be a return to more comprehensive orientations or the increased emphasis will be on specialized, technical practice. Social work has always been recognized for its generic, comprehensive approach to the whole person in treatment. As the specialization trend continues it will be a challenge to maintain a balanced view of the two orientations.

Credentialing

The 1980s saw continued expansion of credentialing of social work. By the end of the decade 47 states had some form of regulation of social work at the state level (Kenemore, 1991:83). Credentialing has direct implications for supervision because there has been a tendency to consider credentialing a substitute for supervision. This is understandable from an administrative perspective since examinations and certification procedures are neat, clear, and time limited. From a clinical practice perspective delivering effective practice is much more complex and time consuming. There is a trend in some agencies to reinstitute supervision practices to provide a balanced approach to ensuring effective and efficient clinical practice.

The expanded utilization of social workers in mental health has led to demand for advanced credentials at the national level, and this has resulted in some confusion as the profession has struggled to determine what would be the best way to provide a credential that would be a clear national standard for third party payors to recognize. Clinical social work developments over the last three decades gave rise to the need for credentialing as third party payors demanded standards for payment. Currently most certification of social workers is generic and there is concern that the existing forms of certification are not specific enough. This trend will most likely continue, and consideration is being given to develop more specialized credentials and multi-levels of certification. Appendix 3 is a graphic presentation of the different forms and types of regulation of clinical social work.

THE 1990s

We are too close to the recent events to describe them with any objective accuracy. Instead the trends in clinical practice and supervision will be explored.

Trends

The second half of this century has produced dramatic changes. We have had an explosion of theory and knowledge. We have learned an enormous amount about the origin and nature of mental illness. There has been refinement of the diagnosis and treatment of mental disorders. The medications to alleviate mental distress have improved and increased significantly. Mental health services have expanded dramatically since the 1950s. Licensing and certification of the mental health professions have been refined and expanded. Administrative supports for clinicians have grown, especially in the area of computer technology.

The advances have improved the lives of the mentally ill and enhanced the practice of professionals. The advances should not deflect our attention from the problems that continue to face us. In some cases the advances have presented us with new problems. Listed below are the ten major problems facing clinical supervisors from the author's perspective.

Clinical Administration

Clinical practitioners and supervisors are increasingly required to become clinical administrators in many settings. This is typically viewed as integrating practice and administration, but frequently it is the result of funding cuts and managing workloads by combining functions. This practice can result in clinical solutions being applied to administrative problems with detrimental results for clients, practitioners, and supervisors. The problems associated with this dual role have received little attention. We know very little about the advantages and disadvantages of these role mergers and how clinicians reconcile the two roles. Supervisors can get caught between the organization and the clinicians. This is not new, but the ways supervisors are getting squeezed has a new and novel twist. One can begin to feel like a Ping-Pong ball if he or she becomes a mediator between the clinicians and the administration. This new development will require attention. Clinicians are rarely trained to fill clinical-administrative roles. If the trend continues, educational programs will need to include curriculum content and internship experiences that prepare for effective performance in this role.

Fiduciary Regulation

Medicaid, Medicare, and insurance reimbursement policies and procedures are a having tremendous effect on clinical practice and supervision. There are numerous requirements that must be met before these organizations will reimburse agencies and practitioners. Some have argued that unreasonable rules and regulations are utilized to cut costs by denying claims. Others argue that such policies are merely designed to ensure quality of treatment. The larger issue is one of control. Who is determining what is proper treatment? Many financial providers now dictate the timing of diagnosis, who does the diagnosis, who is qualified to provide treatment, and the length of treatment.

In addition, the format and timing of social history data (IDB), treatment plans (ITP and RTP), and progress notes are mandated by these funding sources. The role of the clinical supervisor in assisting workers to develop IDBs, ITPs, RTPs, and progress notes is undergoing change. Some funding agencies are demanding the right to review treatment plans before paying. In some settings they require a periodic meeting with the therapist to evaluate patient progress. Some require the therapist to provide a copy of the treatment plan.

Reimbursement by external sources has increased record keeping significantly. In addition to financial records, treatment records are mandated by the funding sources. While based on the premise this will produce accountability, there is little evidence there is any effort to use the clinical record to evaluate utilization of funds and treatment outcomes. The increased record keeping by clinicians has become a significant part of the clinician's workload. Studies indicate that practitioner time devoted to record keeping can be between 30 and 40 percent, and that much information is recorded as many as seven different times in each record. Clinical supervisors have a responsibility to work toward more effective and efficient record keeping. Caution is necessary in this area because a plan to review record keeping methods can result in the opposite of the initial objective and lead to more recording, rather than less.

Clinical supervisors complain of being confined in planning programs, and creative, innovative programming is de-emphasized for fear of funding loss. Some express concern that administrative mandates are dictating clinical judgments that are not always in the best interest of the client. If we are to continue to evolve our understanding of mental health, we will need to find ways to mediate the demand by financial providers for accountability and the clinical need to plan treatment and to utilize innovative interventions.

Privatization

In public programs there have been suggestions that funding issues be addressed by privatization of services. This is viewed as a cost-effective way to provide treatment. There is a trend in the corrections field and health care to privatize institutional programs. The pressure for privatization of mental health services will increase as other social service areas demand increased funding. There are increasing calls for such programs in the mental health field for both institutional and community based care. Traditionally, mental health has not fared well as various service programs engage in the political struggle to receive portions of federal and state appropriations. This has implications for clinicians and supervisors. The clinical issues are quite complex and beyond the scope of this chapter. The clinical supervisor plays a very different role in a private setting.

There are issues of job security, benefits, and working conditions that can be compromised and can produce ethical dilemmas for the clinical supervisor. Much needs to be considered as we drift toward a new model that will most likely be a more equal mix of public and private services than has been the case in over 50 years. In some ways this is a return to a pattern of the past, and some of the literature from that earlier era might offer us some helpful insights.

Task Versus Relationship

The intrusion of administrative and funding considerations in clinical practice and supervision has caused treatment to be increasingly dominated by behavioral and task orientations. We seem to be losing sight of the importance of relationship as a powerful curative factor. A major challenge for the next decade is to develop a model that integrates therapeutic task and relationship phenomena. Until now we have proceeded as if one had to be articulated at the expense of the other. This does not have to be the case, and there needs to be a merging of the two perspectives to maximize treatment outcome. The task that faces us in this area is the essence of the real function of the clinical supervisor.

Diagnosis of Mental Conditions

The issue of who is qualified to do a mental diagnosis needs clarification. In some states nonphysicians can do a diagnosis, but in most states the law requires the diagnosis to be done by a physician or psychologist. Because nonphysician staff do intake in most settings, clients are required to make several visits to get an official diagnosis. This is time consuming, costly, and confusing. At the same time, mental health professionals are being required by agency procedures to enter a DSM III-R Diagnosis in their initial data base (social history) reports. This is confusing for some practitioners and creates much turmoil for staff who have not been trained in the DSM III-R system. The clinical supervisor faces a major challenge in working to promote the use of sound professional practice principles when establishing and revising policies on diagnostic procedures.

DSM III-R is to become DSM-IV in the early 1990s. There are predictions that it will undergo major revisions, and conjecture that it will be more medically focused and less socially oriented. The most interesting speculation about the DSM-IV evolution is that it will provide recommended treatment plans. Some are concerned this could limit the sphere of mental health professionals offering intervention. Clinical supervisors need to closely follow the evolution of DSM-IV and take a major role in training nonmedical staff in DSM III-R and DSM-IV diagnosis. If non-physicians gain acceptance in doing diagnosis, educational programs will need to improve instruction that prepares students to do diagnosis.

Learning Assessment

Due to the growth in the number of mental health practitioners, there has been more reliance on objective tests as the basis of credentials and to promote quality. The use of testing is increasing at the same time there is increased awareness that practitioners cannot be infused with competence through a 150-question multiple-choice examination, and that sound supervision cannot be replaced with a computerized test for the same outcome. As testing emerged as a competence concept, the belief developed that supervision could be replaced with examinations, just as we perceived we could substitute for relationship with behavioral tasks.

We are beginning to differentiate what we can expect from examinations and what to expect from supervision. There is a return to the idea that educational assessment is essential to good supervision planning with students as well as beginning and advanced practitioners. There is serious research effort to develop effective, thorough, accurate, and precise assessment scales. This research pursuit will need continuation and expansion if we are to enhance learning at all professional levels and all stages of practice experience.

Ethics

Ethics have become the focus of general concern in our society. Whether there is more or less unethical professional conduct than in the past is a moot question. There are sufficient reports of problems regarding ethical misconduct to warrant the attention of all clinical supervisors. There are agencies that have considered videotaping all therapy sessions in case there are allegations of misconduct by practitioners. Such actions will present special challenges for clinical supervisors.

As practitioners operate under increased pressure, stress will increase and lead to poor judgment and ethical breaches. Most ethical violations are not committed by devious or malicious people, but by average practitioners who, because of stress, used poor judgment. Stress leads to frustration, decreased coping strategies, and ultimately poor judgment. The clinical supervisor can play an important role in combating stress-induced poor judgment. This will be expanded under the next heading.

There is research indicating that a substantial number of mental heath professionals are not familiar with the mental health ethical codes under which they function. The supervisor has a responsibility to ensure that practitioners are aware of the ethical sanctions of their profession, their licensure body, and their agency or organization.

Stress

Stress is the disease of our age. As all forms of organizations search for ways to cut costs, workloads increase and clients as well as practitioners suffer more stress. A stressed practitioner cannot effectively counsel a client who is experiencing emotional turmoil.

There has been limited research on stress reactions among mental health professionals, but the research that has been done clearly indicates that good supervision is the best preventative measure in coping with stress. There are good programs and literature on how to effectively reduce stress and increase coping strategies. It is hard to sort out all of the literature and programs. For every good resource to deal with stress, there are ten poor ones. Clinical supervisors have a responsibility to be informed and knowledgeable about stress, its manifestations and prevention and be able to assist supervisees develop coping strategies. Research suggests that supervisors currently are ignoring stress reactions in supervisees. This will have to change if service delivery is to be strengthened. Top administrators must be supportive of programs to reduce and prevent stress of clinical supervisors as well.

Proximity

Practitioners are increasingly fearful of touching clients. They are afraid the touch will be misinterpreted and result in a grievance action or lawsuit. The author worked with a therapist who would not close his office door when interviewing a child or female client. He has stated that the proximity issues, as well as the confidentiality issues, are of secondary concern to him. Clinicians reflect the general societal confusion about touch. We have gone from a low-touch society of the 1950s and before, to a high-touch society of the 1960s and 1970s, and back to a low-touch society of the 1980s primarily because of the fear about sexually transmitted diseases, especially AIDS. We remain a society conflicted about proximity. Our clients suffer from lack of closeness, and if practitioners keep them at a distance, how are people ever to recover? This is a challenge for the clinical supervisor to assist clinicians develop reasonable, balanced strategies regarding touch and closeness. Clinicians can touch people in nonsexual ways. Clients know when they are being touched and when they are being fondled.

AIDS

Most workers and supervisors are ill-equipped to deal with the AIDS fear-threat-potential in our caseloads. While casual transmission has been ruled out, many remain skeptical and do not hold rational views about the disease. Clinical supervisors face tough educational as well as practice issues regarding AIDS. We have clients who are putting those close to them at risk by engaging in high-risk activity without revealing it to others with whom they are intimate. What is the role of the clinician in honoring the client's confidentiality and at the same time assisting the unknowing who are put at risk? Practitioners need to be trained to counsel people who lack knowledge and engage in high-risk behavior. This is especially the case when counseling adolescents and children, because research indicates sexual activity is occurring at an increasingly younger age. There are many practitioners who avoid any discussion of sexual activity because they admittedly lack knowledge and experience discomfort with the topic.

There are reports that homophobia is fairly high among mental health professionals. This is a critical issue for the clinical supervisor who needs to assist practitioners in development of nonjudgmental attitudes. Forming and practicing a nonjudgmental attitude takes more than reading or being lectured about it. Some clients bring to treatment very strong prejudices about homosexuality, and practitioners are vulnerable to subtle manipulation if they are not able to distinguish their own personal and professional values. Clinical supervisors can help inexperienced and experienced practitioners to clarify and understand these issues. Supervisors will have to be bold and honest with themselves as they work with these issues because they are subject to the same prejudices and weaknesses as the clients and practitioners.

SUPERVISION ISSUES

During such eras, supervision issues have diminished. This is one of the unexplained ironies of our profession. If our science is real and our theory an extension, reflection, and guide of our practice, then supervision should have been associated with much of the debate. Supervision seems to get put aside during periods of intense theoretical adjustment and to reemerge in times of theoretical dominance and security. It could be that supervision or control must be removed to advance theory through creative practice efforts and that when a new theoretical perspective is accepted and applied widely, supervision and the control it provides are useful in indoctrinating new practitioners and standardizing the theory. If this hypothesis is valid, we need to reconceptualize supervision because it should foster creativity and not block it. What is clear is that cycles of concern with supervision and conflict over theoretical practice have been occurring for decades.

CONCLUSION

I am neither a general historian nor a social welfare historian. I am a social worker who has an interest in social welfare history generally and social work practice history specifically. When historians write about social work practice history, they bring an objectivity that is refreshing, but at the same time they lack a professional insider's perspective. However, when social work professionals write about their profession from an historical view, they lack the skills, tools, and techniques of a trained historian. As a result, to date, a definitive history of the social work practice profession has not been written. This is a major challenge that faces our profession. Our history has much to teach us that we have not explored.

In this chapter I have tried to establish some guidelines for the uncovering of our rich practice heritage. All that we do in our present practice actions, including supervision, is connected to our practice history. The idea used here was to identify the threads of some of these connections, and at the same time keep in mind an old dictum:

> The craving for an interpretation of history is so deep rooted that, unless we have a constructive outlook over the past, we are drawn either to mysticism or to cynicism. (Powicke, 1955:174)

I have tried to keep "a constructive outlook" and avoid the extremes of "mysticism" and "cynicism." I look forward to additional efforts to explain and interpret our history. I am not merely promoting a personal idiosyncrasy in this effort. Instead, my interest is based on the belief that supervisors have a responsibility to know, understand, and convey to their supervisees a sense of our heritage. This heritage need not be conveyed in a technical sense; it can be transmitted in a philosophical and practical manner that provides the practitioner with a sense of mission that is part of an ongoing historical movement. Practitioners who experience supervision from this perspective, I believe, will be inspired in a way that will make them more effective and more immune to the despair, disillusionment, and isolation that erodes pride in our professionalism.

A quote from over 40 years ago about an incident that occurred at the turn of the century can serve as a metaphor for the modern supervisor:

The Survey says that years ago in a midwestern orphanage was a ten-year-old girl, a hunchback, sickly, ill-tempered, ugly to look at, called Mercy Goodfaith. One day a woman came to the orphanage asking to adopt a girl whom no one else would take, and seeing Mercy Goodfaith, exclaimed, "That's the child I'm looking for." Thirty-five years afterward an official investigator of institutions in another state, after inspecting a county orphans' home prepared a report of which the following is a résumé. The house was exquisitely clean and the children seemed unusually happy. After supper they all went into the living room where one of the girls played the organ while the rest sang. Two small girls sat on one arm of the matron's chair, and two on the other. She held the two smallest children in her lap, and two of the larger boys leaned on the back of her chair. One of the boys who sat on the floor took the hem of her dress in his hand and stroked it. It was evident that the children adored her. She was a hunchback, ugly in feature, but with eyes that almost made her beautiful. Her name was Mercy Goodfaith. (Fosdick, 1943:72)

To put it less dramatically, the modern supervisor has a responsibility, a heritage, a philosophy, a set of values, and knowledge to pass along to the next generation, represented by their supervisees.

SUGGESTED READINGS

Walter Barton. *The History and Influence of the American Psychiatric Association*. Washington, DC: The American Psychiatric Press, 1987.
    Interesting historical account with many references to social work and parallels to emergence of clinical social work.

Florence Whiteman Kaslow (ed.). *Supervision, Consultation, and Staff Training in the Helping Professions*. San Francisco: Jossey-Bass, 1979.
    The first two chapters of this book give a very good overview of the history of supervision in medicine and social work.

Katherine A. Kendall. "A Sixty Year Perspective of Social Work." *Social Casework* 63 (September 1982), pp. 424-428.
    A brief, but good, decade-by-decade summary of social work from 1920 to 1980 based on a review of articles that appeared in Social Casework during this period.

Herbert S. Strean. *Clinical Social Work: Theory and Practice*. New York: The Free Press, 1978.

    The first chapter of this book has a good general summary of some aspects of the history of clinical practice.

Francis J. Turner. *Psychosocial Therapy: A Social Work Perspective*. New York: The Free Press, 1978.

    Chapter 1 of this book contains a good summary of the history of social work practice from a psychosocial perspective.

> In the whole of philosophy, there is
> no subject in greater disarray than
> ethics.
>
> E. F. Schumaher
> *A Guide for the Perplexed*

Chapter 3

Values and Ethics

Values and ethics are discussed in relation to the supervisory process. Values and ethics are distinguished as concepts and the relationship between values and knowledge is explored. There is discussion of research on the knowledge level of supervisors regarding ethical tenets. Specific sections of the 1990 NASW Code of Ethics are covered.

INTRODUCTION

Values and ethics are difficult to discuss under any circumstances. There are divergent views about the nature of ethical beliefs in this country currently and historically. Interestingly, ethical behavior and beliefs have not been surveyed or researched. A national survey conducted by Patterson and Kim (1991) found a startling lack of research on people's beliefs. The survey revealed that either people are shifting beliefs, or they never really held to the cherished traditional values. For example, the researchers found that people believe that America has no moral leadership; people are making up their own rules and laws; lying is viewed as permissible and most lying is done to those closest to us; crime is 600 percent higher than government estimates; one in seven adults have been sexually abused as children; there is general loss of belief in marriage as an institution; people believe that malingering and drug use in the workplace is substantial; the majority of people would lie, cheat, steal, and kill for money; there is loss of respect for property of others; and greed is accepted and advocated by consensus. At the same time that these responses were received, Patterson and Kim also found that people deeply love America and would make sacrifices to improve the country, believe ethics and values should be taught in schools, and that 90 percent believe in God. Ethics are no longer viewed as black and white, but are a large gray area where there is much latitude and doubt (Patterson & Kim, 1991).

It is not known what social workers believe as a group. Do we hold the values and beliefs revealed by Patterson and Kim, do we constitute a subgroup with very different personal values, or do we hold these same beliefs but distinguish between our personal and professional beliefs? These are questions that remain to be answered by research. Merdinger (1982) in a study of 367 students found significantly different global values for social work majors and non-social work majors. For the social work majors no significant differences were found on global values for students at different points in the program. Measures of attitudes toward public dependency produced significant differences for social workers and other majors, and students did develop more positive attitudes toward public assistance recipients as they progressed through the educational program. Much more research is needed before we can draw conclusions about the values and beliefs of social workers and what implications they have for **clinical practice.**

Values in relation to supervision have received limited attention in the supervision and practice literature. There are two areas that should be of major concern: first, the supervisor's role in orienting practitioners to values and ethics of the profession, and second, the guidelines for ethical supervisory practices. Although the general field of ethics is in disarray, as Schumaher (1977) has observed, the problem of the field of specific professional ethics is somewhat different. Professional ethics are reasonably clear and concise. In an era of renewed concern with professional ethics, violations are on the increase. Although official reports of ethics violations are increasing, unofficial complaints about ethical breaches are heard in even larger numbers. These "minor" breaches undermine professionalism as much as sensational violations that result in criminal charges and negative publicity. "Minor" breaches can be cumulative and can lead to the more dramatic cases. This chapter covers the major theoretical aspects of values and ethics and draws on the results of empirical research to cover guidelines in the areas of practice and supervision regarding ethical and value sanctions and dilemmas.

VALUES

Values are frequently viewed as such complex concepts and behaviors that, when one attempts to explore these areas, it is tempting to throw up one's hands in despair or to forget the issue until it becomes problematic (Jones, R. W., 1970:35). The view taken here is that the literature regarding values does demonstrate an evolutionary process and that a unified, clear conceptualization of these values for use in practice can be documented. The articulation of values has evolved from the general to the specific. Early conceptions were based on global statements derived from such societal values as democratic participation, basic human rights of the individual (Hamilton, 1951:6-11), the importance of the family to individual growth and development, the role of religion in development of moral values and convictions (Towle, 1965:3-11), and the assumption that all individuals are concerned with biological and psychological survival as a basic necessity (Perlman, 1957:6-11). These conceptions were given more specificity by identifying concern for the well-being of the client, the uniqueness of the individual, the acceptance of the individual, the right to self-determination by the client (Hollis, 1966:12-13), and noncoerciveness on the part of the worker and avoidance of social control of clients (Hamilton, 1951:6-8; Hollis, 1966:12-13). As society has become more complex and diverse, emphasis has been on value conflicts encountered by the helping professions (Briar & Miller, 1971:32-52). To deal with these value conflicts, more attention has been devoted to flexibility in professional activity and recognition that values constantly change and differ culturally and ethnically (Boyer, 1975:13-14).

Recent treatment of values in the literature has turned to operational referents and behavioral manifestations. This effort has led to identification of who possesses which values. In a sense, workers are surrounded by values: the worker's own personal values, the worker's professional values, organizational values, client system values (the values of the client as well as the values of those in his or her environment, such as employers, friends, relatives, etc.), and prevailing societal values. Through interaction, people communicate these various value systems directly, indirectly, and symbolically (Goldstein, H., 1973:90-98). Conflicts frequently result. In interrelating values behaviorally, discussion has turned to ideas of social responsibility, how people are similar and different, means of achieving self-realization (Pincus & Minahan, 1973:38-39), group survival, recognition, security, identity, belonging, self-respect, competence, and privacy (Siporin, 1975:65-68). In explicating values more precisely, study has been focused on how and why people develop values. Values are a result of complex socialization processes, and serve as a means to introduce order into the world and provide a way of coping with it (Siporin, 1975:66; Jones, R. W., 1970:37).

Once the origins and functions of values have been defined, the question remains how they can be identified, changed, and reinforced in the worker-client relationship. There is disagreement about how to categorize values in practice. Distinctions have been made between values and knowledge (Feibleman, 1973:14; Marsh, 1971:132-133) and values and beliefs (Scheibe, 1970:41-42) by writers who have studied functioning from purely cognitive and perceptual perspectives. The study of values in practice settings has tended to view values, knowledge, and beliefs without making clear distinctions. Pincus and Minahan (1973:38) hold that values are beliefs that cannot be verified as knowledge, and Bartlett argues that values are qualitative judgments that are not empirically demonstrable and are invested with emotions that represent a purpose toward which the worker's actions are directed (1970:63). Bloom (1975:109-110) believes that values can be studied empirically as persistent patterns of choice among alternatives. Practitioners are confronted with these patterns of choice based on values daily in practice.

Inexperienced workers frequently, and experienced workers occasionally, encounter value issues in practice that must be worked through in supervision. This is especially true in settings where the practitioner is confronted with clients who deviate from the generally accepted norms and values of the society. It is not always the younger worker who needs assistance with value conflicts. For example, older workers can experience significant value conflicts when confronted with the behaviors of adolescent clients.

VALUES AND KNOWLEDGE

Values and knowledge are interconnected through the choices people make. Although scientific knowledge alone is not sufficient to produce change in behavior, values in practice and supervision can be used to develop awareness of options, predict outcomes for each option, assess the importance of each outcome to the client, combine the outcomes, and measure the degree of goal attainment associated with the choice made (Bloom, 1975:102-113). It is important for the practitioner and supervisor to take into account this distinction between values and knowledge and their interrelatedness. For example, through lack of scientific knowledge of substance and alcohol abuse outcomes, a practitioner can subtly succumb to the client's belief that there is a distinction between drug use and drug abuse, and may come to accept the client's self-generated value stance that casual drug use does not produce negative physical, psychological, and social outcomes. There is much evidence that even casual use can produce serious consequences, and the practitioner who does not find a way to communicate this to the client can contribute to the deepening of the client's problems.

Lack of possession of such knowledge does not have to produce a value impasse between the worker and client or between the worker and the treatment organization, but knowledge is essential to the process of value clarification in the relationship. Through such value clarification, the worker can operationalize a belief in the client's right to self-determination (since the concept is based on the assumption that the client does have alternatives among which to choose) but the worker has to make the value judgment that the client does have viable alternatives (Briar & Miller, 1971:42). This process of values clarification is basic to supervision, and the supervisor has a responsibility to explore carefully client and practitioner options and alternatives in any given situation.

Similarly, knowledge and values merge in relation to confidentiality. Frequently, private interview rooms are not provided in practice settings, resulting in constrained conversations when others are within hearing distance. Knowing this and at the same time wanting to ensure confidentiality, the worker can be placed in value conflict. The supervisor needs to assist the worker with reducing this conflict so that it does not disrupt the entire intervention process. In this same context, little is being done regarding clarification of privileged communication in the case of the practitioner. A client who shares content in confidence can be offered little assurance that the information he or she provides will be held in confidence in relation to law enforcement and criminal justice systems. The supervisor's role in these situations is to clarify values and provide accurate, unambiguous information to the practitioner about safeguards and rights of the client so that these can be guaranteed.

Training programs for drug-abuse counselors conceptualize the drug-abusing individual as having a medical-social problem (Trader, 1974: 100). This is another illustration of how values and knowledge intersect. When counselors internalize this conception as a value, the result is quite often an impasse in the counseling situation. This situation was reported in a study of 224 addicts in which the staff viewed the clients as physically and mentally ill, while the clients did not perceive themselves as having either form of illness. Such disagreement was depicted as a serious block in staff-patient communication and was aggravated in cases in which cultural conflict existed. The researchers argue that successful drug counseling depends on complementary views between the two groups and similarity in background and experience of counselors and clients (Ball et al., 1974). This value stance is somewhat of a dilemma for practitioners in relation to acceptance of the client, because other studies have demonstrated that dissimilarity of interactants leads to higher levels of verbal accessibility between the participants (Tessler & Polansky, 1975).

There are indications that dissimilarity between client and practitioner contributes to the change process. Halmos (1970:91) discusses this aspect of relationship by calling attention to research on Homans' hypothesis that interacting individuals tend to become more alike over time. If the therapeutic relationship is to promote change in the client, the worker must offer the client a different model of values, attitudes, beliefs, and behaviors at given points in the relationship. This view deviates in part from the traditional belief of professionals that the more similar the worker is to the client, the more likely the client will be to invest in the relationship. It also deviates from the tendency among paraprofessional counselors to mistrust their intuitive feelings, to minimize their street knowledge, and to resist imagined professional control of their activities (Dalali et al., 1976). **What seems to be needed in supervision is more clarity about which differences and similarities between practitioners and clients need to be minimized and maximized to produce positive therapeutic outcomes.**

A supervisor's failure to offer help to the practitioner with conflicts in identification with the client or the employing organization can lead to increased strains. But this negative outcome is not inevitable, especially if the supervisor is innovative rather than traditional in orientation and is accepting of cultural differences in values and beliefs (Kaslow, 1972:58). Those who are responsible for supervision have an obligation to articulate clearly organizational and program values for practitioners as well as clients so that the participants can understand expectations as well as make choices about the degree to which they want to participate.

Such openness and acceptance within the organizational context permit the practitioner to fulfill the advocate role that has been identified as appropriate to social work (Trader, 1974:101). The role of advocate must be clearly defined for the practitioner. Role clarity is important to effective functioning of the practitioner (Kaslow, 1972:62-67), but advocacy is one of the more poorly defined functions in the helping professions. Values are important in providing role clarity for the advocate. The role of advocate has been argued from a value stance as being one of total commitment to serving client needs and interests in a social conflict (Grosser, 1965:18; Brager, 1968:6). If the practitioner perceives the advocate role as a one-sided struggle against an alien system and identifies with the frequently held client belief that the professional treatment system is not to be trusted, both the client and the practitioner are placed outside the system. The values of the advocate identified here differ from the conceptions of the role identified by Grosser and Brager. For example, drug-abusing clients often are in conflict with institutional systems or are totally out of contact with them. That substantial numbers of drug abusers are outside the system is illustrated by the wide discrepancy in demographic characteristics between clients surveyed in drug treatment programs (Ball, 1974) and patients treated for drug abuse in a hospital emergency room (Weppner, 1976). This difference is especially glaring in the case of women, who made up a much higher proportion of the drug patients in emergency room cases than in drug treatment programs (Weppner, 1976:172).

To bring about involvement, the practitioner in some instances will have to be the client's advocate in other systems. At times the worker will have to confront the treatment system, the educational system, the law enforcement system, the client's family system, the drug culture system, and the economic system (e.g., employers) to bring about engagement, reengagement, or disengagement, depending upon the circumstances. At other times, the role of advocate will involve supporting and confronting a resistive client in relation to one or more of the above-mentioned systems. In both cases the advocacy role requires providing information, and the practitioner must have substantial and accurate knowledge for his or her values to have genuine meaning for the client. In the first instance, the information will be used to interpret the needs of the client to the system. In the second instance, the client must be informed about what will or can happen or what will be done to him or her.

Through provision of information, the advocate can often promote more equity in interaction between the client and the given system. This promotion of equity is one of the primary values of practitioners in general and advocates specifically. This kind of education is emerging as a significant variable in health and longevity (Comstock & Tonascia, 1977), and the application of these findings to social work settings needs exploration. To be successful in these tasks, the advocate must possess a great deal of knowledge about the functioning of treatment, education, family, law enforcement, drug culture, and economic systems. Practitioners who attempt advocacy roles without thorough knowledge will contribute to further resistance, hostility, and increased anxiety on the part of the client. The supervisor will need to be prepared to aid supervisees with these adjustments.

ETHICS

Generally, values relate to what one believes, and ethics relate to how one behaves. Although our values are hard to codify, social work ethics have become progressively more precise. A general one-page code of ethics adopted in 1960 by the National Association of Social Workers was superseded in 1980 by a longer document including a preamble and six major topical areas. (For a complete statement of the NASW Code of Ethics see Appendix 4.) The social work supervisor has a responsibility to be thoroughly familiar with the NASW Code of Ethics and to ensure that supervisees also understand and adhere to the Code of Ethics. The code should be discussed and reviewed with new supervisees and referred to at points in the supervision process when value dilemmas or ethical issues emerge. The supervisor cannot assume that supervisees have become acquainted with the code as part of their educational program, orientation to the profession, or prior work experience. Many problems can be resolved and much learned about practice from studying the code. The supervisor should approach such discussion in a sensitive, constructive manner, but at the same time not accept practitioner resistance to or defensiveness about such discussion on the grounds that their ethics and professionalism are being questioned. Such exploration is mandated by the code in Section I-B: "The social worker should strive to become and remain proficient in professional practice and the performance of professional functions."

There is no separate code of ethics for supervision, but there are a number of passages in the NASW Code of Ethics that relate directly and indirectly to supervision. The sections that deal directly with supervision are summarized below.

1. *(II-F-8) "The social worker should seek advice and counsel of colleagues and supervisors whenever such consultation is in the best interest of clients."* The supervisee is obligated to seek assistance when he or she encounters problems. Although the code leaves latitude regarding seeking "consultation" of "supervisors" and "colleagues," it recommends that to avoid potential conflict the supervisee consider the supervisor as the first source of assistance with difficulties.

2. *(III-J-9) "The social worker who serves as an employer, supervisor, or mentor to colleagues should make orderly and explicit arrangements regarding the conditions of their continuing professional relationship."* This provision relates to much of the content in this book. The supervisee has a right to know how he or she will be supervised, what the expectations will be, and how performance will be judged.

3. *(111-J-10) "The social worker who has the responsibility for employing and evaluating the performance of other staff members should fulfill such responsibility in a fair, considerate, and equitable manner, on the basis of clearly enunciated criteria."* This section is discussed in detail in Chapter 9. The statement is a clear and direct mandate to which supervisors must adhere rigorously.

4. *(III-J-11) "The social worker who has the responsibility for evaluating the performance of employees, supervisees, or students should share evaluations with them."* Supervisors have an obligation under this section to share with supervisees oral or written results of evaluation of the supervisees' performance.

Several other sections of the code have indirect applications to the supervisor. For example, Section V-M-2 states, *"The social worker should take action through appropriate channels against unethical conduct by any other member of the profession."* Since supervisors are the first level of "appropriate channels" to receive and hear such charges by practitioners in many settings, supervisors must be prepared to deal with such complaints openly, objectively, and with a serious, sensitive approach. Also, since supervisors are in a position to be aware of the practices of their own supervisees, they must be prepared to act when confronted with or observing unethical conduct.

Another broad statement of the code that relates indirectly to supervision is Section V-O-2, which reads, *"The social worker should critically examine, and keep current with, emerging knowledge relevant to social work."* The supervisor has a responsibility for fostering such critical examination and for encouraging practitioners to keep up with and contribute to new knowledge about practice.

ETHICS KNOWLEDGE

The supervisor and worker must have a thorough knowledge of the code of ethics under which they practice. This can be confusing because many social workers are licensed under several statutes and national bodies of professional sanction. It is common for practitioners and supervisors to be unaware of some of the codes. Most social workers are aware of and believe they should be guided by the NASW Code of Ethics. Fortunately, most of the lesser known codes are quite similar in content to the NASW-Code.

Before we can deal with complex ethical and value issues, it is important to determine how much practitioners know about the ethical guidelines under which they operate. There is an assumption that practitioners read, remember, and act on the tenets of the NASW Code of Ethics. The supervisor needs to evaluate this rather than assume the supervisees have such information and knowledge.

Research (see, Munson, 1986) consisting of a fifty item, true-false test to measure knowledge of the NASW Code of Ethics has provided some significant information about the knowledge and use of the Code. The questions were simple, single reference statements covering all major principles in the NASW Code. The instrument was given to a random sample of field instructors. The highest possible score was 100, and the mean score on the knowledge scale was 59.3. On the average respondents were able to identify Code items with just under 60 percent accuracy. Thirty-two percent of the respondents answered fewer than 50 percent of the questions correctly.

Given the importance of the Code in guiding clinicians' behavior, it is discouraging that 40 percent of the items were answered incorrectly by the respondents. There were no significant differences in the mean scores based on sex, religion, or perceived stress associated with work. Several groups have administered this survey to professional social workers, and the results have been similar. This same instrument was administered to several groups of graduate students, and the mean scores were consistently 11 points higher than the average scores of the field instructor groups (the mean score for the student groups was 71.1). Thus it appears that supervisees may actually have more knowledge of the NASW ethics code than the supervisors.

A copy of the instrument used in this study is in Appendix 5. Supervisors are encouraged to administer this instrument to all supervisees who practice under NASW sanction, and the results should be discussed. To do this will ensure a basic exposure to the elements of ethical practice. The NASW Code of Ethics can be a rich source of discussion of elements critical to effective clinical practice. Much of the content of the code refers to the specifics of practice and can serve as a guide for practice activity. By administering the ethics scale the supervisor has a basis for discussing specific aspects of the code with the supervisee, and avoids merely reviewing the different sections of the code.

The results of this survey suggest that there is much that needs to be done regarding the level of knowledge of the Code of Ethics. One question raised by the findings of this survey is: What would be considered an acceptable level of knowledge of the Code? Although it is not reasonable to expect that all respondents would score 100 percent on such a survey, it can be argued that practitioners should possess a higher level of knowledge of the Code than was demonstrated in the survey. If supervisors are to contribute ethical models of practice for supervisees to emulate, they will need to possess a thorough knowledge of the ethics codes.

There is much confusion about ethics and ethical behavior. This is related to the failure of educational programs to systematically teach values, ethics and statutory-mandated behavior. For example, in the survey it had been three and one-half years since respondents had read the Code of Ethics, and the results show they lack accurate knowledge of the Code's behavioral requirements. Even though 49 states now have statutes regulating social work practice, it is rare to encounter a practitioner who has read the statute under which he or she is licensed or certified. Many of these statutes mandate certain ethical behavior. This raises the question of what ethical guidelines practitioners and supervisors use when facing unusual or questionable situations. There are indications they rely on what they consider common sense, logical, reasonable conceptions, and vague remembrances and interpretations of the Code of Ethics. Often judgments based on such recollections are risky and at variance with Code requirements and statutory mandates.

Instead of relying exclusively on common sense, the practitioner can turn to codes of ethics to aid functioning in a complex practice world where there are conflicting practice demands and legislative and court ordered actions that create ethical dualisms. Legal mandates are often contradictory to ethical codes. For example, duty to warn laws and child abuse reporting laws can create confidentiality conflicts. Technology can create ethical issues not covered by ethical codes. The use of video and audio tapes of clients and the practice of leaving messages on phone answering machines when trying to reach clients raise privacy issues. Even modern practice theories raise ethical dilemmas. This is illustrated by the practice of paradoxing techniques. In paradoxing the practitioner may be called on to advocate that the client take some action that would put the practitioner in violation of some codes of ethics. Paradoxing is viewed by some as "tricking" clients to do certain acts. Under the NASW ethics code, clients are to be told the "extent and nature" of services that are available to them and are to be told of the "risks" associated with services. If one tells a client about paradoxing, the intent of the technique is subverted. Some therapists use the paradox of suggesting suicide to a depressed patient in order to prevent the attempt. This is risky and counter to the NASW code of ethics.

The supervisor's role in these difficult situations is to present ethical codes as a guide, and the supervisor must be ready to assist supervisees' work through ethical conflicts. Practitioners need to become aware that laws regulating social work practice are not evolved in any logical manner and legal actions are not taken with professional ethical codes in mind. Becoming aware of this fact can be extremely helpful to the bewildered practitioner confronting complex practice demands.

EXTENT OF ETHICS VIOLATIONS

The extent of ethics violations is hard to determine for a number of reasons. An informal survey by the author revealed that people believe ethics violations have been committed against them at fairly high levels, but there is reluctance to pursue these breaches. However, such reactions could be highly distorted because research reveals that awareness of provisions of the Code is at a fairly low level. People could be the victims of ethics violations and not know it, or they could feel that they are victims of unethical acts when, in fact, those acts are not covered by the Code.

Most professionals view ethical issues as internal to the profession, but increasingly, ethical issues are externally driven as private organizations determine much of the nature of our practice. This trend is actually a return to the pattern of an earlier era in that social workers are being employed in for-profit settings. Social workers are frequently ill-prepared for the ethical compromises they have to make as marketing and profits become the primary guiding principle. There are indications that this trend will continue into the next century. For example, large hotel chains are using billions of dollars in excess profits to buy up nursing homes. It is expected that by the end of this century, the majority of long-term care facilities in this country will be owned by profit-making companies offering what they call "entrepreneurial compassion." Many times the reaction of long-term care facilities and private-for-profit hospitals to adverse publicity is to simply counter with massive marketing campaigns that counter the accusations that have been made against them. As we move toward this form of care and helping, the old free enterprise concept of "caveat emptor" — let the buyer beware — is most relevant. In addition to the individual ethical issues, practitioners in for-profit settings will have to develop coping strategies for dealing with organizationally induced ethical compromises.

ADVANCING ETHICS KNOWLEDGE

How can practitioners and supervisors have more substantial grounding of their practice guided by ethical principles? Professionals should read, reread, and become familiar with the Code of Ethics. They should become thoroughly familiar with the statutes under which they are licensed. Supervisors should require that supervisees become knowledgeable about the Code and statutes. One way to do this is to administer the ethics knowledge scale contained in Appendix 5 to new supervisees and discuss it with them. The supervisor cannot assume that the worker has read and understands ethics requirements.

Supervisors should insist that educational programs and accrediting bodies ensure there is curriculum content regarding orientation to ethics codes and state statutes. Professional organizations should be contacted and encouraged to require knowledge of ethics codes as a condition of membership. Redundancy and repetition of exposure to ethical mandates should be encouraged rather than avoided. It is unusual to encounter a practitioner who has been overexposed to ethical principles.

SUGGESTED READINGS

Frank Lowenburg and Ralph Dolgoff. *Ethical Decisions for Social Work Practice*. Itasca, IL: Peacock, 1988.
   Good survey of ethical issues in social work practice.

National Association of Social Workers. *Code of Ethics*. Washington, DC: NASW, 1990.
    Should be read and studied by all practicing social workers.

James Patterson and Peter Kim. *The Day America Told the Truth*. New York: Prentice Hall, 1991.
    A national survey of attitudes that can be used to generate discussion of personal and professional beliefs.

Fred Reamer. "AIDS and Ethics: The Agenda for Social Workers." *Social Work* 33 (5), 1988.
    Discussion of AIDS and ethical issues for social workers.

Ronald H. Stein. *Ethical Issues in Counseling*. New York: Prometheus Books, 1990.
    Overview of ethical issues in several helping disciplines.

> The capacity to shuttle between levels
> of abstraction, with ease and with
> clarity, is a signal mark of the
> imaginative and systematic thinker.
>
> C. Wright Mills
> *The Sociological Imagination*

Chapter 4

Supervisor Styles

Style is a term that has been used indiscriminately in referring to aspects of supervisors' and practitioners' behavior. In this chapter the term is defined and described in a manner that permits the supervisor to use it to promote learning and guide interaction in supervision. General styles of supervisors are explained as *active* and *reactive*. The supervisors who use these styles can be further described as *philosophers, theoreticians,* and *technicians.* In addition to exploring these classifications and subclassifications of style, information is provided on how supervisors can use the concept to identify their own style which might be beyond the general categories identified.

INTRODUCTION

Style is a concept that is usually taken for granted and is rarely defined or explained on a general or individual basis. This is unfortunate because we can learn much and become more effective by considering our style as supervisors and practitioners. Like the use of the word "art" in social work, the use of the word "style" frequently conceals more than it reveals about one's practice. The following statement epitomizes this flirtation with the idea of style:

> We view social work practice as an art that combines professionally mastered knowledge and chosen values with the individual attributes and style of the practitioner. (Kahn, A., 1973:98)

The writer leaves to speculation the operational meaning of this statement. In order to operationalize this conception we would have to ask several questions: What knowledge? How do we know what has been mastered? What are the chosen values and how were they chosen? What individual attributes? When we explore style with practitioners these questions frequently get answered as part of the process. This is the reason the concept of style is so important to practice supervision.

Style is simply *the patterns we use in attempting to communicate with others*. A refinement of this definition is that style consists also of the consistent focus supervisors emphasize in supervision, the manner in which they articulate the theoretical orientation they hold, the philosophy of practice and supervision they hold, and how they convey it to their supervisees. In addition to using style as a generalized descriptor, it is also common to break one's style into components. For example, the "evaluative style" (Eldridge, 1982:489) of the supervisor one discrete component of style.

Some aspects of our styles are conscious and well-known to us, but we are not aware of other major elements. Common elements of our styles are voice volume, voice tone, facial expressions, posture, use of arms and hands, examples we use, questions we ask, ways we respond to questions, interpretations we give, organization and structure of sessions, physical setting of sessions, theories we use, points we choose to intervene in discussion, how we make suggestions, and what suggestions we offer.

Research by Handley (1982) has demonstrated that cognitive styles of supervisors and supervisees have an effect on the interpersonal relationship in supervision, but similarity of cognitive styles is not associated with supervisor rating of supervisee performance or competence. Handley concludes that it is important for supervisors and supervisees to develop awareness of their cognitive styles early in the supervision process in order to understand better the supervisory relationship and to enhance satisfaction with supervision. This study by Handley is one of the first empirical studies of style in supervision. It supports my own research, reported in this chapter and Chapter 5, regarding the importance of style in producing a positive outcome in the supervisory process.

OBSERVING STYLES

The best way to observe our own style of supervision is through viewing audiovisual recordings of our supervisory sessions. Supervisors should observe themselves often to understand and improve their styles. During observation, the lesser-known aspects of our style will be the most apparent to us and the most surprising. It is common to hear embarrassed supervisors say, "I didn't realize I do . . . ," or ask, "Do I always do that?" when observing themselves in action for the first time.

Supervisors should be exposed to the work of other supervisors in order to develop their own styles, just as practitioners develop their own styles from working with and viewing other practitioners. We need to put more emphasis on the provision of supervision or consultation for supervisors for this purpose.

The supervisor needs to develop an orientation or frame of reference to supervision that incorporates his or her style. This relates to the focus of the supervisory interaction. The supervisor should consider his or her primary responsibility in relation to the patient (Langs, 1979:18). If the supervisor keeps this focus, he or she will prevent the supervision from becoming vague or pointless, and will avoid frustration for the supervisor and the supervisee. Use of this frame of reference also helps to prevent the supervision from becoming focused on the practitioner rather than the treatment. Any interaction concentrated on the practitioner should be in the context of the work with the client. This is important because many practitioners who are having difficulty in their work with clients and are getting lost in their therapeutic efforts attempt to deal with it by discussing themselves and their personal actions or motives with supervisees. (The implications of this are discussed in detail in the section "Self-Analysis" in Chapter 5.)

Also, practitioners who are having difficulty in their work may attempt to deal with it by attributing it to problems they are having with the supervisor. The supervisor should minimize such discussion and always relate it to what it has to do with the client or clients under consideration. It is the supervisor's responsibility to keep the focus on the client under discussion. When therapy and the resulting supervision get difficult, it is to the supervisee's advantage to shift the focus.

STYLE AS A RESOURCE

Supervisees and supervisors frequently use the term style indiscriminately and as a generalization. This is illustrated by a supervisor's comment in connection with a problem she was having with a supervisee: "Her style and mine are different; the problem of style is the way she talks about her cases." The supervisee responded to this comment by agreeing that the styles were different, and said she had difficulty visualizing how this could be reconciled. Before such a problem can be confronted, both the supervisor and supervisee must be asked to specify the behavioral components of their style.

An example of how style is differentiated by practitioners is illustrated by a comment made by a worker in an acute care hospital who was trying to explain how her style differed from that of her supervisor. The MSW practitioner explained the difference by stating:

> When I get a referral, I like to meet face to face with the spouse of the client as soon as possible. I arrange an interview. I want to see how the spouse is reacting. I want to get the spouse's impressions of how the client functioned before and after the initial onset of the disease. Usually, in our situation, the onset is an event, specifically a stroke. I see the spouse or family member's information as important to my assessment before seeing the client. Mary, on the other hand, likes to see the client first. She will visit with the client and then contact the family member by phone. She gathers information over the phone, and sets up a meeting with the family member.

This illustration demonstrates a difference in structural or procedural style. Ultimately, the outcome is the same. Both the client and the family member are sources of information for the assessment. This is the case in most instances in which there are differences in style. Frequently supervisors and supervisees get so focused on stylistic differences that they are unable to see that the outcomes are often the same regardless of style.

Structural differences exist within the interview format. For example, the two workers mentioned above had different styles of note-taking during the interviews. One took brief notes during the interview; the other wrote notes about the session immediately after the interview. The workers stated that they had tried the other's style of note-taking without much success.

Another difference in style can be in the interactional component. This relates to how the worker interacts with the client or family member during the interview. Again, different interactional styles can result in similar outcomes regarding assessment and intervention efforts. The supervisor needs to help the practitioner identify his or her style in practice and understand how it affects the outcome. In supervision, the supervisor should identify his or her style and explain how it affects achievement of the goals of the supervision.

The purposes for which the concept of style and categories of style are intended here are not necessarily the same as they would be in research. They can be used in research and given very precise definitions. However, to get very detailed in their contexts here would defeat the purpose, which is to explore interactions in a wide range of ways, rather than narrowly focusing people in precise categories, like research does, thus leaving no room for deviation, error, adjustment, alteration, or even complete reversal.

Supervisors who elicit feedback from supervisees about their supervisory style can gain much insight into their performance as supervisors without threatening the supervisee. Also, supervisors can gain insight into whether their supervisees perceive them in the same way as they view themselves.

STYLE AS A CONCEPT

Style as a means of understanding behavior is receiving more attention in the behavioral sciences. Sternberg and Davidson (1982) have identified the "impulsive" and "reflective" cognitive styles in problem solving. It is their view that effective "problem-solvers are those who manage to combine both impulsive and reflective styles." Harrison and Bramson (1982) have developed a comprehensive view of styles of thinking based on the five styles: synthesist, idealist, pragmatist, analyst, and realist. They give an example of a casework supervisor and how the difference between her style and that of her supervisees can be problematic.

Jane, a social work supervisor with twenty years' experience in community agencies, tells of a problem she has with her younger caseworkers. The conversation goes something like this:

JANE: I can't seem to convince them to do the job properly.
WE: They aren't performing?
JANE: Oh, they work hard. I can't say they're not performing.
WE: But they cause you problems anyway.

JANE: It's their attitude. They bring up all these ideas about case-
        work that just aren't right.

WE: Such as?

JANE: Well, I was trained to practice nondirective counseling
        methods. Clients should be given the chance to work out
        their own problems. Caseworkers are there to help them do
        that.

WE: But your younger people do it differently.

JANE: Sometimes I can't believe what I hear. They act like Dutch
        uncles. They will tell a client what to do.

WE: Do they do it all the time?

JANE: Oh no. Just now and then.

WE: Do they get results?

JANE: Well, yes. For the short run, anyhow. But I wonder some-
        times about the long-range effect on the client.

WE: *(persisting)* But the results they get are generally satisfac-
        tory? They meet agency standards?

JANE: Mm—yes. I can't really criticize them for that. But I just
        wish they would do it the right way.

Jane was trained in an idealistic, supportive casework method. Her
younger employees sometimes take a more pragmatic or realistic,
direct approach. Jane's training and her preferred way of thinking
about casework (and probably about many other things in her life)
make it difficult for her to acknowledge that anyone could succeed
as a caseworker using another set of strategies.

   At the heart of Jane's problem is a commitment not only to a
certain method and approach, but to a set of basic values. The
method and the values go hand in hand. In effect, they define Jane as
a professional. She is uncomfortable when others use methods different from her own, because that is a violation of her value system.
To the extent that others succeed while using such methods, Jane's
discomfort is increased.

   Notice, that is true of all of us. The importance of the individual
value system as one determinant of behavior and attitude is not peculiar to idealists, such as Jane. What is peculiar is the weight given by
idealists to their values, to value judgments, to moral questions, and
ethical principles. (Harrison & Bramson, 1982:39-40)

From this example we can see how style, the concept of intervention, and
values all become integrated in a way that can dramatically influence what
gets done in supervision and what people think about supervision (see

Chapter 1). It can lead to positive outcomes, negative outcomes, or, as in the case of Jane, an ongoing sense of adequacy but frustration.

Beels and Ferber were the first to identify therapist styles after studying videotapes of family therapists at work. They labeled two main styles: conductors and reactors. Conductors are more active in the treatment and direct the interaction. Nathan Ackerman, Virginia Satir, Salvador Minuchin, and Murray Bowen were classified as conductors. Reactors are viewed as "less public personalities who get into families playing different roles at different times." Carl Whitaker, James Framo, Jay Haley, and Don Jackson are examples of reactors (Guerin, 1976:17).

Main Styles

This led me to ask the question: Do clinical supervisors manifest styles that characterize their interaction in supervision? Based on content analysis of supervision, I was able to establish that they do (Munson, Study B). Supervisors generally adopt one of two styles that I have identified as *active* and *reactive*. The active style consists of being direct with the supervisee and asking pointed questions, answering questions directly, and offering interpretations. Active supervision is problem-focused, based on exploring alternative interventions, focused on client dynamics, and speculative about outcomes. The reactive style, on the other hand, is more subdued and indirect. The reactive style involves asking limited general questions and not giving answers. Reactive supervision focuses on the process of treatment, explores issues about interaction, and tends to focus more on practitioner dynamics.

Being active or reactive is not necessarily good or bad. It is merely a way of behaving. The style can become negative if someone experiences it as negative. For example, as some of the respondents in the research told us, the quiet, passive supervisor who uses the "my door is always open" style is not always the best supervisor. The open-door policy often results in infrequent, inconsistent supervision that remains unstructured and operates on a crisis basis. This is a poor way to promote learning in supervision: it can lead to resentment on the part of the responsible practitioner; or it can be graciously accepted by the insecure practitioner who is quite willing to let well enough alone. However, in this latter situation, the clients will be deprived of the quality services they are entitled to receive.

The first step in identifying supervisor style involves this general categorization. In a survey of graduate students, I found that the majority of supervisors were viewed as being reactors (Munson, Study A). For the total group, 64 percent of the supervisors were identified as reactive and 36 percent as active. An interesting finding was that 74 percent of first-year students perceived their supervisors as reactive, while 66 percent of the second-year students perceived their supervisors as active. From the logical standpoint, the reverse should be true. Beginning students would appear to need more active direction of their work, while advanced students could benefit more from the reactive style as they emerge as independent practitioners. Since style is such a new concept in analyzing supervision, more research is needed to refine how these styles are differentiated.

Substyles

In my research, after identifying the main styles, I wanted to subclassify the styles. When doing my early research, I had difficulty conceptualizing how to describe supervisors. That is: How could you characterize what they do? How could you compare differences? At first I tried to classify styles on the basis of personality, and found such conceptions inadequate. Some respondents would say, "My supervisor is anal retentive," because they had been trained predominantly in psychoanalytic settings, and terms like "anal retentive" were readily available for expressions of hostility about supervisors. Such terms were not very descriptive of what supervisors actually do. They might be poor supervisors, but calling them anal retentive does not describe their behavior toward the supervisee.

My second strategy was trying to determine styles on the basis of job description or on the basis of task. That is: How could you organize what supervisors do? Do their tasks fit into any pattern? They did not, because the tasks are very diverse. Only later did I realize that it is necessary to analyze the interaction that takes place in supervisory sessions. That is: What does the supervisor talk to the supervisee about? How does the supervisor talk to the worker? The word "how" from this perspective means that some supervisors ask a lot of questions and never give any answers, whereas other supervisors give a lot of information and never ask any questions. They never give any answers even though they give a lot of information, but the information they give does not necessarily answer the questions that the worker asked.

When I analyzed and categorized the interactional process that took place in supervision, patterns began to emerge. Some general categories of how supervisors tend to be described became apparent. Also, some ways the supervisees responded to supervisors could be categorized. **There are three basic substyles of supervisors in addition to the main** styles: *philosophers*, *theoreticians*, and *technicians*. Observation of supervisors at work revealed that each has an overall pattern of working that fits these styles. The combinations of the main style and substyles are shown in Visual 4-1. Some of the more renowned practitioners, when in a teaching or supervisory role, illustrate these styles. For example, I would characterize Carl Whitaker as a philosopher, Murray Bowen as a theoretician, and Jay Haley as a technician. Occasionally, one encounters a practitioner-supervisor who effectively combines components of all three styles. Descriptions of the early days of the Vienna Psychoanalytic Society (Clark, 1980:218-219; Roazen, 1974:176-179), lead me to believe that Freud, in his role as leader of this group, assumed all of the styles as theory, philosophy, and techniques were explored. Although this was not a supervision group as we know it today, it was a precursor of most approaches to group supervision and consultation currently in use. The same varied stylistic effectiveness can be documented in Freud's individual work with his pupils (Freeman, 1980).

APPLYING STYLE

Any time an attempt is made to categorize people, error is committed to a certain degree. People do not fit into categories completely, and there are always deviations. In terms of listening to the interaction and listening to the descriptions of the workers, I found that supervisors generally fit into one of these three categories-philosophers, theoreticians, or technicians-based on what they do over time.

Before describing the three individual styles, the notion of style itself needs some elaboration. In social work we have placed much emphasis on the importance of self-awareness and use of self, but often we have no idea about what we really mean by these terms. The question is: How would one actually be self-aware in a session with a client? The same is true in supervision: How is the supervisor actually aware of what it is that he or she is doing? One way for the supervisor to be more aware is simply by asking himself or herself: What is my style? The answer to this question should not be found in the categories above, but in self-description.

I asked this question recently of a supervisor who has been in social work for over 40 years, has worked in the same agency for 33 years, and has been director of the agency for 14 years. When I asked her this question, I thought I was going to have to get a fan and revive her. No one in her career had ever asked herthat question. She was taken aback, and said she would have to think about it because she did not know what her style was. She thought about it and came up with some words that she believed were descriptive of what it is she does and how she operates. In subsequent consultation visits, she has injected the idea of style into the conver-

VISUAL 4.1. Conceptualization of Main and Substyles

sation repeatedly. She has thought about it and uses it to determine how she is relating to others and how they relate to her.

When asked to analyze their own style, to consider how they perform in a given situation and to put a label on it, people assess what they have done in the past. Their answers have immediate impact on their present and future behavior. I developed the idea of style originally in relation to treatment and teaching people about treatment. I found that after I asked people, "What is your style?" (which practitioners do not think about while doing treatment) it later affected what they did with clients. The practitioners were spending more time trying to determine what their style was than they were concentrating on what the client was doing. Eventually, the practitioners overcame this and became consciously aware of their style. In the long run, going through this process benefits the client more than the temporary distraction of concentrating on practitioner styles may harm them. Many practitioners and supervisors never stop to consider what it is that they are doing. By simply talking about style, we can affect behavior directly.

In addition, the substyles of philosopher, theoretician, and technician are convenient models for describing techniques used in supervision practice. The idea of a philosopher substyle as a generalization can be transformed into the concept of philosophical abstraction to explain a specific segment of supervisory interaction, the theoretician style can be translated into theoretical speculation, and the technician style can be translated into technical strategy. The difference is that when talking about a supervisor's overall pattern of interaction, we use the concept of style, but when talking about a specific unit of interaction in supervision, we can use the terminology of a technique. Using this dual focus gives the concepts much more utility.

SUPERVISOR STYLES

Supervisors tend to respond in three substyles that can also serve as specific techniques. The forms of supervisor substyle/technique are:

- philosopher/philosophical abstractions,
- theoretician/theoretical arguments,
- technician/technical strategies.

These forms of response can be appropriate or inappropriate, depending on the practitioner's response to the supervisor (see Chapter 5). Each of these supervisor forms of interaction is discussed separately below.

Philosopher/Philosophical Abstraction

Rarely do supervisors use philosophy in its pure form — a profession of inquiry (Feibleman, 1973:14). Philosophy in its pure form has been described as "a difficult subject that uses ordinary words in queer ways and has no practical application whatsoever" (Feibleman, 1973:11). Philosophy can be used to intensify life and to support everyday activities. But sometimes supervisors launch into philosophical abstractions that have little or no application from the practitioner's standpoint.

Practitioners will present everyday material from their practice that concerns them, and the supervisor will become philosophically abstract in response to such content. Although this type of discussion might be interesting and stimulating, it frequently has no immediate practical value for the clinician. In some instances, it can be very helpful even though it takes years for understanding to emerge. Supervisor responses can be lengthy explanations or brief, global statements. One example of a global statement of this type occurred when a practitioner "was bemoaning some ineffectiveness in [his] work as a therapist," and received the response, "It takes ten years before a therapist begins to know what he's doing." It took the practitioner involved "many years" to see the wisdom of this statement, and that "ten years" was a metaphor for "a lifetime" (Kopp, 1976:94). This example illustrates a philosophical abstraction of long-range impact that proved useful.

However, at times supervisors will respond with lengthy statements of this type that the practitioner finds of limited use, finds frustrating, and views as a supervision strategy for avoiding the case material. An excerpt from a clinician's summary of her supervision illustrates this situation:

> We began today by discussing my patient, Arlene, who is undergoing resistance to family of origin work with her mother. My supervisor suggested I request the mother join the therapy for awhile. He mentioned that some people will do it on their own and some won't. I said, "Yes, like me," thinking to myself about parallel process in supervision and treatment. He asked me to repeat what I had said, and after I did, this led to a lengthy conversation which was philosophical in nature about family of origin material versus other ways of dealing with such material. We went on to talk about our own family of origin material. The discussion got heavy, and I think he sensed this and switched back to supervision. I started talking about another case. Afterwards, I felt frustrated and concerned that I did not get supervised on the original material.

Some supervisors make philosophical abstraction their major form of response. Such supervisors frequently preface their remarks with, "I had a case like that once" or "That reminds me of a case where I . . ." If this becomes the major focus of the supervision, the practitioner will become frustrated and resentful after a while, especially when he or she actively seeks help with technical skill. If this cannot be worked out and more congruence brought about between the supervisor's style and the practitioner's needs and expectations, consideration should be given to switching the practitioner to another supervisor.

The reactor/philosopher style of supervision is illustrated by the following description by a supervisee whose supervisor is much older than she:

> My supervisor, being the same age as my father, often treats me like a daughter instead of a social worker, which affects the structure and style of supervision he gives me.
>
> When I asked my supervisor about his style of supervision, he said, "I am eclectic." It is a cop-out; it is a way of avoiding a commitment. He is really a philosopher in supervision. He does not deal directly with my cases. He does not give me feedback. He does not take an active role. We have no specific times for supervision. He never gives straightforward answers.
>
> My supervisor often engages in small talk by discussing his graduate school experiences and earlier times and work in the field of social work without directly relating any of this to my cases. I don't gain insight about my cases through this method of discussing his past experiences, and he never gives me a clue to the connection between the two. When I ask him to explain the relationship between his past experiences and my cases, he replies, "Well, what do you think the connection is?" I often try to make up a connection to avoid looking and feeling stupid. My supervisor usually agrees with my reply no matter how off-the-wall I feel it is. This style of supervision is very frustrating and confusing, and it creates a feeling of incompetency about the supervisor.
>
> In addition, my supervisor maintains a very relaxed and casual manner throughout supervision. He is rarely direct; he doesn't offer explanations or examples. Often I'm disappointed, angry, and frustrated with my supervisor as a person, [and] I don't perceive him as being a competent supervisor. I feel he has much knowledge and information to offer, but he has difficulty explaining what he does and why.
>
> There are several characteristics that I truly like about my supervi-

sor. For instance, my supervisor stands by me and offers me security and reassurance when I feel anxious due to the emotional impact of my work. In addition, I'm comfortable with my supervisor and feel free to ask questions, intervene in treatment, try new methods of therapy, express myself, and come and go as I please. Furthermore, I respect my supervisor because he tries his best to work independently from the larger system. Most importantly, I admire my supervisor because he enjoys his clients, and he's concerned about helping them. My supervisor finds hope in an elderly client when most people would give up. His clients often improve because he gives them hope and reassurance which motivates them to recover.

This is a typical response to this type of supervision. The supervisor is liked and disliked, is irritating in some respects and comforting in others. This excerpt illustrates how style is interrelated with the way supervision is structured and how authority is exercised. It also exemplifies how the philosopher style is problematic only when it is a consistent pattern of relating to the supervisee. This practitioner identifies how the philosopher style is helpful when she is feeling distress associated with her work. If this supervisor could shift into the other styles at different points in the supervision, he could avoid the supervisee's perception of his being incompetent.

Supervisors should think twice about using philosophical abstractions. When they are used they should be brief, to the point, and clearly stated. To ensure that the practitioner has benefited from the philosophical abstraction, the supervisor should give the practitioner time to think about it and ask him or her to attempt to make some connection between it and the case. To guard against the overuse or misuse of philosophical abstraction, the supervisor should reflect about the supervisory interaction and its content. Through such a conscious process, the supervisor can shift style to become more effective.

Theoretician/Theoretical Arguments

The use of theory in therapy is the primary focus of many supervisors. These supervisors believe mastery of theory leads to good practice. Some supervisors use case material as a means to the end of understanding theory. According to this style of supervision, once the theory has been mastered, the practitioner can deal with future case material on his or her own.

Theoreticians tend to be logical and orderly in their approach to case material. They are about evenly divided when it comes to being active or reactive. They are usually respected by their supervisees and are frequently viewed as "taskmasters" when it comes to dealing with clinical material. The only time the theoretician is viewed negatively is when he or she talks about theory in the abstract and does not relate it directly to case material and learning. Supervisees become upset if the theoretician tends to ramble from theory to theory or does not remain consistent to a theory after proclaiming it.

The following is a practitioner's description of an active/theoretician supervisory style:

> My perception of my supervisor's style was that she was primarily a theoretician. She loved to discuss theory and at the time was taking a course on family theory. On numerous occasions she would point out to me various instances of maybe a client resistance or a triangulation. She was logical and organized in her approach. She would ask specific questions: . . . Did I observe how the family was triangulating? or Did I pick up on the fusion in the family? I remember I was in awe of her style.

Not all theoreticians are active. Some stay focused on theory but remain reactive to the supervisee. The following account illustrates the reactive/theoretician style:

> My supervisor's style is that of a psychoanalytic theoretician. She fosters a growth environment as much as possible in our relationship. When I go in to discuss issues, she usually leaves it up to me to decide what I want to do. There are times when I know from her facial expression or body language that she does not agree with my conclusions or techniques. Unless she feels it's very important for the patient's well-being, she won't say anything.

Practitioners undergoing such supervision soon learn that the cases they present are secondary to the goals of the supervision, and any immediate help they get with presented cases is incidental. Practitioners adapt to this form of supervision and select cases for discussion that are amenable to theoretical speculation. The most difficult cases the practitioner has will be worked into the supervision, and the practitioner will present questions or theoretical comments that he or she hopes will lead the supervisor to present some tangible ideas for dealing with these troublesome cases. We have encountered several instances where supervisees have deliberately **misinterpreted the theory** or feigned lack of knowledge of the theory when presenting difficult cases with the hope of getting some tangible help from the supervisor attempting to "straighten the therapist out about the theory." This same pattern occurs in the philosopher style of supervision, but is much more common in the theoretician style because there is a better chance for getting the supervisor to be case specific.

Supervisors who rely heavily on this form of interaction frequently use the Socratic method, asking questions that directly or indirectly cause the practitioner to see the connection between theory and practice. Such questions usually are not related to a theory as a complete set of propositions, but deal with specific concepts from a theory. Questions take the form: How can you help this client develop ego strengths? Are you sure you are showing unconditionally positive regard for this client? How are you going to use the here and now to lay the groundwork with this client? This form of questioning is viewed by such supervisors as shaking the concepts out of the theoretical rug. It is important to note that all three of these questions, derived from different theories, relate to the same dynamic of showing acceptance of the client and establishing a positive relationship, so that the conceptually based questions are related to the broader theoretical implications of the case. All of the questions are oriented to future actions of the practitioner rather than to strategies for dealing with problems already presented in the treatment.

There are instances where conceptual questions based on theoretical orientations are necessary and helpful, but only when the practitioner is specifically asking for assistance with the broader implications of the case or when the supervisor has determined that this is the needed focus in supervision. The use of this type of question is generally of limited help in response to a specific question about problems in a case. This can be understood when we come to realize that theories are not wrong, theories are not uncertain, and theories do not make mistakes. Only practitioners and supervisors commit these acts. Often supervisors will help practitioners to circle the theoretical wagons to defend against practice mistakes. For example, it would be difficult to envision how the supervisee could give answers to any of the three questions listed above that would be considered wrong. Questions need to be worded in ways that require the practitioner to explore alternatives of actions and to select the best or potentially most productive alternative.

It is important to recognize that in supervision the practitioner will often use inductive logic, while the supervisor tends to use deductive logic. In other words, the practitioner uses case points to derive a conclusion, and the supervisor uses a conclusion to identify case points. This produces learning gaps that must be overcome. Dealing with differences in orientation is not as difficult as it seems. The important factor is to identify which form of logic is being used and to have the supervisor and practitioner use the same form of logic. The supervisor and practitioner can openly discuss the direction they want the logic to take, and both can work at moving in the same direction.

We have made the mistake of thinking that it is the theory that is important in practice. What really is important is the way we use the theory, how well we understand it, how well it works, and that we recognize its limits. Theory in supervision should be viewed as a tool of knowledge. In turn, knowledge developed in supervision should be treated as both a dependent and an independent variable. This duality gives both the supervisor and the practitioner much more flexibility.

After the discussion of theoretical implications and the resulting knowledge in a case, the supervisor and practitioner are still left with what to do about the case from a practical standpoint. This is similar to activity in the scientific method—you must still explain the implications of a hypothesis after it has been found to be statistically significant. Rather than ending supervision with the theoretical significance of a case, this should be considered only the beginning, and the practical steps to be taken should be identified. (The purpose here has been to give an overview of the theoretician style and technique. For a detailed discussion of theoretical approaches, see Chapter 8, in which the use of theory is the focus of the entire chapter.)

Technician/Technical Strategy

This style of supervision is vastly different from the two styles just explained. Instead of being philosophical or theoretical in orientation, the supervisor deals almost exclusively with details of case problems and relates them to technical skills. In philosophical abstraction, the emphasis is on what ought to be known; in theoretical argument, emphasis is on the "why" of doing; and in technical strategy, the emphasis is on what was or is to be done. This style is problem focused and interactionally oriented.

Good technicians are not cold, calculating bureaucrats. Good technicians are sensitive persons who can ask highly specific and focused questions in skilled, empathic ways. Without confrontation or threat, they can pressure supervisees to deal with difficult material. They have patience and respond in ways that encourage practitioners to find their own answers. These supervisors are respected by their supervisees, but are also viewed as demanding and having a no-nonsense approach to supervision.

Technical strategy takes three forms: explanation, description, and planning. These forms are described below.

Explanation

This subcategory takes the form of the supervisor actually telling the practitioner what to say to the client. At first consideration this would seem to be completely unsound educationally and to promote dependence. However, there are situations in which the practitioner will present specific concerns about what to say to the client, and the supervisor makes the judgment that explains the appropriate and most efficient way to convey certain strategies to the practitioner.

Occasionally supervisors will be so concerned that their supervisees make a good impression and be successful within the organization that they will "coach" them extensively in exactly what to say in treatment. This occurs most often in settings where all practitioners have high visibility and do much cotherapy or collaboration. Such "coaching" at best is selectively ignored by practitioners (i.e., used only when they are in doubt and ignored when it is considered impractical), and at worst leads to practitioner frustration and eventual confrontation with the supervisor.

Description

Technical strategy based on description rests on after-the-fact exploration of case material. Most supervisors and practitioners describe their skills by describing processes rather than by focusing on behavior that occurred in the situation. Skill is more than description of practice, more than saying the client did better as a result of the interventions used. Skill involves timing in the situation and being able to articulate why a given intervention, action, or verbalization was used and how it promoted insight or moved the interaction into a helpful realm. It is only when the practitioner can differentiate the intent and the actual effect of any given intervention that learning and understanding have occurred. Most supervision is done in this context. It primarily involves learning from what has already taken place or is already known. The individual case conference or group conference is where most descriptive technical work takes place.

Some people hold that although the case conference remains a primary method of teaching in psychotherapy supervision, there is no evidence that this contributes anything to client improvement and that this method is relatively ineffective in producing learning (Bergin & Garfield, 1971: 896). We should use the case conference method when appropriate. Very little attention has been devoted to teaching in supervision, how the results of that teaching show up in practice, or how it ultimately gets acted upon by clients. This is a very complex, multilevel process that will require sophisticated research strategies. In the meantime, we must strive to improve educational supervision techniques and to be more specific about what and how we teach.

Planning

This component of technical strategy is organized around working with the clinician to plan strategies and techniques of intervention that will be used in general, as well as in specific individual cases. In many instances this will be based on discussion of case material from past sessions and cases, but what distinguishes this from the descriptive form of technical strategy is that it is almost exclusively focused on future actions of the practitioner, rather than reflection about past events. The chief focus of planning is teaching technique.

Technicians are usually active, although if you watch good technicians at work you can get the impression that they are reactive if you simply count the frequency of their verbalizations. Good technicians are listening, planning, and then strategically asking questions or making comments. When technicians do poorly it is because they have become too active and are controlling the practitioner. The technician must be on the alert about this problem and guard against it. Here is how one practitioner described her active/technician supervisor:

> When we discuss a particular case my supervisor is very methodical, and she stays with the case material. We have a format. We talk about the client's appearance and feeling tone. We focus on the purpose of the session, topics introduced by the client, topics introduced by the practitioner, therapist interventions, and the client's response to the interventions. We talk about goals, about feelings. We explore possible questions, problems, and observations for the future. We talk about my resistances and how to unblock them. We always discuss where to go next in the treatment. We discuss themes, topics, and key issues in the treatment.

The primary style and the predominant substyle can be identified for analysis. Certain patterns of the main styles and substyles usually emerge. For example, reactive supervisors tend to be philosophers; active supervisors show a propensity to be technicians. These classifications are always just approximations, and are designed only to help focus the supervisory interaction. As other research on style has indicated (Sternberg & Davidson, 1982:44), it appears that supervisors who are effective at combining and moving back and forth among the main styles and substyles at appropriate points in the supervision are the most successful.

It has been difficult to establish that supervisors adjust their style to accommodate the needs of individual supervisees. Since thinking about styles of supervisors as presented in this book is relatively new, it is possible that further research could lead to developing ways of adjusting to individual needs. For this reason, discussion of the supervisor's style is important, regardless of how the style is described or labeled. If supervisees are encouraged to discuss supervisory styles they prefer, supervisors can work at adopting variable styles based on individual need.

In exploring supervisor styles, one is not limited to the styles that have been identified in this chapter. Exploring the concept of style will enhance supervisory interaction regardless of the label that is used. It is important to understand that assigning a label is necessary, but not sufficient. The supervisor must give a description of the behavior that is associated with the label applied to the style. When a supervisor describes his or her style as "a teacher," for example, the supervisor, in order to become more aware of this style and what it means to the supervisor and the supervisees, must answer the questions: How do you teach? What do you teach? How do you determine what should be avoided in teaching? What do you do when teaching fails to achieve the desired result? These are just a few of the key elements that make up one's style, and making one's style known to oneself or to others is much more than using a label to describe it.

STYLE AND THEORETICAL ORIENTATION

Guerin (1976) has speculated about the relationship between the idea of style and theoretical orientation. He has asked whether theory sets limits on the clinician's style. He observes:

> Beginning family therapists inevitably go through stages in which they mimic the styles of the masters. Only if this remains a fixed phenomenon does it become an obstruction to the development of the therapist as a clinician. It is my belief that a well-defined, open-ended theory does allow a family therapist to evolve his or her personal style of operating with a family. (Guerin, 1976:17)

We do not know enough about this process to make any definitive statements. Questions that should be explored are: Do supervisors develop supervisory styles similar to the styles they use in treatment? Do supervisees copy the styles of their supervisors? What role does theory play in contributing to and determining styles of treatment and supervision?

SUGGESTED READINGS

Jay Haley. *Problem-Solving Therapy: New Strategies for Effective Family Therapy*. New York: Harper Colophon, 1976.
   A good discussion of techniques used in practice as well as a good chapter on supervision.

Allen F. Harrison and Robert M. Bramson. *Styles of Thinking: Strategies for Asking Questions, Making Decisions, and Solving Problems*. Garden City, NY: Anchor Press/Doubleday, 1982.
   This book describes five styles of thinking. The book is a good introduction to the concept of style from a cognitive perspective, with some good ideas for the supervisor on how to approach styles and thinking processes.

Elizabeth Webster and Paul Haler. "Effects of Two Types of Direct Supervisory Feedback on Student Clinicians' Use of Consequation." *The Clinical Supervisor* 7 (Spring 1989), pp. 7-26.
   Report of student reactions to different supervisor styles.

It has required 20 years of supervisory work to generate these current discoveries. Interacting with direct observations of patients and the unfolding of an interpersonal-intrapsychic theory of both the treatment experience and emotional disturbance, the detachment of a supervisor studying the therapeutic experience offered by student therapists to unknown patients proved to be indispensable. (It is impossible to learn how to do psychotherapy without such supervisory help.) However, insight emerged only because these student therapists would present the details of their therapeutic exchanges in strict sequence. This permitted not only observation and formulation, but also prediction and validation. It embedded the supervisory work in interactional considerations.

Robert Langs
The Psychotherapeutic Conspiracy

Chapter 5

Practitioners' Reactions to Supervisor Styles

Supervisees generally develop interactional reactions to supervisory styles. Supervisee reactions can be positive, or they can become problematic if they form patterns that thwart learning. Eight major reactions the supervisor must be conceptually aware of and prepared to handle are: (1) reasoned neutrality, (2) perceived organization constraints, (3) overwhelming clinical evidence, (4) persistent diagnosis, (5) oversimplification response, (6) pseudo criticism desire, (7) theoretical speculation, and (8) self-analysis. Each of these reactions is explained, and suggestions are offered for dealing with them. A set of three basic supervisory questions is presented for use in organizing ways of focusing supervisory interaction that can offset the negative effects of supervisee reactions.

INTRODUCTION

Although supervisors develop styles, practitioners generally do not develop styles in their role as supervisees that are unique or unrelated to the supervisor's style. In fact, most practitioners' styles in supervision are reflections of the supervisors' styles. There is evidence practitioners change styles when they change supervisors. Some practitioners who have had two different supervisors simultaneously use different styles with each supervisor. It was while working with practitioners in this unique position that I first discovered that the styles practitioners adopt in supervision are reflective of the supervisor's style. These workers were able to adapt quite well to the differing styles encountered in dual supervision.

Further study of practitioners' style in supervision revealed that their personal style or professional style as a practitioner had little correlation with their supervisee style. The key to the worker's style in the supervisory setting was the style of the supervisor. Supervisors must remember that they have power by virtue of their position; therefore, they do not have to work as hard as the supervisee to establish the supervisory relationship. Regardless of the practitioners' personal or therapeutic styles, in supervision they followed the lead of the supervisor. This probably accounts for the high levels of satisfaction with supervision that have been reported in a number of research studies.

SUPERVISEE EXPECTATIONS

In a study by Webster and Haler (1989) the style of the supervisor produced different interactional response from supervisees. Supervisees expect that the supervisor will set the style for the supervisory interaction, and they follow that pattern with a high level of acceptance. This interactional congruity is not always consciously planned or directly recognized as the supervision process unfolds. In other situations supervisees are aware of their reactions, as the following remarks by a supervisee reveal:

> My supervisor tends to use me as a sounding board. Maybe that is because he sees a lot of patients and doesn't have anyone else to talk to. I have some difficulty because I never know what role I'll be playing when I go in for supervision. So what I do is just adjust my mood to his. If he is laid back, I'm laid back. If he is hyper, I'm **hyper. If he is reflective,** I become reflective. I take responsibility for this behavior, but it's not comfortable sometimes not really being myself.

When the practitioner is unable or unwilling to conform to reflecting the supervisor's style, difficulty develops in the supervisory relationship. If, for example, a supervisor is a philosopher and the practitioner assumes a style of technician, difficulty will soon follow if both persist. Failure to work through varying perceptions of supervisor and practitioner can lead to conflict and frustration. The following summary of a supervisee's perception of his supervision illustrates this problem:

> I never knew where I stood with her. Everything was a power issue with her. She told me to take more initiative, and when I did, she accused me of "usurping authority" and "resisting direction." She also saw my time as having no value. What I mean by this is that when I was late for supervision sessions, it was a crime and I was told I was avoiding supervision, but when she was late, and that happened often, "it was just one of those things." I think she is really too busy as a therapist to have supervisees, but I never dared say that to her. When the situation got unbearable, she decided I should be evaluated by the staff. I agreed to this, but the problem with this was that I wasn't involved with the other staff. They really didn't know me. When the evaluation took place, I felt "ganged up on" and got defensive, so I didn't come out looking too good.

When this kind of difference in style occurs, it rarely gets recognized or discussed as an interactional stylistic problem. The problem is attributed to many other factors—most commonly, personality clashes, theoretical differences, or authority struggles. If the participants could recognize and explore the differences in styles covered in this book, much frustration, conflict, and lost learning opportunities could be avoided. I have assisted many supervisors and practitioners in overcoming their relationship problems by identifying the clashes of style. In doing so, I avoid personality variables, theoretical conflict, and authority struggles, since this type of difference is rarely reconciled. With some genuine efforts, styles can be altered and made more compatible. Understanding and recognizing styles in supervision are also important because practitioners who eventually become supervisors usually adopt the style that was predominantly used in their most significant supervision. This leads to particular styles' being perpetuated in supervision, and is the chief reason for weak and ineffective practices being repeated and passed along.

Although the practitioner mirrors the style of the supervisor, the practitioner does develop different interactional strategies at times to deal with the supervisor. Within these styles, practitioners utilize what I define as *interactional reactions* that occur periodically and episodically and often become patterns that can be identified and addressed.

INTERACTIONAL REACTIONS

The supervisor, as well as the practitioner, must be aware of and alert to the fact that these interactional reactions lead to obstacles to learning in supervision. This does not mean that clinicians deliberately avoid learning. Most of the resistances are unrecognized as clinicians are required to develop new techniques and new strategies in treatment. It is safer and easier to rely on familiar methods even when they are therapeutically naive or neutral.

The adjustments in style made by supervisees, either for encounters with different supervisors, or as distinct from the supervisees' practice styles, are quite subtle, but they can have major influence upon the supervisory interaction and outcome. Our fairly limited ability to adapt has been described by Harrison and Bramson:

> When we approach problems or decisions, we employ a set of specific strategies, whether we know it or not. Each of us has a preference for a limited set of thinking strategies. Each set of strategies has its strengths and liabilities. Each is useful in a given situation, but each can be catastrophic if overused or used inappropriately. Yet almost all of us learn only one or two sets of strategies, and we go through life using them no matter the situation. (1982:1)

Although our predominant cognitive styles and resulting interactional styles used as coping strategies are limited in range, the techniques or specific interactional reactions we employ in adjusting to supervision are somewhat broader.

In considering the supervisee reactions explained below, it is not intended that these responses be viewed as negative. Each one can be positive when employed rationally, logically, and specifically in a case situation. The categories of reactions can be considered resistances, but this is the case only when they become an inhibiting pattern or a block to learning.

The forms these interactional reactions take are varied, but the most common ones that practitioners manifest are:

1. reasoned neutrality
2. perceived organizational constraints
3. overwhelming clinical evidence
4. persistent diagnosis
5. oversimplification response
6. pseudo criticism desire
7. theoretical speculation
8. self-analysis.

Some practitioners repeatedly use one or two of these reactions, although in cases of severe blocks to learning, the practitioner will use all eight forms—and usually in the order that they have been listed. Each of the obstacles is discussed separately below.

Reasoned Neutrality

In this form of resistance, the practitioner will balk at a supervisor-suggested intervention on the basis that it will make the practitioner appear to the client as if he is "taking sides." This is a quite reasonable response since there is general agreement in treatment training on the importance of impartiality on the part of the practitioner. However, when it is used in response to a supervisor's attempt to deal with a specific segment of clinical intervention, it is a distortion of the practice dictum. Patterns of activity and consistency—not single episodes of intervention—are important to the neutrality rule (see Haley, 1973:36). When reasoned neutrality is invoked by the practitioner, the supervisor needs to make the distinction between patterns and portions of interaction in practice.

Perceived Organizational Constraints

Often practitioners will resist implementing certain interventions on the basis that the agency would thwart or not permit a recommended intervention. For example, a 24-year-old woman sought help in a mental health center at the insistence of the man she was living with. It was the worker's assessment after the initial diagnostic interview and supervisory exploration that the woman was functioning quite well and that the boyfriend was really the one in need of help, but he refused to enter the treatment. The supervisor suggested that the worker share this with the woman in a subsequent interview and not offer further treatment unless the boyfriend agreed to participate. It was the supervisor's view that to offer the woman treatment individually would confirm the boyfriend's motives. The practitioner agreed with this reasoning, but was reluctant to implement such a strategy because this would be against agency policy of offering treatment to those who desired it. This view was reinforced and voiced by the agency director frequently in staff conferences. The supervisor pointed out to the practitioner that the client was not being denied treatment, that conditions were merely being set on the treatment contract, and that such a strategy could be defended. The practitioner could make a case for the view that he was acting in the best interest of the client, and he reluctantly implemented the strategy. Two weeks after the follow-up interview, the woman phoned the worker to set an appointment for herself and her boyfriend. This resulted in a successful course of joint therapy. If the supervisor had not supported the practitioner in overcoming this perceived organizational obstacle, this woman could have been destined for a course of therapy that would have perpetuated her perception of a nonexistent individual dysfunction.

The supervisor must be prepared to deal with perceived organizational obstacles. The practitioner should be allowed to identify any organizational constraints he or she can, but the practitioner should also be required to search for ways to overcome them. Since there are no supervisory injunctions in educational supervision, the practitioner has a wide-open clinical field to explore freely. Although the field may be surrounded by an organizational fence, it is the responsibility of the supervisor to keep the practitioner moving rather than permitting him or her to climb the fence. This does not mean that organizational constraints should be discounted. They need to be separated from clinical material so that the emphasis can be placed on the clinical issues. Although more information is often needed and organizational rules are often real obstacles, it is interesting how often practitioners find things they can do when they focus solely on understanding the client's needs.

When viewing supervision as a learning enterprise and dealing with organizational issues, it is often easier to explore organizational dynamics through what I call *office pathology* and *office rationality*, rather than talking in abstract and theoretical terms associated with organizational theory. Freud is reported to have applied clinical concepts to organizations (Freeman, 1980:91). Practitioners think best in clinical terms, and at times it is easier to provide understanding through using familiar concepts and theories to aid learning about unfamiliar material. Clearly, there are limits to such a strategy, and organizations do not in reality take on characteristics of humans or operate on a rational basis. There are many glaring and tragic examples of this. It is in this area that the supervisor can help the practitioner to see the distinction between organizations as entities and the individuals that make up the organization. Practitioners are trained to do treatment and to work with clients, and many times are naive in their understanding and expectations of organizations. Perhaps more emphasis should be placed on understanding of therapeutic organizations in training programs, but supervisors will still need to work with practitioners as they encounter organizations in their therapeutic efforts.

Overwhelming Clinical Evidence

This reaction takes the form of the practitioner's presenting the supervisor with a series of symptoms, problems, and behaviors that make the case seem hopeless. When the supervisor offers help with a portion of such complex situations, the practitioner responds with more dynamics that seem to put the case out of therapeutic reach. The supervisor can become overwhelmed by such cases, and such feelings of hopelessness should be an indicator to the supervisor that this reaction is occurring. The supervisor should work to get the practitioner to organize and categorize the problem areas, then to assign priorities, and finally to explore a strategy for dealing with the specific problems selected for intervention. The supervisor should aid in the selection of problems to be treated by thinking in terms of which ones cause the most pain or impairment of functioning but at the same time have the best chance of amelioration.

Also, in some cases it helps simply to confront the practitioner with the hopeless nature of the case. Simply to ask if the case is hopeless usually results in a "no" answer. When this occurs, the supervisor can move to having the practitioner identify what leads him or her to believe the case is not hopeless. This strategy breaks up the interactional sequence of clinical hopelessness and transfers it from a negative to a positive approach to the case. If the supervisee responds with "yes," the supervisor needs to explore with the supervisee the basis of such an attitude. Such exploration can lead to a philosophical abstraction form of discussion that can open other insights into the case for the supervisee.

Persistent Diagnosis

Persistent diagnosis occurs when the practitioner continues to gather in treatment and provide in supervision information about the case, as if a point will be reached at which enough information will be accumulated to make interventions and solutions apparent. This is especially a problem in group supervision, and it is also a reaction to which the supervisor is highly susceptible. It is interesting to discover facts about cases and to speculate about the meaning of events. The supervisor needs to make a judgment about how much information is enough in order to move to planning intervention strategies. There are no easy answers to knowing when this point is reached. This is why it is so easy to get caught up in persistent diagnostic interaction.

The supervisor must remember that it is frequently necessary to act on the basis of insufficient information. There will never be as much information available as one would like to justify an intervention. Once the judgment is made to press the practitioner to move from diagnostic effort to intervention planning, this can and should be done simply and directly. The supervisor should keep in mind that practitioners cling to persistent diagnosis tenaciously. Often, even though they have been asked by the supervisor to move beyond diagnostic activity, they will respond briefly, but will return to it. It is common for a supervisor to have to confront persistent diagnosis several times in one supervisory session.

Persistent diagnosis can result in speculation about patient behavior that remains undocumented and in unfair judgments of the client. For example, in group supervision a case was presented and the group persisted in asking questions about the client and speculating about a diagnosis. One group member commented, "It sounds as if she is a potential drug abuser." Now the practitioner not only had a problem that was not clear, there was unsupported speculation about a potential problem. This is unfair to the client, and causes the practitioner to pursue a course that can be damaging to the treatment and the therapeutic relationship, as the practitioner becomes concerned with potential problems rather than existing problems in the case. The supervisor has a responsibility to guard against such speculation and to focus the supervision on identified problems that constitute the basis of treatment.

If persistent diagnosis is allowed to continue for a protracted time, it can lead the participants to conclude that there is *overwhelming clinical evidence* that moves the case into the realm of hopelessness. When these two categories of interaction are combined in this manner, it can be seen how some cases can be subtly dropped from supervision attention without ever being considered from the perspective of interventions to be attempted to help the client.

Oversimplification Response

Oversimplification response occurs when the practitioner presents a complex case. The worker is bewildered by all the dynamics, and the supervisor has some difficulty in gaining a comprehensive view of the case or in locating specific and appropriate points of intervention. In such a situation, supervisors will often focus on a specific piece of clinical material that is the most troubling to the client and that can be used for focus, or they will integrate less significant aspects of the case. The practitioner is offered simple strategies to guide initial intervention.

The oversimplification response occurs when the practitioner responds to the supervisor's comments and suggestions with, "I think your response is an oversimplification of what is taking place in this case." Timid and inexperienced supervisors will often be intimidated by such a response, withdraw from their initial observations, and launch back into the quagmire of clinical complexity. This often leads the supervisor and practitioner to revert to the earlier categories of *overwhelming clinical evidence* or *persistent diagnosis* and a stalemate. Practitioners use this strategy and supervisors succumb to it easily; as Scheflen (1972) has pointed out, middle-class Americans seem to have a tendency to engage in oversimplification when explaining behavior. Supervisors must be prepared, when faced with such responses, to articulate that they are not oversimplifying, but are merely offering points for initial intervention in a complex situation. The practitioner must be asked to suspend judgment of oversimplification until the proposed intervention is attempted.

Not all suggestions made by the supervisor will be valid, but this can be known only after intervention is attempted. The supervisor can concede that the practitioner might be right, but neither the supervisor's attempt at simplification nor the practitioner's perception of oversimplification can be determined until the strategy offered is tested out in the practice situation. However, if the worker persists in the belief that what is being offered is oversimplification, he or she might influence the patient to view the use of the strategy in practice as an oversimplification. The supervisor should point this out, stand firm if committed to the need for use of the strategy, and remind the practitioner to avoid being defensive about the supervisory response.

Pseudo Criticism Desire

Practitioners will at times take the stance that they want more critical analysis of their work by the supervisor, usually with the implied assumption the supervisor is failing to give them sufficient feedback. Often this is the case, and the supervisor simply needs to spend more time doing case analyses with the practitioner. However, when more case analysis is done, the practitioner frequently will become defensive of therapeutic action. The supervisor becomes confused and frustrated because he or she thought this is what the practitioner was asking for. Even when practitioners ask for criticism or evaluation, they are often seeking confirmation of their work. When, instead of complete support, genuine criticism and evaluation are offered, the practitioner resists.

This practitioner reaction occurs as a pattern over time rather than being episodic. Supervisors will often withdraw from such conflicted communication and respond only when necessary and in a positive way. This lessens the conflict and gives practitioners what they were seeking—no real evaluation of their practice and predominantly positive feedback, even when it is inappropriate. When this state of affairs is reached, the supervision is stalemated and learning ceases.

To reinstate a learning process in the supervision, the supervisor must reorient the focus of the interaction. The supervisor needs to place responsibility on the practitioner for bringing to the supervision case material that is troublesome. (The self-assessment form explained in Chapter 9 is a good way to initiate this.) However, if the supervisor assumes responsibility for identifying the problem areas, the practitioner is more likely to become defensive and to shift the focus on the basis that these are not the real problems.

Theoretical Speculation

More intellectual and academically oriented practitioners are likely to derive satisfaction from theoretical speculation about cases. They will be interested in the exploration of the theoretical implications of case dynamics or demonstrating how patient behavior is illustrative of theoretical concepts. These practitioners are delightful to work with in supervision, and are especially welcomed by the supervisor who uses the theoretician style or theoretical speculation technique. The use of theory in supervision is important, but the supervisor must avoid it becoming the major focus of supervision, causing both participants to lose sight of the client's efforts to change. The practitioner and supervisor can easily move away from the clinical material at hand and shift to a debate over the meaning and significance of theoretical concepts.

Sometimes young practitioners want to use supervision to learn more theory, but limits must be placed on this activity by the supervisor. The use of theory in practice is important, but it can become a dangerous obstacle. Many practitioners have difficulty boiling theoretical water. Theoretical discussions often lead to speculation about concepts the practitioner marginally understands, has difficulty precisely defining, and difficulty relating to theoretical origins. The supervision in such circumstances can lead to intriguing, but lengthy, continuing, unresolved debates. The supervisor must limit the discussion of theoretical material that is indirectly and inconsistently applied to the case material. (For more detailed discussion of how to deal with discussion of theory, see Chapter 8.)

Self-Analysis

Self-analysis is a common response among practitioners. Practitioners are taught throughout their education and supervision the importance of self-awareness to being a good practitioner. Unfortunately, there has been little attention devoted to how much self-awareness is enough and what kind of self-awareness is appropriate. The pattern has been: the more self-awareness, the better. There are limits to self-awareness that practitioners must be taught in order to avoid becoming therapeutically immobilized. Just because practitioners indicate a desire to develop more self-awareness, does not necessarily mean this is what they need. The supervisor must ask: What kind of self-awareness? For what purpose? Development of self-awareness in the practitioner promoted by the supervisor should be case specific. Encouraging self-awareness outside the context of practice material increases the risk of placing the practitioner into therapy, a situation that should be avoided.

Given the emphasis placed on the importance of practitioner self-awareness to treatment, it is understandable that many practitioners will fall back on self-analysis when faced with a difficult case in supervision. Supervisors trained in the same way find it easy to deal with practitioner dynamics rather than relating to client dynamics. The practitioner is present in the supervision, and his or her behavior is directly available for observation and interpretation; the client is once removed and only presented through the eyes of the practitioner, giving the supervisee more knowledge and control than the supervisor.

For unclear reasons, supervisees tend to block out positive feedback from the supervisor about their work. In some cases this is due to inconsistency between the worker's self-image and the supervisor's feedback. This causes the worker to retreat psychologically from the positive feedback. The supervisor can overcome this by making sure that the supervisee has heard the feedback and requiring the worker to give some response to it. In supervisory interaction, exploration of client dynamics should precede discussion of practitioner dynamics. That is, practitioner dynamics should be discussed only in the context of case material. Orienting discussion in this manner prevents practitioner behavior from becoming the primary focus of the supervision. When worker dynamics become the predominant area of exploration, the practitioner can develop the belief that supervision is a form of being put on the hot seat and can become defensive.

Self-analysis can take several forms, but the result is always the same — an avoidance of treatment issues. One form of self-analysis is focusing on worker "burnout" or distress (see Chapter 10). The supervisor should separate such discussion from discussion of case material.

In supervision, therapy should be avoided even if the practitioner asks for it directly or indirectly. Supervision is supervision, and therapy is therapy. There is limited value to a practitioner's learning to do treatment from being in therapy. Haley has taken a strong stand on this issue by stating: "There does not appear to be a single research study showing that a therapist who has had therapy himself, or understands his involvement with his personal family, has a better outcome in his therapy" (Haley, 1976:178). Therapy is education, but it does not necessarily follow that education is therapy. This is a mistake in logic that supervisors sometimes make when attempting educational efforts in supervision.

I feel that there should be some personal reference in supervision, but the supervisor must be careful how this is done and how it is stated, and must ensure that it is always related to the practitioner's own work. It has been known for quite some time that when practitioners are placed in therapy in their supervision, they will begin to act like clients, especially in group supervision (Beukenkamp, 1956:82).

Ambush Interaction

Some practitioners who are having difficulty in supervision or who are resistant to it will engage in what I call *ambush interaction*, using any or all of the reactions just covered. The practitioner will set the supervisor up with case material that he or she knows cannot be effectively dealt with, and each attempt to assist the practitioner will be met with an excuse or an explanation that the strategy being suggested has been tried to no avail. Practitioners who have a craving to know and master theory in supervision are at times avoiding committing themselves to an intense set of practice relationships. The interactional reactions of supervisees do not have to be identified or discussed as such, but the supervisor must be aware of them conceptually and, when they become problematic, find ways within their own style to deal with them.

CONCLUSION

In general, all of the reaction categories just discussed can be in part guarded against, dealt with, and overcome by focusing on the following three questions:

1. What are the major areas in which the client needs help?
2. What are the genuine problems the client has encountered?
3. What are the positive and negative patterns of relating that the patient demonstrates?

These three questions alone can be very helpful in focusing large segments of supervision.

In addition, all of the suggestions for developing effective supervisory styles discussed in Chapter 4 can be helpful in dealing with all the practitioner reactions covered in this chapter. Finally, a matrix of supervisory styles and the supervisee reactions is provided in Visual 5.1, which also indicates the outcome when each two factors interact. Both supervisors and supervisees can use this visual to assist in overcoming or enhancing styles and reaction combinations. For each style there is a corresponding listing of the supervisee reactions. The supervisor can identify a given style and connect it with a particular style that the supervisee is prone to use in order to determine a likely outcome. If the outcome is limiting the learning the supervisor may want to shift style slightly or organize the supervision so that the supervisee will be required to shift reactions. For example, if a supervisor uses the philosopher style and the supervisee frequently responds with clinical helplessness this can result in duplicity. In this context duplicity means that the style and the reaction are compatible but the combination results in mutual floundering and lack of focus, usually leading to frustration for the supervisor and the supervisee. When this occurs the supervisor should shift to another style. If they shift to a technician style this could be more helpful to the practitioner if he or she remains in the clinical helplessness mode.

SUGGESTED READINGS

To date, there are no books or articles devoted exclusively to the role and function of style as an interactional process. The only related book I am aware of is on cognitive styles of thinking, and I recommend it highly to the supervisor interested in the concept of style. The book is:

Allen F. Harrison and Robert M. Bramson. *Styles of Thinking: Strategies for Asking Questions, Making Decisions, and Solving Problems.* Garden City, NY: Anchor Press/Doubleday, 1982.

VISUAL 5.1. Matrix of Supervision Styles and Supervisee Reactions

SUPERVISOR STYLE

SUPERVISEE REACTIONS	Philosopher	Theoretician	Technician
Reasoned Neutrality	Moderately helpful if justification is avoided	Helpful	Helpful
Perceived Organizational Obstacles	Can be helpful when rationalization and justification of inaction are avoided	Moderately Helpful	Helpful
Clinical Helplessness	Can be helpful if duplicity that leads to mutual frustration is avoided	Can be helpful if duplicity that leads to mutual frustration is avoided	Helpful
Persistent Diagnosis	Avoidance of genuine Clinical issues can result	Can result in avoidance of genuine Clinical issues and narrow focus	Helpful
Over-Simplification Response	Can be helpful if unclear, frustrating, and defensive interaction is avoided	Moderately helpful when used to move beyond supervisee reaction	Very Helpful
Pseudo Criticism Desire	Use to avoid genuine Clinical issues should be guarded against	Can result in distraction from clinical issues, conflict, and distortion of treatment	Can result in avoidance of genuine Clinical issues
Theoretical Speculation	Use to avoid genuine Clinical issues should be guarded against	Can result in avoidance of genuine Clinical issues and distraction	Helpful
Self-Analysis	Can result in duplicity and mutual frustration	Can result in distraction from clinical issues, conflict, and distortion of treatment	Helpful

The processes and the changes in
processes that make up the data
which can be subjected to scientific
study occur not in the subject person
nor in the observer, but in the
situation which is created between the
observer and his subject.

Harry Stack Sullivan
The Psychiatric Interview

Chapter 6

Technique in Supervision

This chapter focuses on the concept of technique in supervision. It
is not a listing of techniques supervisors can use but an orientation
to the idea of supervisory technique, along with some general examples that can act as guides for individual supervisors to use in
developing their own techniques. Case material and technique are
explored through ten basic questions that can serve as a starting
point for any supervisor. Guidelines for case presentations as well
as sources of distraction in case presentations are identified. The
importance of focus is illustrated through discussion of four sets of
patterns that can be utilized to guide supervisory discussion. Questioning is one of the chief techniques that the supervisor can use,
and guidelines are given for developing good questioning technique. Contracts are being used more in supervision, and are discussed as a form of technique. Even good supervisors resist performing certain functions at times, and a way in which this
resistance can be turned into a positive technique is explained. As a
conclusion to this chapter, nine elements of good supervision and
eleven techniques to encourage learning in supervision are listed.
Much of the discussion in this chapter is oriented to the development of supervisory techniques that promote good practice techniques.

INTRODUCTION

Certain supervisory techniques can be used with each of the supervisory styles mentioned in Chapter 4. It should be kept in mind that each of the supervisory styles can also be used as a technique when applied to a specific unit of interaction in supervision. A host of techniques is included throughout this book. This chapter is devoted to general techniques that can be helpful in a broad range of situations.

EDUCATIONAL ASSESSMENT

There is renewed interest in supervision within many disciplines that make up the helping professions. An aspect of this trend is new interest in the role of educational assessment. That is: What does the student or new supervisee know as he or she enters the new situation? What does he or she need to learn? Years ago this was referred to as "educational diagnosis," but this terminology was abandoned when it was felt it suggested doing therapy with the learner.

In the past there was a tendency to focus the educational diagnosis on the personal aspects of the learner's functioning. When this approach was eliminated, there was a tendency to do very little assessment of the new supervisee. There was a belief that the learner was a blank slate, and it was assumed that the program staff or the supervisor knew what the supervisee needed to learn without much review of the supervisee's level of functioning or knowledge. When assessment began to reemerge, it took the form of relying almost exclusively on strengths and weaknesses identified by the learner. There was a general belief the learner was the person best qualified to establish what was needed to enhance learning. In other words, we shifted from the view that the learner knows little about his or her own needs to the position that the learner knows precisely what was needed to promote learning.

When educational assessment as a concept began to be formulated, a more balanced view of what constituted a good assessment evolved. The focus now is aimed at a mutual evaluation of the goals of the learning experience. There has been an effort to identify the major areas that are basic to a good educational assessment. The major areas are covered below.

1. Previous experience. It is important for the supervisor to know exactly what work and volunteer experiences the supervisee brings to the situation. This has become more important as supervisees increasingly come to the practice situation with substantial experience. It is common to encounter supervisees who have held several practice positions prior to entering an advanced educational experience. In most educational programs, almost three-fourths of the students are part-time and hold some form of employment associated with the helping professions. It is true that learners today have significant experience in positions related to the learning situation. At the same time, however, the supervisor cannot assume that the learner has mastered all the elements of a position that he or she has held. In this age of specialization, the exposure of a practitioner in a given position can be quite narrow. For these reasons the supervisor needs to explore thoroughly all past positions the learner has held.

2. Ethical awareness. Ethical practice is of paramount concern in most aspects of our society today. There is much confusion about what is ethically appropriate behavior in many settings. All disciplines have some ethical code that guides practice. It is the supervisor's responsibility to determine the learner's knowledge of the ethical code or codes he or she is required to conform to while in the educational environment. It is a good idea for the supervisor and learner to engage in a detailed review of the relevant codes that apply to the situation.

3. Theoretical knowledge. There has been an explosion of theories of behavior and intervention in the past two decades. The practitioner may have varying exposure to theories from past educational and work experience. Educational programs and agencies place varying emphasis on theories and theoretical knowledge. The supervisor needs to know what theories the practitioner has knowledge of and the depth of the knowledge of each theory the practitioner identifies. The supervisor needs information regarding what theoretical orientations the clinician is currently exploring and how the clinician is integrating the theory in practice.

4. Assessment and diagnosis. What experience and skill has the clinician accumulated regarding assessment in general, and in a given treatment area or speciality specifically ? In-depth assessment involves more than being able to do a social history or initial data base. Assessment involves the ability to integrate knowledge of behavior, personality, social functioning, educational development, health, economic, and spiritual activity. The specialized aspects of assessment can be troublesome for practitioners. For example, in mental health agencies the supervisor needs to know the practitioner's level of knowledge and skill in using the *DSM III-R* and manuals used to reference medications. Some clinicians resist developing knowledge in these areas even though there are increasing demands to be skilled in these areas of assessment.

5. *Organizational understanding.* Supervisees usually have some degree of experience in organizations. The supervisor needs to learn how the practitioner has come to view organizations and their formal and informal structures. Clinicians can have unique perspectives on their own experience in an organization. One of the author's supervisors wisely stated that a person can have ten years of experience in an agency or one year of experience repeated ten times. In this example the practitioner with ten years of genuine experience can build on the cumulative insights he or she has gained, and the clinician with one year repeated ten times will need to be assisted in developing a broader perspective on the significance of experience in an organizational context. It is critical for the supervisor to determine what type supervisee he or she has in order for an effective organizational educational experience to evolve.

6. *Agency functioning.* Organizational understanding is more comprehensive and global than agency functioning. The supervisor needs to assess the supervisee's knowledge regarding the nature of the agency he or she is about to enter. Each agency has a unique structure and atmosphere. A practitioner can have general knowledge, but the clinician has to be able to apply this generalknowledge to an individual setting.

7. *Attitudes and values.* Supervisees with work experience have undoubtedly developed values and attitudes toward working with clients. It is not just social agency experience that gives rise to attitudes and values about clients. The supervisor needs to be aware of negative attitudes and conflicting values as the supervisee enters the agency so that accommodation can begin to avoid problems for clients and the practitioner. Such practitioner attitudes are often subtle and unconscious. Once identified, clinicians are usually able to change these attitudes and remove them as barriers to effective relationships with clients.

8. *Goals and objectives.* It is important that the supervisor know about the practitioner's general goals. Frequently clinicians have difficulty identifying specific skills and knowledge they want to acquire, but are able to state their career goals. Through identifying career goals the supervisor can learn much about what the practitioner hopes to achieve as part of the placement experience. The types of interventions, modalities, methods, and speciality areas that are of interest to the clinician are factors the supervisor can explore to help the practitioner refine precise learning goals.

9. *Previous supervision.* Practitioners have usually undergone some form of supervision in helping professions and general employment areas. The supervisor should explore with clinicians their perception of the qual-

ity of past supervision and as well as its duration and structure. Past experience shapes the person's expectations. Supervisees who were given much independence in a past position may resist meeting regularly with the supervisor. Supervisees who have been oversupervised may make excessive demands on the supervisor's time. By knowing the past supervisory experiences, the supervisor is in a much better position to establish current expectations.

10. Learning impediments. Practitioners have very active lives. Balancing all of life's demands becomes a juggling act for the person. When demands become too great the job is usually the first area to be compromised, and family the second. The supervisor needs to have accurate information about the overall functioning of the practitioner. The supervisor should avoid intruding or imposing on the practitioner's life outside the agency, but does need to be aware of events that could influence educational functioning.

The supervisor should cover these general areas with any practitioner before he or she begins practice. After completing an assessment, the supervisor is much better prepared to develop an educational plan for the supervisee. Developing educational plans that are not based on information in these areas puts the supervisor in the position of blindly assuming what the practitioner does and does not know.

Different supervisors have varying ways of doing educational assessment. The most common method is to interview the person and evaluate the practitioner's responses to a set of loosely organized questions. Some supervisors have the practitioner make a list of strengths and weaknesses. These are effective ways of doing an assessment, but there needs to be some record of the practitioner's participation in the process, as well as a way to review with the clinician periodically the degree to which the educational program and supervision are meeting the learning needs.

An instrument that can be used to organize educational assessment is printed in Appendix 2. The instrument focuses on the ten assessment areas identified above. After the practitioner completes the instrument, it is discussed and becomes a part of the supervision record. It is reviewed at key evaluation points during the educational experience.

CASE MATERIAL

Case material is the foundation of supervisor clinical techniques. Case material should be the focus of supervision and most techniques in some way derive from this focus. In considering case material, the supervisor should use some general areas for practitioner reflection that can help the supervisee gain a comprehensive perspective of the case regardless of the supervisee's specific concerns. The supervisor can help the practitioner in a general way to think about future treatment sessions by asking some form of the following questions:

1. What do you like about this client?
2. What do you think the client likes about you?
3. How much of yourself do you see in this client?
4. What do you feel inside yourself when you are with this client?
5. Where in your body are these feelings concentrated?
6. Theoretically, what is the basis of what you have presented about this client?
7. On what basis did you decide to use the techniques you did in this session with the client?
8. What was the major focus of this session?
9. What worries you the most about this case?
10. What are you going to do next with this case?

The supervisor needs to cover these areas in some format. The supervisee needs to grapple with these questions, but the supervisor should assist the practitioner when the response is "I don't know."

The question "What do you like about this client?" might be dismissed by some as insignificant, but this question can elicit a great deal of helpful information about the client to which the practitioner has not given much thought. This is very similar to Harry Stack Sullivan's observation:

> Psychiatrists know a great deal about their patients that they don't know they know. For example, caught off guard by the offhand question of a friendly colleague — "Yes, but damn his difficulties in living! What sort of PERSON is this patient of yours?" — the psychiatrist may rattle off a description that would do him honor if he only knew it. (1954:14)

This example relates to the idea of the "level of knowing" in practice, and the ten questions relate to knowing that goes beyond professional knowledge. The questions are designed to be clear, simple inquiries that go to the essence of the treatment relationship.

CASE PRESENTATIONS

Practitioners who are asked to present cases or share their practice are being expected to take risks, and can feel threatened. This anxiety can be lessened when the supervisee is given time to prepare, organize questions, and consult with the supervisor in advance. The practitioner may have two fears: fear of not meeting expectations and fear of losing existing autonomy. The supervisor must support and reassure the practitioner to lessen both fears. When supervisors accept that they cannot be responsible for the practitioner's performance, but are responsible only for clarifying the expected standards of performance, the door is opened to interaction that allows the supervisor and practitioner to engage in a process of genuine growth and development.

To help the practitioner who is struggling with a case, the supervisor should identify with the client and assist the practitioner in understanding what the client may be experiencing and how the client may be responding. If the supervisor has difficulty identifying with the client, he or she should ask the practitioner to describe and imitate or role play the client. Through this process the practitioner will be forced to identify client patterns of relating, and the supervisor will gain access to client characteristics which he or she can then feed back to the practitioner. Langs strictly adheres to this view of supervision, seeing the central focus of supervision as the therapist-patient interaction, and considering all else to be peripheral. He says: "I spend much of my supervisory time attempting to identify with the patient and what he is experiencing both within himself and from the therapist . . . because I . . . wish to experience the therapeutic interaction as it unfolded for the supervisee" (Langs, 1979:15).

Any presentation of a case for supervision should result in the supervisor's asking the practitioner to explain all efforts to deal with the problem before giving assistance. This helps avoid the practitioner response: "I tried that, and it didn't work."

Not every act of the practitioner can be scrutinized in supervision, and not every case can be explored. Priorities must be set for which cases and which case material will be reviewed. Priority should be given to areas of practitioner concern, but there should be provision for reinforcement of the practitioner's strong points to avoid an exclusive focus on areas of weakness and vulnerability.

The following guidelines for case presentations are offered to assist supervisors and supervisees in keeping presentations focused. Remember, case presentations can be threatening. Anxiety about case presentation can be lessened by the following:

1. The supervisor should present a case first.
2. The supervisee should be granted time to prepare the case for presentation.
3. The presentation should be based on written or audiovisual material.
4. The presentation should be built around questions to be answered.
5. The presentation should be organized and focused.
6. The presentation should progress from client dynamics to practitioner dynamics.

There are also several common distractions that occur in case presentations that the supervisor must be alert to:

1. presentation of several cases in a short session;
2. presentation of a specific problem rather than the case in context;
3. presentation of additional problems in a single case;
4. therapist dynamics preceding case dynamics during discussion;
5. intervention expectations beyond the capabilities of the therapist.

LEVEL OF KNOWING AND TECHNIQUE

Level of knowing can be generally divided into two types—technical skill and perspective (Lachman et al., 1979:4). Technical skill in this context relates to specific units of activity; perspective deals with understanding the relationship among sets of units of activity that allows comprehension of the whole. A bus driver can be a good driver without understanding the total functioning of a mass transit system. By the same token, the director of a mass transit system can understand the complex operation and large-scale issues without being a good bus driver. Technical competence is possible without perspective, and perspective is possible without technical skill. It is helpful if one has both, but it is not always a necessary condition. Practitioners can develop technical skill without a great deal of perspective about treatment, and supervisors can supervise with perspective while having limited technical skill, although this is much harder to accomplish. It is important to promote both levels of knowledge in both supervisors and practitioners.

In treatment-oriented supervision, problems can arise when the practitioner and supervisor are aiming at different levels of knowledge. Practitioners are more often interested in technical competence—in improving their practice skills—while supervisors frequently focus their attention on perspective—on philosophical and theoretical issues. When the practitioner's level of knowledge or inquiry is different from the level at which the supervisor wishes to work, supervision becomes at best benign and ineffective, and at worst frustrating, tense, and conflictual.

In order to avoid this mismatch of knowledge development, the supervisor must be sensitive to the fact that the two levels exist and aware of how each is presented in supervision. There are times when it is appropriate to focus on one level in supervision so that learning can be maximized. For example, younger, inexperienced practitioners are more likely to be interested in learning technical competence; older, experienced practitioners are more interested in perspective from a philosophical and theoretical stance and will be annoyed when supervisors force them to focus exclusively on technical skills. At the same time, practitioners will at times raise perspective issues to avoid discussing technical competence. This is not always a deliberate shift of focus. Sometimes it is a more subtle erosion of the appropriate learning process to which the supervisor must be alert and against which he or she must guard.

It is a good general policy to begin with technical skill learning and then move to perspective learning. One helpful way to picture this in supervision interaction is to view technical learning as the *horizontal* aspect of supervision, and perspective or philosophical and theoretical learning as the *vertical* component of supervision. Technical competence, then, relates to activity on a horizontal level with individual cases, and perspective or insight comes as one moves up the scale of complexity and integrative understanding in a series of cases.

It is best to begin with development of technical skill, because traditional learning theory has taught us that technical obstacles must be removed (in therapy this translates into mastery) before the higher-level of perspective learning can occur.

CONTINUITY

Supervision should have continuity, just as treatment does. A case should be presented sequentially, beginning with identification of patient dynamics and problems, a tentative diagnosis, alternative intervention strategies, selection of a general intervention approach, and follow-up of the case. Supervision that focuses only on specific problems will not be much of a learning experience for the practitioner. Observation of supervision sessions often reveals that the supervisor failed to follow a comprehensive process, which results in confusion and frustration for both supervisor and practitioner. The supervisor cannot perform the supervisory function effectively if one of the elements listed above is missing or slighted.

Most often, follow-up is the missing component. Failure to do follow-up deprives the supervisor of an opportunity to evaluate the effect of the supervision on the practitioner and the treatment. When follow-up is not done, the supervisor has no way of knowing if the efforts of a considerable amount of supervisory time were ever applied.

Thorough follow-up can serve as ongoing evaluation of the practitioner, the therapy, and the supervision. Some strategies worked out in supervision are wrong and inappropriate, and this needs to be made known. Many errors of supervision are repeated because of failure to do follow-up.

TREATMENT PATTERNS

In supervision it is important to focus on patterns that occur in the treatment. It is only through identifying patterns that the supervisor and practitioner can be confident that they have a comprehensive grasp of the client and his or her life situation and problem. Focusing on isolated behaviors of the client can lead the treatment astray and cause it to become fragmented and frustrating. There are four forms of patterns in the patient that can be identified and interrelated:

1. patterns of personality or behavior;
2. patterns of life events and interaction;
3. patterns of interaction during a single treatment session; and
4. patterns of the treatment process.

MECHANICS OF TECHNIQUE

For the supervisor who wants to learn the mechanics of how to teach technique to practitioners, there are several factors to consider. First, techniques cannot be taught in isolation or without regard to the total therapeutic process. Techniques are never entities in and of themselves. A technique taught as a self-contained activity will leave the practitioner holding the bag interactionally once it is introduced or used in the treatment.

Therefore, the second factor is that techniques must be identified and taught as a series of actions so that the process of beginning with a client includes developing techniques for setting up the initial session, greeting the client, putting the client at ease, discussing fees, explaining how treatment works, gathering information, helping the client verbalize difficult material, formulating a diagnosis, setting priorities for problems, and mutually establishing treatment goals. Techniques for accomplishing these tasks can be taught and practiced individually, but this must be done within the context of initiating the treatment process.

Third, a series of techniques should be arranged from the simple to the complex. It is difficult to identify the ordering of techniques because some techniques will be difficult for some practitioners and quite easy for others, depending on their level of experience, training, self-awareness, and emotional orientation.

In discussing practice skill, most practitioners and supervisors give descriptions of process rather than talk about skills developed and used around behavior that occurred in the situation. This is what Haley is referring to when he states, "the therapeutic process is such that one cannot go directly from the problem at the beginning to the cure at the end" (Haley, 1976:121). Skill is more than description of practice, it is more than saying that the patient did better as the result of the techniques used or the skills applied. The supervisor can be the instrument through which the practitioner develops awareness of skills he or she possesses.

Finally, teaching technique can be like the job of a swimming instructor teaching small children. The supervisor who wants to learn how to teach technique should observe this process of teaching swimming. The instructor demonstrates basic arm strokes, leg action, and head movement individually out of the water, and then each activity is demonstrated and practiced in the water individually. Head movement and arm strokes are practiced while the learner walks in shallow water. Leg kick is practiced using a kickboard for buoyancy. In many respects, the kickboard is to swimming instruction what audiovisual teaching aids are to supervision. The students then put all these strokes together while the instructor observes them from in the pool and outside and offers comments about incorrect use of movements. Sometimes the instructor will swim alongside the students and point out misapplications. Then the students practice, practice, practice.

OVERCOMING DIFFICULTY

There are many parallels between what the swimming instructor does and what the supervisor needs to do to teach a series of techniques for mastery of an intervention strategy. The supervisor can learn much about style and technique from observing how technique is taught in other disciplines. Musical instruction, dancing classes, dramatic artists rehearsing, painting classes, and baseball and football clinics are some of the more common learning situations that can be helpful to the social work supervisor in treatment-oriented settings.

Any technique worthy of the term can be described and explained. More effort needs to be devoted to describing and labeling techniques we have used. We need to focus on why we used a particular technique, how it was used, what the response was, and the outcome of its application.

If practitioners use any technique in treatment long enough, it will eventually backfire on them. Because of this, in supervision there should be emphasis on developing alternative strategies in advance.

Practitioners can go sailing along in a treatment session with their style and technique serving them effectively, but then they enter a difficult interactional sequence that is sufficient to get them completely out of style and cause them to lose sight and command of their most reliable techniques. When this occurs practitioners usually withdraw verbally, ask questions that are not relevant, or become supportive of the client regardless of the appropriateness of such support. If such sequences can be identified and explored openly in supervision, the practitioner can be helped to develop strategies for overcoming such situations rapidly, and can readjust more quickly.

Many sessions that have been headed toward a productive outcome have been totally altered and have floundered when practitioners failed to work their way out of such setbacks. Generally, this pattern occurs more frequently or has more potential for occurring as the number of clients in the treatment increases. Cotherapy activity is one good safeguard against this pattern.

We know that clients resist change and will consciously and unconsciously attempt to thwart the worker. The practitioner is way behind the client when treatment begins with respect to the problems, feelings, concerns, and conflicts. This remains the case throughout the treatment. The client has more knowledge and information than the practitioner, who learns only what the client chooses to reveal. At the point when powerful interventions are taking place, the client will resist with strategies equal to the practitioner's best interventive efforts. Practitioners frequently underestimate the power of the client to resist. The practitioner's reluctance to recognize the client's pattern of efforts to maintain dysfunctional behavior can severely retard the progress of treatment.

When practitioners are distracted by difficult material, discussion of what happened, why it happened, and how it can be prevented in the future can take many forms, and creative suggestions are limited only by the practitioner's and supervisor's ability to dissect the material. Several **general guidelines can** be offered to practitioners when they sense that their style is shifting or disrupted because of discomfort or overwhelming content:

1. Stop the interaction and focus on analyzing the meaning of the most recent interaction.
2. Withdraw temporarily and think of an alternate way to return to the difficult content. This must be accomplished fairly quickly. The therapist must develop skill at thinking fast.
3. Avoid admitting to feeling uncomfortable or overwhelmed. This can diminish trust in the therapist or reinforce the patient's dysfunctional pattern in the treatment. It is better to attempt to relate in some way to the possibility that the patient is uncomfortable or that the focus of the interaction is in some way upsetting.

TECHNICAL DIFFICULTY

Supervisors who use technical strategies periodically experience *technical difficulty*, and this is to be expected. There will be times when the strategies they use fail to work or are completely effective. This should not immobilize the supervisor. When good supervisors encounter such difficulty, they shift to another strategy, and continue to shift techniques until they reach their objective.

Practitioners are prevented from accomplishing goals or applying techniques through interventions if they are unable to practicably carry them out or control the treatment. For example, a practitioner cannot do intensive intervention with the family of a terminal cancer patient if the practitioner works on an open cancer ward and has no private office to interview the family. The good technician will be sensitive to this kind of issue.

The "if-then" proposition is a good linguistic and interactional technique to approach much case material explored in supervision, especially when technical difficulty is encountered. Statements should be in the form of "if the client is this way, then this technique should result in . . ." Every statement of the practitioner should be well thought out and incisive. Each comment should elicit more than one possible response. The practitioner, like the good writer, must be precise to stimulate a variety of responses. As Thomas Wolfe said of Hemingway, he "says one thing and suggests ten more . . . ."

Supervision of cases on a weekly basis provides continuity and follow-up of specific techniques and is well suited to individual supervision; cases reviewed only periodically or during one session are better suited to theoretical and conceptual learning, and this can be better achieved in group supervision.

QUESTIONING TECHNIQUE

Questioning is one of the chief techniques supervisors use to help practitioners reflect about their own work. Limited attention has been devoted to the use of questioning in supervision. When and how a question is asked can be one of the most valuable forms of interaction used in supervision. Supervisors attempting to evaluate their questioning technique should review tapes of supervisory sessions and evaluate their style of questioning on the basis of the following guidelines:

1. Questions should be general in nature, but the practitioner's answer should be specific. This should be a basic rule of the questioning that is made clear to the supervisee. A general question avoids locking the practitioner into a predetermined perspective held by the supervisor. A general question allows the practitioner to answer in one of several ways, usually in relation to a specific of the case.

2. A general question that is answered in a general way can be repeated. The supervisor can repeat and rephrase the question again and again until a mutually agreed upon response is achieved.

3. When the supervisor wonders whether the practitioner has adequate knowledge of the case (diagnosis) to make treatment decisions, the supervisor needs to move from general to specific questions. If the practitioner demonstrates lack of knowledge, it is appropriate to delay discussion of the case until the practitioner becomes more familiar with the case. Too often supervisors pursue cases for which adequate information is not available, and this can lead to idle speculation, misguided treatment, and poor learning. This is important because the more the practitioner knows about the case, the less likely it is that errors in treatment will be made.

4. When general supervisory questions result in answers that reveal thorough knowledge of the case, the supervisor can move to questions related to treatment and intervention strategies. If diagnostic questions repeatedly reveal lack of knowledge of cases, the supervisor needs to shift the focus of the supervision temporarily to deal with problems the practitioner is having in grasping the dynamics of cases. Excuses or substitution of speculation for lack of knowledge of cases is unproductive in supervision.

5. Questioning is one of the best techniques the supervisor has available to help practitioners articulate knowledge (both manifest and latent) of cases.

6. Questions related to diagnostic understanding should be more specific than questions related to treatment strategies and techniques. Usually diagnostic questioning will require a series of specific questions that will

result in a generalization or conclusion about the case. A treatment-oriented question should be general and singular, resulting in a series of answers that will reveal various techniques or strategies.

7. Questions should be simply stated, clear, and concise. The supervisor should avoid prefacing a question with a lengthy introductory statement. Good questions stand on their own.

CONTRACTING AS A TECHNIQUE

Contracting in human services has come into vogue during the past two decades, and this has carried over into supervision to the point that most schools of social work require student-field instructor contracts, and some agencies require contracts for professional-level supervision. There has been some emphasis on the procedures in negotiating supervisory contracts (Wijnberg & Schwartz, 1977). Most of the contracting literature has failed to take into account the power difference in the supervisory relationship that places serious limits on the ability of the supervisee to negotiate. Any structure, technique, or issue the supervisee wishes to negotiate must always be judged in advance by the supervisor as to whether it is essential to learning and, therefore, nonnegotiable. Under these circumstances, anything that is deemed nonessential to learning is negotiable, but any item that falls into this category can be easily perceived by the supervisee as unimportant. It is hard for a supervisee to take such a contract negotiation seriously.

The advocates of contracting in supervision have been strangely silent about what to do when conditions of the contract are not followed. If contracts are to have any value, they must be honored. The supervisor must confront supervisee failures to meet conditions of contracts, or they risk loss of authority and respect. The situation gets much more complex when the supervisor fails to live up to the contract. Most supervisees feeluncomfortable confronting supervisors about such failures. For this reason, supervisees regard contracts as rather one-sided documents. Given these problems, it is a good idea to include in the contract what procedures can be used if either party fails to meet the conditions of the contract. Also, contracts should be fairly general and limited to short periods. Six months is an appropriate time period.

Contracts in clinical settings should include at minimum reference to:

1. *Timing element.* This section should include items such as frequency of supervision, length of sessions, duration of supervision process.
2. *Learning structure.* This would include any learning structures the supervisor may use such as joint interviews, audiovisual techniques, consultants, continuing education, etc.
3. *Supervision structure.* This section would include the type of supervision to be used such as individual, group, or a combination.
4. *Agency conformity.* Items such as dress codes, listing of phone numbers, licensing requirements, and work hours and days should be covered in this section.
5. *Special conditions.* These are usually requirements that are unique to the setting such as requirements to do DSM-III-3 diagnosis, to be familiar with medications, to provide legal testimony, or any requirements that the practitioner many not have training in or be familiar with. In such cases the contract should state how the agency expects the practitioner to acquire the knowledge and skill required.

READING AS TECHNIQUE

Reading books is rarely associated with supervision. Supervision has always been perceived as highly personalized teaching with a "hands-on" and "learning by doing" approach. Reading about practice has been reserved for the more abstract classroom aspects of learning. Even continuing education programs have focused mostly on practical, rather than "bookish," learning. Supervisors rarely use books in supervision and express reservations about trying it. With some supportive discussion, and suggested techniques for how to begin, the resistance subsides. The reluctance is mainly due to lack of assistance and encouragement in using this as a teaching method.

This is interesting since supervisors, when discussing their own development as a practitioner, comment on cherished and truly integrative learning resulting from books that their supervisors had suggested they read. Passages, concepts, and ideas from some of these books still guide their clinical and supervision practice at different times. One supervisor commented:

> I draw on my reading that my supervisor suggested. It is not extensive, a few very essential books and articles. I cannot say I remember or use any of the textbooks from my classroom days. I cannot recall any of the reading my supervisor suggested turning out to be a negative. I realize now the supervisor reading assignments were em-

bedded in and grew out of the supervisors' own practice. For example, Sidney Jouard's *The Transparent Self* and *Disclosing Man to Himself* are two books a supervisor introduced me to that deepened and expanded my learning and continue to influence my understanding. Another book I go back to often is Wilhelm Reich's *Listen, Little Man*. This is a book about freedom, oppression, and authority that can promote understanding of practice, the clients we see, and some of the inherent conflicts supervision produces. I have found that it is the small, clearly-written books that are the most helpful and memorable. The books do not have to be serious to make a somber point. This is the case with Greenburg and Jacobs' *How To Make Yourself Miserable*, which I sometimes recommend to supervisees and to clients. I customize my book suggestions to the individual.

Supervisors should frequently suggest that supervisees read books that can supplement their learning. If supervisors promote reading as a learning method, supervisees will come to associate reading with their own self-development long after teachers, supervisors, and educational programs become a fond memory. Practice, even in an agency, can be a very lonesome endeavor. While colleagues and continuing education programs can be a rich source of stimulation and learning, the act of reading and discovering commonalties with other's experience, and applying the techniques and thoughts of others to your own practice, can be the most rewarding and comforting form of growth.

A nice feature of reading as a supervisory technique is that it does not require a lot of formal mastery of educational methods or techniques. It emerges out of your own past or present reading experience. There does have to be a logical connection between the circumstances surrounding the supervision and the books you suggest. There should be some follow-up of connections made between the reading and the supervision or practice dynamics. This is essentially all one has to do. Of course, there are many variations on the theme.

This form of learning is present to us at all times. It is only as far away as pulling a book off the shelf. Learning through reading does not have to wait until the next supervisory or consultation appointment, the weekly staff meeting, or the continuing education workshop next month. This is a form of learning that is truly convenient and completely under the control of the practitioner. By promoting reading in supervision, the supervisor can genuinely contribute to giving rise to the "self-directed" practitioner who has a research orientation to practice.

This form of learning is not the passive learning of the traditional model utilized in training programs and continuing education programs. We have so ritualized the teacher-student model that self-induced learning is foreign to and difficult for many practitioners. This is not the fault of the practitioner. It is a systemic problem. For example, licensing and certification bodies do not have provisions to provide continuing education credits for reading. Credits for such learning would be very difficult to monitor. The irony is that the most significant learning usually grows out of experiences that cannot be monitored by organizations and teachers. It seems we have become too dependent on externally monitored learning. Supervisors can assist in overcoming such attitudes through aiding supervisees by using reading to enhance learning.

LATENT SUPERVISION

There are forms of what I call "latent supervision" that supervisors must be aware of and take into account in their supervisory interactions. Latent supervision refers to any aspect of the supervision in which the supervisor makes decisions or judgments about the practitioner's work in which the practitioner has no say, or of which he or she is unaware. This occurs, for example, when the supervisor reviews the case summaries or tapes of the practitioner's work. Another example is when the supervisor discusses one of the practitioner's cases with another clinician or another supervisor. Although such activity can be beneficial to the practitioner under supervision, in the long run it can also lead the supervisor to unsubstantiated and unjustified evaluations of the practitioner and his or her work. In any judgment or evaluation of a supervisee's practice, the supervisor should ensure that the supervisee has had a fair opportunity to defend the action taken in the case or to document its basis.

A more subtle form of latent supervision occurs when the supervisor holds a particular philosophical or theoretical perspective that the practitioner finds alien. In this situation the supervisor can indirectly and unknowingly foster discussion in a way that will force the practitioner to present cases from the supervisor's preferred orientation. In some instances, simply the choice of cases the supervisor asks the practitioner to present in supervision can shape the nature of the supervision.

In order to promote supervisee creativity, flexibility, and adaptability, supervisors need to monitor their own actions to ensure that practitioners are not being "pushed" or "pulled" into viewing their work in a manner not of their own choosing. Practitioners at times will be aware of such latent supervision without the supervisor's recognizing that this form of suggestion is taking place.

Supervisees who experience discomfort about raising such issues with their supervisors will develop a sense of frustration, and adjust their activity in supervisory sessions by presenting material in a framework that the supervisor finds pleasing. When this occurs, the supervision becomes a game for the practitioner and the focus shifts from genuine learning to a secondary purpose of developing congruence with the supervisor's style. By encouraging open discussion of the supervisor's and the practitioner's respective orientations, and by identifying points at which these orientations converge and diverge, this form of latent supervision can be decreased.

SUPERVISOR RESISTANCE

In my work as a supervisor there is at times a tendency to resist teaching what the young, struggling practitioner needs to know. There is a withholding of knowledge, an unwillingness to share one's style, techniques, and strategies. Other clinical supervisors have shared similar feelings when asked about this phenomenon, but they have not been able to offer much help in identifying the reasons for this vague reluctance in teaching. This withholding occurs more in group than in individual supervision, and is usually experienced just after a supervisory session when I am reflecting on some difficult case or some clinical process with which we were struggling. At these times I realize that I was aware of much information that could have been helpful but that I did not share it. Sometimes this occurs during the supervisory session. Even though I am aware of this pattern, it has happened to me repeatedly and still happens to me. Grotjahn has hinted at this reluctance by saying, "I have had a terrible time revealing group interaction and the private life of the group and its members. It feels like being disloyal to one's own family" (1977:6).

I think at times it occurs because I recognize the complexity of the situation, and the time and energy that would be required to make it understandable and useful to the supervisee would be greater than I am willing to invest. Rather than attempting to explain, understand, or overcome this supervisory weakness, I have devised a way to make up for it. When it occurs, I immediately make detailed notes about the material and bring the information to the supervisees at the beginning of the next session. The first time I have to come back to a particular supervisee with such an admission, I explain what happened and present the new information. Often this has led to supervisees' sharing a parallel process that occurs in their own therapeutic work, and my strategy has served as a model for developing a similar technique to use in their own practices.

GUIDELINES

As a summary set of guidelines for the supervisor to keep in mind in relation to techniques used in supervision, the following elements of good supervision and methods to encourage learning insupervision are provided.

Elements of Good Supervision

1. Supervision should be based on the needs of the practitioner.
2. Supervision should be based on the premise of education for what to do.
3. The supervisor should stand for and manifest commitment to good practice. Practitioners have difficulty committing themselves to something to which the supervisor is not committed.
4. Give answers when the situation demands it.
5. Authority should be de-emphasized rather than explicated.
6. Avoid relying on nonverbal communication. *Spell it out!*
7. Limit teaching through analogies or stories.
8. Use case material as a teaching tool, not as a threat.
9. A key to practitioner unity and understanding is adequate interaction with the supervisor.

Techniques to Encourage Learning in Supervision

1. Allow the practitioner to select material on which to work.
2. Encourage practitioner self-development of learning material.
3. Focus on skills in which the practitioner is strong, and then move to weaknesses.
4. Give recognition to the practitioner for overcoming weaknesses.
5. Remove technical obstacles to practice and supervision.
6. Develop strategies to simplify complex material.
7. Use varied learning techniques.
8. Encourage lively discussion.
9. **Set goals.**
10. Use positive control.
11. Stress the enjoyment of doing treatment.

SUGGESTED READINGS

Jay Haley. *Problem-Solving Therapy: New Strategies for Effective Family Therapy*. New York: Harper Colophon, 1976.
An excellent book on family therapy that is consistent with the technician style of supervision covered in this text. Contains an excellent chapter on "Problems in Training Therapists." Haley discusses "Orientation A" and "Orientation Z," which parallel the conception of style covered in this book.

Gordon M. Hart. *The Process of Clinical Supervision*. Baltimore: University Park Press, 1982.
A good overview of clinical supervision.

Allen K. Hess (ed.). *Psychotherapy Supervision: Theory, Research and Practice*. New York: Wiley, 1980.
A collection of 31 original papers on a broad range of supervision topics. A good reference book for the supervisor.

Alfred Kadushin. *Supervision in Social Work*. New York: Columbia University Press, 1976.
A good overview of basic social work supervision.

Robert Langs. *The Supervisory Experience*. New York: Jason Aronson, 1979.
A broad-ranging discussion of psychoanalytically oriented supervision.

Carlton E. Munson (ed.). *Social Work Supervision: Classic Statements and Critical Issues*. New York: The Free Press, 1979.
A collection of 31 articles that serves as an introduction to the history and current practice of social work supervision.

Roberta G. Sands. *Clinical Social Work Practice in Community Mental Health*. New York: Macmillan, 1991.
Excellent coverage of clinical practice in mental health.

> The difficulty in elaborating this intuitive sense of authority is the idea of strength on which it is based. I have never known a bad or inept musician who managed to preserve his authority over an orchestra for very long.
>
> Richard Sennett
> *Authority*

Chapter 7

The Role of Authority and Structure

This chapter covers the basic concept of authority and how it relates to the supervisory process, as well as its role as an inherent part of organizations. The interactional manifestations of authority are explored along with the ways in which authority orientations vary with respect to different supervision structures. Some guidelines are provided for appropriate use of individual and group supervisory structures.

INTRODUCTION

The quote from Sennett's excellent study of authority epitomizes the essence of what supervisors must keep in mind as they embark on the supervision process: *never attempt to direct the work of others when you are not good at doing that work yourself.* This rule is the basis of this chapter.

Authority has always been troublesome. Perhaps, as has been observed, Don Quixote expressed a universal desire with the words, "I would have nobody to control me, I would be absolute" (Marcus & Marcus, 1972: 234). But at the same time, Don Quixote was depicted as a man who had "lost the Use of his Reason" (Cervantes, 1605; 1950:3). Freud expressed the other side of this desire when he wrote, "The great majority of people have a strong need for authority which they can admire, to which they can submit, and which dominates and sometimes even ill-treats them" (Freud, 1939; 1967:139-140).

Balancing these two opposing desires is a dilemma that is a part of the human condition. Clinicians, in their lives and in their supervision, have not been spared this dilemma. Practitioners and their supervisors overtly and covertly grapple with independence and accountability issues daily in practice and supervision. The personal and professional struggle with authority has been described in the literature by Endress:

> In examining my own professional identity, I found that when I first entered the professional field, in a mental health center, I had no clear-cut guide or idea of what it meant to be or become a professional. I had no professional identity, and what is more, I was not even sure if I had any respect for the so-called professionals. Perhaps the reason for this feeling was that in the past, my early childhood, my marriage, and my battling with the welfare system left me feeling that the professionals or authority figures were always trying to control my life . . . . Because of my past experiences, I chose the profession of social work. As I began my professional career . . . I experienced a feeling of conflict between my personal self and my professional self. Because I had often viewed myself as the underdog in the past, I began to overidentify with clients of similar socioeconomic standing or concerns. In my attempt to help them acquire autonomy, I rebelled against my fellow professionals, seeing them as authoritative parental figures, out to exploit my clients as was done to me throughout my childhood. (1981:306-307)

Endress points out that "exhorting a beginner to model himself after the experts can prove to be more discouraging than motivating" (1981:305). Instead, workers must be helped to discover a style and method of their own. Because the authority issues were handled in a sensitive manner and Endress had an effective role model, she evolved a different perspective:

> I am no longer a scared, rebellious little girl; instead I see myself as being free from poverty and dependency. I see the world around me filled with opportunity. . . . Because I am not out to prove I am the best, I can be more relaxed with my clients, listen to them more effectively, and give of myself in a way that encourages them also to give of themselves. (1981:308)

That a student has to point this out to us is indicative that we have forgotten something over the years. In 1929, the same statement about the idea to "let learn" was apparent:

> Students who are given responsibility as an opportunity for them to learn will themselves provide teachers with plenty of opportunity to teach. We believe it to be true that students learn more from teaching which they have sought because of a consciousness of need than from any offered by a teacher because he knows something which he thinks the students ought to know. (Lee & Kenworthy, 1929:187)

ORGANIZATIONS AND AUTHORITY

The growth of organizations and the formalization of the profession of social work has led to the dilemma of the modern-day practitioner as a creature of organizations. The nature of authority and autonomy have evolved through Durkheim's belief that the division of labor would not destroy the notion that "to be a person is to be an autonomous source of action" (Durkheim, 1933:403) and through Weber's earthy description, as organizations emerged, in which:

> the principles of office hierarchy and of levels of graded authority mean a firmly ordered system of super-and subordination in which there is a supervision of the lower office by the higher ones . . . [but] hierarchical subordination . . . does not mean that the "higher" authority is simply authorized to take over the business of the "lower." (Schuler et al., 1971:348-349)

The vivid description of the "Social Ethic" is William Whyte's way of defining the struggle of the individual for autonomy in organizations. Whyte gives a summary overlay that fits professionals in organizations:

> If individualism involves following one's destiny as one's own con-science directs, it must for most of us be a realized destiny, and a sensible awareness of the rules of the game can be a condition of individualism as well as a constraint upon it. . . . I speak of individ-ualism WITHIN organization life. . . . Every decision he faces on the problem of the individual versus authority is something of a dilemma. . . . We do need to know how to cooperate with The Organization but, more than ever, so do we need to know how to resist it. . . . Organization has been made by man; it can be changed by man. (1956:3-14)

We have come a long way since Don Quixote, and this chapter deals in part with ways of changing the organization with respect to supervision of professional practice so that authority and autonomy become less of a dilemma. Supervisors tend to overlook authority issues until they become seriously problematic, but authority is increasing in organizations rather than decreasing. In addition to all the traditional areas where authority is exercised most often, such as record keeping, statistical reporting, work hours, case load size and type, and case management, there is increasing authority associated with peer review, utilization review, accreditation, and third party payors (Rock, 1990:29). This increased control is occur-ring at a time when the profession is again raising concern about its degree of professionalism because autonomy is limited and shrinking (Veeder, 1990:33). This requires supervisors to be skilled at dealing with authority issues and comfortable with their own degree of authority and autonomy.

AUTHORITY AND SUPERVISION

Supervision is the arena in which a great deal of the knowledge regard-ing the limits of and creative capabilities in practice are worked out. The definitions of professionalism associated with practice come from exter-nals such as status, esoteric training and knowledge, sanction through licensing, remuneration, and professional organizations. Little attention has been focused on the interactions that constitute professional behavior among participants within the professional group. Elements of this aspect of professionalism can be identified and articulated through the exercising of authority in supervision.

Authority issues repeatedly have been overlooked and pushed into the background in the social work literature and in actual practice of supervision for quite some time. In some instances group supervision (Munson, 1976) and the more recent development of peer group supervision (Hamlin & Timberlake, 1982) have been used to sidestep authority issues, but these issues remain and can erupt in these forms of supervision (Hamlin & Timberlake, 1982:87). Supervisors must remember that they have power by virtue of their position; therefore, they do not have to work as hard to establish the supervisory relationship as do supervisees. Some hold that anxiety in the supervisee grows out of the fear of emotional dependence on the supervisor. Supervisee anxiety can just as easily grow out of lack of mechanisms to cope with problems encountered in practice. In general, the use of authority in supervision of clinical social work practice should recognize the role of authority and its limits while placing emphasis on the function of creativity in practice.

Hughes epitomized the issue of authority in supervision when he asked the question: "What orders does one accept from an employer, especially one . . . whose interests may not always be those of the professional and his client?" (1963:658). The problem of control in conjunction with the teaching and evaluation functions in supervision of professional practice leads to a number of important questions. What are the limits of control in teaching and evaluation through supervision? What are the best means of carrying out the teaching and evaluation function in relation to professional autonomous practice? What is it appropriate to teach and evaluate, and how is supervision to be designed to help experienced and inexperienced practitioners differentially? These are some of the questions covered in this chapter.

Social workers have always functioned predominantly within the confines of organizational necessities (Barber, 1963:678-682). Supervision is the arena in which much of the conflict regarding professional autonomy versus organizational authority is confronted. Mandell (1973) has pointed out that this conflict has increased within the profession in conjunction with the "equality revolution" that has taken place at the societal level, and sees only limited opportunities for more autonomous social work practice. Epstein (1973) holds the same view, but argues that limited qualified autonomous practice is possible if authority can be decentralized and teaching de-emphasized in supervision. Levy (1973) has suggested that the question of authority can be partially resolved through application of a code of ethics to supervision. Kadushin (1968) has related authority problems to interactional games played by supervisees to avoid risk and loss of control; Hawthorne (1975) has applied the same framework to supervisors who play games categorized as *power* and *abdication*. Most of these writers describe the process that takes place, but not much progress has been made to reduce authority conflicts substantially, and only limited theoretical and practical models have been developed to resolve the issues. I have developed a dual model of supervision and consultation (Munson, 1979a:336-346) as an attempt to decentralize authority and to maximize professional autonomy in organizational settings to deal with some of these issues.

The question of authority and autonomy in practice through supervision is an issue that is on the minds and in the discussions of most workers who are in active practice. Scott Briar has summarized the issue that faces the social work profession:

> Ninety percent or more of all caseworkers practice in bureaucratic organizations, and the demands of such organizations have a tendency to encroach upon professional autonomy. Every attempt by the agency to routinize some condition or aspect of professional practice amounts to a restriction of professional discretion, and for that reason probably should be resisted, in most instances by practitioners. . . . There are of course, realistic limits to the amount of autonomy and discretion an organization can grant to the practitioner, but no one knows just where that limit is, and we cannot know until we have tried to reach it. (1970:96)

The problem of control in modern professions and organizations leads to a number of questions especially appropriate to social work. Supervision has traditionally been summarized functionally as administration, teaching, and helping (Pettes, 1967:15). If this is the case, what are the limits of control in these functions? What are the best means of carrying out these functions structurally? In some clinical settings there is a growing sense that autonomy is decreasing and much clinical activity is being dictated by third-party payors. Cost, length of treatment, type of treatment, who is qualified to do the diagnosis and treatment, and who is included in the treatment are essentially determined by the payors in many settings. Supervisors must play a difficult role in helping practitioners reconcile these autonomy control issues. They can cause a great deal of confusion and frustration if the practitioner fails to accommodate to the amount of internal and external control of practice that exists in a profession that has been in recent years extolling its autonomy.

INTERACTION AND AUTHORITY

A great deal can be accomplished by applying individual and group supervision differentially according to experience, education, and preference of workers. However, this alone does not seem to be sufficient to bring about optimal congruence between the worker, the supervisor, and the organization. Analysis of the extent and nature of interaction in supervision, regardless of the structure used, is helpful in sorting out authority issues and conflicts. How the supervisor interacts with the supervisees has been demonstrated to be the crucial variable. This has been demonstrated in psychiatric studies of supervision, which are substantially more controlled and empirical than those that have been conducted in social work (see Munson, 1979a:337-338).

The interactional framework can be applied to the structure of supervision in terms of how the supervisor will exercise authority in individual and group supervision. A supervisor can exert a great deal of control in both types of supervision, although it does appear that control is more difficult to exercise in the group situation. Regardless of the model, authority can be dealt with directly by establishing at the outset what the roles of the supervisor and worker will be. Interactional issues that deal directly with authority are: Who sets the agenda? Who establishes the frequency, time, and length of the session? Will emphasis be placed on case discussion, worker growth, or both? Will the supervisor present case material? Who will make which decisions? Who establishes the structure of presentations? Who establishes the content of presentations? These examples can be applied to either individual or group supervision, and have less to do with how the supervisory process is structured in general and more to do with authority and interaction.

Supervisees can use interactional strategies to subvert the authority of the supervisor. This is illustrated by a group supervision situation. A supervisee presented a case in the supervision group of a Mexican-American family, with an acting-out child, who was to come for an initial interview the following week. The supervisee expressed concern because she had never interviewed a Mexican-American family. In setting up the appointment, the father was resistant and noncommittal about coming for the interview. The supervisor and several members of the group offered the practitioner some suggestions for working with Mexican-American families, as well as how to deal with her concerns about the father's resistance.

During the next supervision group session, the supervisor asked the practitioner how the interview with the family turned out. The worker said that it had gone very well, and indicated that one of the members of the supervision group had offered her additional advice after the group session. The worker made it a point to state that the advice she had received from the other worker outside the group was the opposite of the advice she had received in the group. That worker did not offer her comments in the group, but chose to share the information outside the group. The supervisor in this case was good, highly trained, and well-liked by the supervisees. The supervisor felt circumvented in this situation, and the group had some difficulty moving ahead after the worker gave this feedback.

The supervisor chose not to comment on this attempt to subvert the purpose of the supervision group, and did not share her feeling of being undercut and, to some extent, foolish in the eyes of the other supervisees. The supervisor did the best thing by not commenting on this and not making it a direct issue of authority in the supervision. The supervisor moved on to the next case, and was able to recover without much loss of power or respect. However, if this type of worker behavior became a pattern, the supervisor would need to deal with it directly by requesting this individual to share her observations in the group.

It would be best to discuss this privately with the worker and not make it a group issue. The worker might not be consciously aware of the effect her behavior was having on the supervisor and the group. The supervisor can directly ask this particular worker to comment on specific material during group supervision to minimize the possibility of such material being discussed outside the group.

Studies of interactional issues regarding presentation of case material and sharing of clinical material deserve more attention than they have been granted in the past, and can be important to practice outcome. In a study of 89 patients treated by psychiatric residents, Burgoyne and his associates found that there was an inequity in the cases presented in supervision. Those presented differed significantly from others in that the patients were younger, were better educated, had higher incomes, were better liked by the residents, and were given longer-term treatment (1976). Dressler and his associates found that residents showed more warmth toward patients with low suicide risk and limited overall psychopathology, and that they felt anxious about patients with high suicidal risk and significant pathology. The authors used supervision interaction to modify these attitudes, and thus improved the equity of service delivery (1975). These studies involved psychiatric residents. No comparable studies of social work students or practitioners exist, but if such studies did exist, the results most likely would not differ since social workers often work with the same patients and their families. These studies demonstrate the importance that supervision can have for adequate service delivery purely on clinical grounds, and involve interactions that should be shared free of administrative constraints and evaluation.

AUTHORITY AND STRUCTURE

Many of the issues surrounding supervision and development of the profession have focused on the structure of supervision and the use of authority. The arguments regarding structure of supervision have centered on whether group supervision is more effective than individual supervision or mixed models, without much empirical research to support the theoretical arguments. The same pattern has occurred with respect to authority in supervision. With increased emphasis on independent professional practice, there has been debate regarding how much autonomous practice is possible (Epstein, 1973:6). At the same time that the case for control in supervision has been getting more difficult to make (since emphasis on autonomy has increased in education and practice), there has been a trend to license social workers, and the licensing laws mandate varying degrees of active supervision. There is a connection between structure and authority since much of the supervision literature indicates that the structure of supervision has been varied to dilute and redirect authority in supervision. Little progress has been made in resolving these issues, and not much is known about worker attitudes toward authority in and structuring of supervision.

It is difficult to discuss the use of structure and authority in supervision separately, and historically supervision literature has made few if any distinctions between the two concepts. There is a certain degree of authority inherent in the supervisory relationship. Pruger has pointed out that the worker must be attentive to and understand legitimate authority, but that "there still exists significant autonomy for the individual, if he consciously recognizes and uses it" (1973:28). For social workers to grow and at the same time recognize the limits of autonomy, a distinction needs to be made between the structure of supervision and authority. Pruger unites the two concepts by stating that "if . . . autonomy is lost, it must be because it was . . . given up, rather than because it was structurally precluded" (1973:28). The idea that authority and structure in supervision are two different but related concepts is supported by my research, which found that structural models are independent of authority models, that structural arrangements do not produce significantly different outcomes, but that the perceptions of authority models do show major, significant differences (Munson, 1975:131-186).

Although there have been increasing demands for worker autonomy, the research indicates that the struggle for less control has had little impact on the structure of supervision (Mandell, 1973:43). Group supervision has been viewed as an alternative structure to promote autonomy. In spite of the claims for group supervision, there is evidence that group supervision has not been implemented on a broad basis, and where it is used, use of authority is a better predictor of outcome than use of group or individual structures in supervision. Kaslow (1972:117) attributes this to supervisors' lacking the skills or confidence to engage in supervision that requires group methods. If this is the case, the issue becomes one of how competent the supervisor is perceived to be by the worker. The failure to use group methods widely in supervision could be related to the supervisor's fear of loss of control and authority in the group setting. Supervisors can manifest specific behaviors that will promote worker regard for their competence to decrease the resistance to group supervision and increase the degree of autonomy the worker can have through the group approach. This view is consistent with the finding of Cherniss and Egnatios that the ideal supervisor is one who "knows when to ask questions and when to give advice without always doing just one or the other" (1978:222-223).

Widen defined supervision as a creature of agencies rather than as a professional enterprise. It was his view that supervision literature had explored the supervisory process, but little attention had been paid to supervisory structure, which "is particularly sensitive to the life-style of the agency as a social institution," with the result that "each agency that has a formal supervisory structure has a philosophy of supervision" (1962:79-84). Often the problem of autonomy and supervision gets expressed as a conflict between the individual professional worker and the agency. The supervisor, who is usually a member of the same professional group, is put in conflict when expected to mediate this relationship. As long as the issue is viewed as a worker-agency conflict with the supervisor as mediator, little substantial change will occur. Kadushin found that the greatest discrepancy between supervisors and supervisees regarding the role of the supervisor existed around the mediation function. Workers wanted the supervisor to mediate more than the supervisors were willing to (Kadushin, 1974:294). Supervisors' failure to use the mediator model could be the result of a conscious attempt to avoid role conflict and strain since most supervisors in the social work profession know the consequences of such role performance. Nonetheless, at the same time the supervisee is left with the problem of how to confront the organization. Only when the social work profession as a group addresses this issue through its professional organizations will systematic, standardized principles be established to guide agencies in their practices. Organizational issues can be resolved only at the organizational level.

In addressing the issue of supervision at the professional level, the unit of analysis should not necessarily be the structure of supervision itself; it should be the content and means of implementation, regardless of the model used. Autonomy will be achieved best when the worker is free to select the model to be used rather than having one imposed by theoreticians, agencies, and supervisors. Given the diversity in agency resources, agency size, worker education, worker experience, personalities, and worker supervisory preferences, it seems unrealistic to seek one best model of supervision. It is realistic to select a model that is best suited to a given situation. When the supervisor and supervisee are willing to work at it, such a flexible system is attainable.

STYLE AND AUTHORITY

The supervisor needs to strive for a model of exercising authority that will be accepted by supervisees. Supervisee perceptions of how supervisors exercise their authority produces different outcomes for supervisory interaction and satisfaction (Munson, 1975). The styles of authority identified in one study fell into two main types: *sanction* and *natural competence*. The sanction style is the traditional style in which supervisors are perceived as relying on the official sanction and power granted to them by virtue of their hierarchical position in the organization or profession. The competence style was perceived as originating from supervisors' knowledge, skill, and ability as competent practitioners who derived power from their self-confidence. In other words, the sanction style is used by supervisors who view their power as originating externally, and the competence style is used by supervisors who view their power as originating internally from their own performance and skill. Research (Munson, Study B) shows that the sanctioned approach of authority is more often associated with the overall philosopher style of supervision, and the natural approach of authority is more likely to be found in relation to the theoretician and technician style (see Chapter 4). This research suggests that supervisors should strive to achieve a perception of their authority based on competence rather than merely through organizational sanction. Supervisory interaction and supervisory satisfaction are higher in the competence than the sanction model, and the competence model of authority as perceived by workers is the more productive model in all respects.

My research in this area is quite similar to that of a sociological study of supervisory styles of authority in which an association was found between authority styles, verbal aggression toward the supervisor, productivity, and job satisfaction (Day & Hamblin, 1967). If this distinction is valid, agencies, the profession, and supervisors must strive to attain workers' perception of competent supervision to achieve the most effective functioning of the organization and to promote workers' satisfaction. In light of these findings, the most difficult task remains for the profession and agency managers. If the competence model produces the better outcome, we must define what produces workers' perceptions of their supervisors as competent. Worker responses in my research indicate that such perceptions involve personal characteristics that the supervisor most likely brings to the situation; they involve genuine interest and support of what the worker is doing, organizationally manipulable behaviors such as availability and appropriate levels and timing of control, and superior skill and knowledge with respect to the task and position to be supervised. Agencies need to make hard decisions about who becomes and remains a supervisor, and supervisors need to make firm choices about what and when to control and not to control. Authority involves the ability to influence, but the subjective responses of workers indicate that workers should also be able to influence their supervisors. When this is actually taking place, supervisors are viewed as true mediators with respect to authority:

> A greater amount of total control, whereby subordinates can actually influence their supervisors, will heighten, not lower, the organization's performance. However, when subordinates obtain a measure of expertise but are given no control, morale and willingness to contribute to the organization decreases. (Marcus & Marcus, 1972:234)

Workers say that they continue to look for supervisors "who are smarter than we are," and want to feel that "I work for my supervisor, not the agency." At the same time, they contend that supervision is no good if you have to tell a client, "I will have to talk this over with my supervisor and let you know," and they say that good supervision exists "when you know you are supervised, but you are not aware of it every moment."

AGE AND AUTHORITY

Authority can become a problem when there are large differences in the ages of the supervisor and supervisee. Authority problems can emerge when the supervisor is much older or much younger than the supervisee. The problem can originate in the supervisor or the supervisee, but the supervisor has the responsibility to be alert to such issues regardless of the origin. The problem of the older supervisor and younger worker was identified many decades ago by Bertha Reynolds (1942; 1965:193); she assigned responsibility to the supervisor for recognizing and overcoming it.

Less attention has been devoted to the difficulty that arises when the supervisor is much younger than the supervisee. I encountered a 28-year-old MSW who was assigned to supervise a 49-year-old, untrained, but experienced, woman. Although the supervisor was highly competent and had much to offer the supervisee, she felt inadequate to contribute to this older woman's growth and learning. The supervisor became sensitive and immobilized when the supervisee made comments such as, "If I were in charge I would not do it that way." It was suggested that the supervisor handle such a paralyzing comment by asking, "If you were in charge, how would you do it?" This question released the authority blockage in the relationship, providing the supervisee the opportunity to have input into the decision-making process. It also allowed the supervisor to learn that her ideas and the ideas of the supervisee were not as different as she had thought. This approach opened up exploration that led to a more positive relationship. Not all situations can be resolved as easily, but this situation illustrates the major point that such differences must be brought out into the open in order to be resolved.

Paralleling the authority approaches and structures of supervision is the model of intervention that supervisors use. Some supervisors see themselves as antecedent to the practitioner's interventions. Other supervisors view themselves as intervening between the practitioner and the client as the practitioner tries to change. Others see their role as parallel to the ongoing change efforts of the practitioner. Each of these models can be effective if applied in a sensitive and consistent manner. The models are illustrated in Visual 7.1.

AUTONOMY

A significant historical contribution that social work has made is the supervision model. In the early years of social work, the model we picked up on and tried to implement in the schools was a model based on medical

VISUAL 7.1. Models of Supervisory Intervention

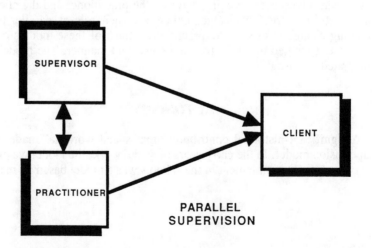

education. We soon deviated from that model, but for a long time had a very strong model with very formal supervision. Initially, social work deviated from the medical model in one significant respect: after people were graduated, we continued the model of supervision in their practice for a year or two, and some people were supervised even longer. There are people in agencies who have been supervised for an hour a week for as long as 15 years. We deviated from the medical model in that we did not recognize people as having the ability to practice autonomously.

In 1956, when NASW was founded, we developed the notion that to become a full-fledged professional one had to function autonomously. We have exploited the term autonomy to promote professionalism. The evolution of autonomous practice has been occurring for over 40 years. Schools and agencies alike have been promoting the idea of autonomy without much regard for its consequences for the practitioner, supervisor, or client. Supervisors and practitioners are confused about the role of supervision in relation to the idea of the fully-trained, autonomous, professional practitioner.

The word autonomy is inappropriately used in relation to the nature of most social work practice settings. There is no such thing as a completely autonomous practitioner. The word autonomy means that one functions without regard for anyone or anything else. Practitioners tend to view the autonomous practitioner as totally out of the control of others. We do not function that way. The majority of social workers are employed in agencies that put severe constraints on their activity. Even private practitioners are required in most states to have their work reviewed by psychiatrists for insurance reimbursement.

We tell our students that upon graduation they will be autonomous practitioners, but indications are that most beginning practitioners do not believe in this autonomous, professional image (Munson, Study A and Study B). The confusion that results from academic portrayal of the autonomous practitioner is illustrated by the reflection of one beginning practitioner several years after graduation:

> What happens is after you have graduated you go to the door of the agency, and you are assigned a supervisor, if you are lucky, and the supervisor will then say, "Well, now you are an autonomous practitioner; you are competent. You've had two years of graduate education, and really, the only thing I'm here to do is to help you if you **have any personal problems**," or "If there is anything I can help you with, just let me know." Nobody is going to admit or own up to the fact that they are not ready to do this all by themselves and that

they need some help. I had a limited number of cases in school; now here I was faced with this. I had five cases my second year of school, and now the supervisor says I'm going to do twelve intakes this week. But I never admitted that I needed help with that. Also, I was led to suspect that I should resent supervision. I should resent that somebody should want to try to tell me how to practice. But they are really not telling us how to practice. What they are supposed to do is help us learn those additional things that we didn't learn in school, but my supervisor didn't say that.

This practitioner's statement illustrates the confusion on the part of the supervisor and the practitioner about the role of supervision and what to expect from it. Most graduates want to develop their skills. They want to test what they have learned theoretically and abstractly. Some have never had a group or family therapy treatment experience.

Autonomy is something we need to be very clear about. The practitioner has to ask: How much autonomy does one really have when functioning in an agency? It is unrealistic to think that you can function autonomously and do only what you want to do. For example, in many public agencies, such as probation, officers are required to have their phone numbers listed in the phone directory. In some agencies there are rules against making home visits, even if the practitioner thinks it is appropriate. So we can quickly dispel the illusion that we have autonomy. We need to recognize the reality that when we work in an agency, we function under the constraints and limits of that agency. Those constraints must be kept in mind when we deal with clients; if we do not, we can get into difficulty. Even in private practice, we really are not autonomous. Insurance companies and other referral services often place constraints on what we do.

Because autonomy has been defined in reaction to authority in the social work profession, authority is often viewed as the opposite of autonomy. This is the most basic issue that faces anyone who enters supervision today—students and practitioners. Supervisors and supervisees can get locked into authority struggles and not see what is happening. Some social workers and agencies do not like authority. It does not go along with our democratic principles. However, our democratic principles have limits in practice, and failing to face up to the reality of their limits in supervision can lead to difficulty, especially in the student-field instructor relationship. Field instructors have authority. They have control over students' destinies to some extent, and this should be recognized by both parties in each relationship. Some supervisors try to avoid authority issues by referring to themselves as consultants. This is not a good practice. There is a difference between a supervisor and a consultant. A consultant gives recommendations or suggestions. When a supervisor makes a suggestion, the worker does not necessarily have the freedom to reject it, for it may be a directive.

In some situations it comes down to the supervisor's having to order the worker to do certain things, saying, "You will do this." From the beginning, supervisors should accept their authority and get on with the job of supervising. The supervisor must not first say, "I'm your consultant, and I'll help you with this, but you are not under any real obligation," and then, when something goes wrong, say, "You have to do this—I'm your supervisor." It is too late to change the rules then. The rules should be set clearly at the outset.

GROUP SUPERVISION

There is not much evidence that the manner in which supervision is structured is changing, but the content is changing. The individual and group models, or a mix of the two models, predominate, while the content of supervision has evolved from a psychological to a sociological orientation in the sense that the emphasis has shifted from supervising the *person* to supervising the *position*.

Most of the material covered in this book can be applied to individual or group supervision, but some factors that are unique in group supervision are covered in this section.

Group supervision can be a valuable and rewarding experience, but a positive outcome is highly dependent upon how it is presented, set up, and carried out. It requires more preparation and organization than is recognized by supervisors. Group supervision often comes about through default, rather than design, in that it is entered into because it seems like the thing to do. Any structuring of supervision should be based on the needs of the practitioners. Group supervision should not be entered into simply to relieve time pressures of the supervisor. When a supervision group is used by the supervisor to learn to do this form of supervision, the supervisor needs to be supervised or provided with consultation.

Supervisors need to be aware that many practitioners undergoing group supervision for the first time have never been in a group, even though they may have read about it. Some have experienced group therapy as clients or practitioners, and may respond to group supervision in the same manner as group therapy. Others will treat group supervision as a class where they are to be lectured or taught didactically. In other words, most practitioners do not know what to expect from group supervision, and the supervisor must make the expectations clear. Many practitioners and supervisors who have not experienced it view group supervision as a sound idea theoretically, but question its utility from a practical standpoint. Once they have experienced good group supervision, this resistance dissipates. When one moves from individual to group supervision, something is gained and something is lost. In group supervision, there is less time for each practitioner's individual cases, but more information is generated for discussion. The supervisor must evaluate which approach is best suited to the practitioner's needs.

It is easier for the individual practitioner to escape evaluation in group supervision. Some practitioners may resist group supervision initially, but later may use the group setting to avoid exposure. The supervisor will need to work with such practitioners to aid them in appropriately using group supervision.

Basic Questions

The supervisor contemplating group supervision needs to think through some basic questions before embarking on such an effort:

1. Will it be defined as supervision or peer consultation?
2. What methods will be used to get practitioners to risk exposure in group supervision, and how will anxiety about such risk be dealt with?
3. How will competitiveness be dealt with?
4. How will overly verbal and reticent members be dealt with?
5. How do you deal with the different backgrounds and skill levels of practitioners in the group?
6. How will case monitoring be handled?
7. What are the assets of group supervision in comparison to individual supervision?
8. How will transference and countertransference material be dealt with?
9. What techniques will be used to initiate the supervision successfully?
10. Who will be supervised in groups?
11. How large will the group be?
12. What day and time will the group meet?
13. What limits will be set on the group, and how will they be presented?
14. How will resisters be handled?

15. What impact will the group have on other elements of the agency or organization?
16. Who will be responsible for setting the agenda?
17. How many supervisors will be in the group?
18. How many groups will be used?
19. What are the main purposes for establishing a group?
20. How will the goals of group supervision differ from the goals of individual supervision?
21. In what different ways will the supervisor interact in group supervision and in individual supervision?
22. How will the supervisor structure the group?
23. How will feedback be channeled?
24. How will group commitment and identity be fostered?
25. What kind and amount of record keeping will be done?
26. How will therapy be avoided, if it is to be avoided?
27. How will the group be used to improve working relationships?
28. Should the supervisor present cases?
29. How will poor presentations be handled?
30. Will the group be time limited or open ended?

Practitioner Experience Level

Even the most skilled practitioners need advice and support at times. Generally, inexperienced practitioners need and prefer individual supervision more than experienced practitioners. This varies with years and types of experience, but often the needs of both groups are not adequately addressed in supervision. The less experienced practitioner usually needs help with the specifics of practice and aid in developing a repertory of techniques; this is often better suited to individual supervision. The more experienced practitioner desires more general evaluation of practice and opportunities to apply different or more complex treatment modalities, which is more appropriate to group supervision. When supervisors focus on the problems of the young, inexperienced, and inept practitioner at the expense of the experienced practitioner in a mixed supervisory group, the potential for innovation in supervision and treatment is decreased.

Experienced and prestigious practitioners should not be denied supervision. If experienced practitioners are to be genuinely autonomous, they do not have to be anonymous and left with no way to make a contribution to the learning of their colleagues and their profession. This should be kept in mind when planning group supervision, especially when the supervisor is responsible for experienced and inexperienced practitioners. Including both types of practitioners in a supervisory group can be beneficial if the supervisor is sensitive to their needs and provides a healthy balance in the content of the group.

Supervisor's Role

The supervisor's chief responsibility in group supervision is to keep the group on task. The aim of group supervision is to present clinical material in an organized fashion so that new and alternative practice strategies can be developed. The whole process assumes that problematic and difficult material will always be before the group. Practitioners resist dealing with difficult material. After the basics of a difficult case are presented, the group will often attempt to gather more information from the presenter or begin telling the presenter what to do. Without assistance from the supervisor, the group will frequently grope for a diagnosis to no avail. The leader must intervene and push the group beyond this point, asking members to relate the case to their own practices. This is why the supervisor has to be more skilled than the group members. In this situation, the supervisor does not give answers, but simply reminds the group of its task, and asks questions that move the group beyond information gathering.

Once the group experiences the freedom to struggle at being clinically competent, a sense of trust will develop. A good indicator of this is the feeling of freedom to externalize concerns about case material. Members will begin to express fears and problems they would not share before. For some, this is the first time in their professional training and career that they will have shared real questions about their practice.

The leader must be careful of what he or she says and how it is stated. Even skilled workers, when discussing difficult clinical material, will take clues from the supervisor. One simple statement by the supervisor, which is designed only to elicit further information about the case, can result in the group's moving in a very specific direction that becomes the major focus for the intervention. Such statements as, "Do you think they have a symbiotic relationship?" or "Has the marriage always been this combative?" can influence the focus of the group so that broader aspects of a case are missed. The supervisor has a responsibility not only to comment on specific material, but also to organize and guide the discussion.

Once trust is established, the supervisor usually has a new problem. Group members tend to become quasi-supervisors. The supervisor must guard against this. The emphasis should be oncontinued sharing, with the presenter articulating the significant material that is applicable to his or her own case. What is being sought is a judgment-free learning environment. The group members must be made aware that they are not at risk with the supervisor or other group members, but are at risk only with themselves and their clients. The client is at risk secondarily in group supervision, but the outcome can benefit both the client and the practitioner. To achieve beneficial learning, the group must go beyond what the case presenter *should do* to what each group member can gain from the discussion and apply in practice. This self-directed, self-selected learning results in independent clinical competence.

When one supervisor works with several practitioners separately in individual sessions, a certain amount of practitioner competitiveness and curiosity frequently develops. This is healthy as long as it does not develop into intense rivalry or game playing. When supervision is done exclusively in a group setting, competition within the group also develops, and the supervisor has a responsibility to prevent this from becoming a negative experience for one or more members of the group. When two supervisory groups exist simultaneously in the same setting with one supervisor, intergroup competition and curiosity can develop, and the supervisor must be alert to this.

CONCLUSION

The supervisor must give some thought to the role of authority in supervision, how that authority will be used, and how it will be perceived by the supervisee. Authority is inherent in the supervisory relationship and must be recognized as such. It should be discussed openly when supervision is initiated and at relevant points in the supervisory process, especially when it threatens the learning component of supervision. Supervisors should not be reluctant to use their authority, but should apply it with caution and sensitivity in the context of the needs of the supervisee. Supervisees welcome constructive use of authority and accept direction from the supervisor when it originates from the supervisor's skill, knowledge, and confidence. The practitioner in fact is under ethical mandate to seek supervisory assistance. Section II-F-3 of the NASW Code of Ethics states, "The social worker should seek advice and counsel of colleagues and supervisors whenever such consultation is in the best interest of clients."

SUGGESTED READINGS

Barry Rock. "Social Worker Autonomy in An Age of Accountability." *The Clinical Supervisor* 8 (Summer 1990), pp. 19-31.
    Discussion of the tension regarding professional autonomy and organizational accountability.

Richard Sennett. *Authority*. New York: Knopf, 1980.

An excellent general study of authority and its origins. The historical analysis of authority can be related to the authority issues that face the social work profession.

Nancy Veeder. "Autonomy, Accountability, and Professionalism: The Case Against Close Supervision in Social Work." *The Clinical Supervisor* 8 (Summer 1990), pp. 33-65.

Summary of the authority and autonomy issues facing the social work profession.

Theory cannot, in reality, create
the world: it can only help in
explaining what we have chosen to be
interested in.

Joe Bailey
Ideas and Intervention

Chapter 8

Use of Theory

The use of theory in practice has long been advocated in the social work profession. This chapter deals with how to use theory in supervision to enhance practice activity. There has been confusion about theory and the terms that are associated with it. To clarify some of these issues, this chapter begins with explanations of the terms technique, methods, modalities, philosophy of practice, theory, ideology, practice theory, and theory of practice. The elements of theory are explained and include a discussion of facts, concepts, and hypotheses. The functions of theory are covered through explanations of the functions of organizing, explaining, and prediction. The components of theory are explained as utility, verification, comprehensiveness, and simplicity. The use of theoretical speculation in supervision is discussed, as is the occasional abandonment of theory to aid learning. Theory application and supervisory interaction are explored along with a list of guidelines for using theory in relation to clinical material in supervision.

INTRODUCTION

In clinical practice there has always been a polarity between the philosophical and the scientific, which in one form or another can be traced to the earliest philosophers and theoreticians. Chessick (1977:81) has described this polarity as the "empirical materialist visible world versus the invisible spiritual world of being," and reminds us of Spengler's thesis that the pendulum swings back and forth between these orientations.

This historical polarity is recreated in supervision, and rather than occurring over decades or centuries, it can take place in a matter of minutes. This is to be expected during an endeavor that grapples constantly with ways of resolving problems in human functioning, while drawing on numerous theories and strategies. In order to avoid confusion and frustration, supervisors must control such rapid swinging of the pendulum in a smooth, orderly fashion that promotes understanding and learning.

This chapter addresses how to bridge the philosophic-scientific polarity in supervision through the use of theory.

THEORY IN SUPERVISION

Theory in supervision is a tool used in making knowledge apparent and understandable. In a sense, we need literally to shake the concepts and examples out of the theoretical rug. We frequently commit the classic mistake of confusing terms by inadvertently referring to a theory as treatment modality.

In practice the practitioner is faced with more data than can be dealt with effectively or efficiently. Consciously and unconsciously, we are selective about the data upon which we choose to act. The data we choose is related to the theory in which we have been trained or to which we subscribe. Thus, to a certain extent, theory has a major impact on the diagnostic phase, and in turn, the diagnosis frequently determines much of the direction taken in the treatment phase.

Practitioners who have been exposed to and know a smattering of theory develop a practice orientation that takes the form of a mixed application of a variety of concepts that can result in therapeutic confusion for the supervisor, the practitioner, and the client. When there is an inadequacy of theory in use in a given practice area, obscure and gimmicky techniques get expanded and elevated to the level of quasi theory. This results in a narrow and limited approach to practice. The elevation of paradoxing techniques in family therapy to the level of quasi theory is an example of this phenomenon.

In supervision we often use theoretical constructs rather than empirical concepts. This is accepted practice in science when we know that something exists but that we cannot explain it completely. If astronomers and physicists can do this in the name of science, so can we. We should use science to free us to learn more, not to lock us into a system that frequently leaves us feeling unable to find solutions.

CONFUSION ABOUT THEORY

It is common for some supervisors to confuse theory with practice methods, modalities, philosophies, and techniques. So that there will be no confusion here, these various concepts are clarified below, as are the definitions of theory used in this chapter.

Techniques

A *technique* is the most basic tool of practice. It is a specific action taken by the practitioner to promote change, give insight, or gather information in treatment. A technique is a highly specific, singular action. It is meaningless to ask a supervisee, "What is your technique?" Practitioners don't use one technique all the time, and if they did, they would be ineffective. A better question would be, "What are several techniques that could be used in this situation?" or, if the supervisor is more interested in the practitioner's general pattern of relating, "What is your style?" Questioning, interpretation, comment, and paradoxing are all techniques. A simple way to separate theory from technique for exploration in supervision is that *what* is said during treatment relates to theory, and *how* it is said is related to technique. This is not a hard-and-fast rule but a quick way to sort out issues in the midst of supervisory discussion.

Techniques can be analyzed on the basis of those that deal with the *structure* of the treatment, those that deal with *content* of the treatment, and those that deal with the process of intervention. Some general categories of techniques related to structure are:

1. composition of therapy (pertaining to clients and practitioners)
2. length and number of sessions
3. **setting in which the** therapy occurs
4. rules related to degree and level of interaction
5. type of therapy itself (i.e., individual, group, or family).

Techniques related to content can generally be categorized as:

1. support
2. confrontation
3. encounter
4. interpretation
5. comment
6. questioning
7. focus
8. reflection
9. recapitulation
10. restructuring
11. sculpting or choreography
12. conflict
13. paradoxing.

Techniques related to process can generally be categorized as:

1. projecting outcomes
2. predicting the future
3. expressions of trust.

Methods

Methods deal with the broad structure of practice and describe practice orientations. Casework and group work are methods. When a person says, "I am a caseworker at the mental health clinic," he or she is describing an overview of the role and the structure of the work.

Modalities

Modalities are more limited forms of practice. Family therapy and group therapy are modalities. Caseworkers and group workers might engage in family therapy or group therapy from time to time, or they may even specialize in these modalities.

Techniques are used in all of these forms of practice. Some techniques are common to all, and some are unique to one form.

Philosophy of Practice

A *philosophy of practice* is a belief system that guides a person's activity. It is a generalization that determines why a person performs in a given way in the practice situation. A family practitioner might say, "It is my

philosophy that people can be treated only in the context of the family."
Their philosophy determines the modality to which they limit their practice. A philosophy is usually connected to both a personal and a professional belief system.

Most practitioners believe it is important to have some philosophy of
life that is applicable to their practice in some general way. Supervisors
need to be aware of these beliefs; in order to be helpful to supervisees,
they must ask them to articulate their philosophy. In asking practitioners
to state their philosophy, supervisors can get access to a great deal of
information that can be helpful in gaining insight about workers and their
level of practice functioning. When practitioners state their philosophy, it
usually contains some variation on a cluster of five elements:

1. Workers have a *motivation* to make a contribution in some way to
   the welfare of humankind.
2. Workers have a degree of *idealism* about people and the belief that
   clients have a desire to do good in life and to grow and change. As
   one supervisor stated, "The practitioner must accept that the clients
   we see lead the best lives that they can."
3. It is important to have a desire to *help* others and to recognize there
   are many ways of helping different clients.
4. Workers have a sense of *caring* about others and genuine concern
   for them and their problems.
5. There must be an element of *suspense* in our practice to keep it lively
   and focused. In this context, suspense is a belief that in the practice
   situation we are always striving to make the unknown known, and
   that this process of discovery will make the treatment effective and
   successful.

These five values, which are the elements of a philosophy of practice, can
be used to promote learning and growth on the part of the supervisor and
supervisee in the process of supervision. These elements can be applied to
the supervision process as well as to the treatment process.

Discussion of philosophy can be brought down to specific issues in
supervision and may be helpful to the supervisor in addressing a particular
problem the worker is experiencing. This is illustrated by a child welfare
supervisor who strongly disagreed with a young, inexperienced worker
about removing a child from the home. The supervisor felt that the child
was in danger if allowed to remain in the situation. The supervisor realized that all the specific points about the situation had been resisted or
rebutted by the worker. The supervisor then asked the worker: "What is
your philosophy about removing children?" The worker gave a lengthy,

but articulate, explanation revealing that she did not believe in removing children under any circumstances. This had not occurred to the supervisor or the worker before, and further discussion revealed that this was due in part to her lack of confidence as a worker. It also helped to explain problems she was having in other cases, and led to insights about negative attitudes the worker had toward the agency, her clients, and her job. The supervisor was then able to focus with the worker on the details of handling a removal and placement, and how to handle feelings about such a drastic step. The worker was then able to accomplish the removal and change many of her attitudes that had emerged about herself and her job. If this philosophical discussion had not taken place, the worker might have left the agency eventually, or even worse, would have gone on for years as a disgruntled practitioner who put many children at risk.

Social workers in supervision operate out of a philosophical stance rather than a theoretical stance. We made this transformation when we applied Freudian theory as a philosophy to the worker as well as to the client, rather than empirically matching it with the client problems that confronted us.

Ideology and Theory

Stevenson makes a fine distinction between theory and ideology, stating that "a system of belief about the nature of man which is thus held by some group of people as giving rise to their way of life is standardly called an 'ideology'" (Stevenson, L., 1974:7). Since Gestalt therapy has been called a form of treatment as well as a way of life by many of its proponents, it could be argued that it is an *ideology* rather than a theory of treatment. There are many implications for this holistic or unified approach of Gestalt therapy that remain unaddressed by many of its advocates. When a theory becomes an ideology and gives rise to a way of life for a particular social group, it is difficult for the members of the group to consider it objectively (Stevenson, L., 1974:12). This lack of objectivity can become problematic in applying theory in supervision. Learning through theory is most effective when the supervisor and supervisee embrace a theory objectively rather than as an ideology.

A *theory* is a set of propositions that are designed to describe, explain, and predict. There are various forms of theory: theories of personality and theories of human behavior. Many of these theories grew out of theorists' experiences working with individuals in therapeutic relationships, and some examples are the theories of Freud, Jung, Adler, Sullivan, Horney, and Rogers (Hall & Lindzey, 1970:526). All of these theories are well codified in extensive literature. In the discussion of using theory in supervision in this chapter, this form of theory is used as well as the unsystematized form of theory referred to as practice theory.

Practice Theory

Practice theory, also referred to as theory of practice, is a highly generalized term used in connection with the individual theory utilized by various practitioners. "A *practice* is a sequence of actions undertaken by a person to serve others, who are considered clients" (Argyris & Schon, 1980:6). Horney observed, "A saleswoman will heed other qualities in a customer than a social worker will in a client applying for help" (1942:115). A theory of practice is a highly individualized set of propositions aimed at communicating how change is produced.

There is a distinction between formal theory and practice theory. Formal theory is the highly organized conceptions that constitute textbook explanations and that practitioners can describe. Practitioners can give articulate accounts of Freudian, Gestalt, existential, and other theories. Unfortunately, or perhaps fortunately, these descriptions bear little resemblance to what these practitioners do in their practice. Although formal theory leads off most clinical discussions, practitioners quickly launch into what they do and how the client acts in treatment. Supervisors must listen closely to these descriptions because supervisees' practice theories emerge from them.

Practitioners have an "espoused theory" that they use when asked how they would behave in a given practice situation and a "theory in use" (Argyris & Schon, 1980) that actually governs their behavior. This distinction is very important for a discussion of supervision and how to manage theory exploration in supervisory sessions. For example, a clinician's espoused theory might be made up totally or in part of descriptions of the various theories of personality and human behavior that exist in the literature, but his or her theory in use, which is made known to the supervisor through direct observation of practice behavior, might be quite different. For the theory in practice to be effective, there must be congruence with the espoused theory. Promoting this congruence is the main task of the supervisor in the theory-exploration component of supervision.

TEACHING THEORY

In teaching theory supervisors tend to use conceptual perspectives at the same time as supervisees are attempting to apply experiential material. There is a natural incongruence built into this situation. The supervisor must find a way to promote congruence. This gap can be lessened, but rarely eliminated, by:

1. *connecting* the conceptual material with experiential material,
2. *translating* the conceptual material into experiential material before presenting it and while presenting it to the supervisee, or
3. *abandoning* the conceptual material, presenting exclusively experiential material, and checking that the supervisee has made the association.

Completely eliminating the gap between the two areas means telling the supervisee what to do and why to do it. This is ineffective because it fosters dependence, and should be differentiated from the third procedure of abandoning.

Learning a theory and learning to apply a theory are two different matters. These two forms of theory learning involve different skills, and it is primarily the application form with which the supervisor will need to deal. In this process there are three salient factors the supervisor must constantly keep in mind in relation to the supervisee:

1. We know only what we can state.
2. We know only what is manifested by behavior.
3. We know more than we can tell and more than our behavior consistently shows. (Argyris & Schon, 1980:10)

Initially there seems to be a contradiction in these factors, but they could be adopted as a functional creed for the supervisor. The supervisor must focus on having supervisees state what they know as well as stating something so that they can know it; exploring supervisees' knowledge about their behavior as well as discussing their behavior will improve their knowledge of it.This is the essence of the supervisory process, and repeated circular discussion of factors one and two leads to that unknowable component of practice contained in factor three.

In discussing practice skill, most practitioners and supervisors give descriptions of process rather than talking about skills developed and used around behavior that occurred. This is what Haley is referring to when he states, "the therapeutic process is such that one cannot go directly from the problem at the beginning to the cure at the end" (Haley, 1976:121). Skill is more than description of practice, it is more than saying that the client did better as the result of the techniques used or the skills applied. Supervisors can be the instruments through which practitioners develop awareness of the skills they possess.

THEORY AND PRACTICE CONNECTION

The connection between theory and practice has worried social work educators and supervisors since the beginning of education for practice. This concern grows out of our desire to have students and practitioners proficient in theory as well as practice. In our efforts to achieve this, we have too often failed to see that attempts to mix theory and practice randomly are more likely to result in confusion than in solutions. Research has demonstrated that educational techniques for the integration of theory and practice are very different. To achieve this integration, which has been called "dynamic intellectualism," requires use of educational models that promote systematic comprehension of both theory and practice (Williams, 1982:168-169).

In part the confusion of the past has been fostered by our direct and indirect use of the term and process of "eclecticism." It is common to hear students and practitioners say, "I don't use any one theoretical orientation; I am eclectic." The word eclectic is a term we have loosely borrowed from the arts. It means "selecting what appears to be best in various doctrines, methods, or styles"; eclecticism is "the theory or practice of an eclectic method" (*Webster's New Collegiate Dictionary*, 1979:356). Eclecticism relates more to techniques or components that go to making up a theory rather than being a theory itself. Once the best components have been organized into a new constellation, they constitute a theory of eclecticism that can be explained and described. This new description is the espoused theory, and the eclectic components are the theory in use described earlier. In supervision it is insufficient for supervisees to say, "I am eclectic." Supervisors must require supervisees to state the set of propositions that make up their espoused theory of eclecticism.

In the past we have made the conceptual mistake of thinking that it is the theory itself that is important in supervision and practice. The real task is the way we use the theory, how we understand and apply it, being able to observe when theory is relevant, and recognizing its limits.

Theory taken alone without connection to behavior or, in our case, without connection to case examples is of little value. The failure to make this connection has been chiefly responsible for our repeated shortcomings in applying theory to practice.

In most social work education programs much time is devoted to talking about theory. Some discussions present theories accurately, but at times there is confusion because what is presented as theory fails to genuinely meet the criteria of theory. Thus, in many instances there is a tendency to confuse students about theory and its relevance to practice. This confusion carries over when graduates begin practicing. Many practitioners say that they use theory, but if you observe their work, there is no connection between the theory that they say they use and what they actually do.

This chapter is an orientation to theory utilization that can be helpful in the supervisory process. In this approach theory is not just an abstraction, not just a set of concepts that somehow get presented in supervision and never get used in the agency or with cases. Unfortunately, there are very few theories that supervisors actually connect with the behavior we see in clients and practitioners. When we manage to accomplish such a connection — when a concept from a theory is used to understand or explain actual dynamics in a case — it is one of the most exciting and fascinating events a supervisor and supervisee can share because it is one of those rare instances in which the abstract world comes together with the real world. This is the essence of learning through supervision.

For theory to be helpful, it must be useful. Practice theory must be at the level of relating everything that is in the theory to what goes on in practice. In order for the theory to be helpful the concepts must be constantly related to behavior. If abstract theory is all the supervisor has to offer, it would be better just to teach people techniques. As supervisors begin to use theory as a learning tool in supervision, they need to know some of the basic, traditional approaches to theory. In other words, we must learn about theory before learning a theory; we must teach about theory before teaching a theory.

ELEMENTS OF THEORY

What is a theory? Theory is the explanation of the interrelatedness of concepts. Some people will define theory in various other ways, but essentially this is what it comes down to for the practicing supervisor. Usually a theory is made up of a set of conventions, and in almost all theories — or, at least, in the theories that we use in the behavioral sciences — there are at least three elements: facts, concepts, and hypotheses.

Facts

Every theory has facts. There are various levels and types of facts. The only level of fact with which we are concerned in terms of practice theories is that they are observations that can be verified. Even very general facts can exist on several levels in clinical practice. You could say that the person you are working with is a 28-year-old white man. That is a set of three facts — 28 years old, white, male — and we could very easily verify that. Another level of fact that we can go to is that this man is having difficulty in his social relationships, especially with his wife and his employer. Most of the time we would accept this as a fact, and it is a form of fact, but it cannot be verified in the same way as that he is 28 years old, that he is white, and that he is male.

At another level one could say that this man seems to have suicidal tendencies. Some would declare this statement as a fact, but facts can get fuzzy in supervision. Does this mean that the person has to commit suicide before we can verify his tendencies as a fact? No, that would be absurd. There is a certain general level of fact that we accept in practice as we go about using theory in supervision. The critical point is that any "statement of fact" accepted in supervision should be able to be verified from the practice activity. To accept suicidal tendency as a fact in supervision and theory, there must be observations and statements from the treatment session that verify such tendencies.

If something cannot be verified, it is an assumption. If a supervisor and supervisee do not agree on the verification the supervisee offers regarding a case dynamic, it remains an assumption until they can agree on an alternate verification. This is an important basic process that the supervisor and supervisee engage in as they go about amassing factual information that becomes the foundation for theory application.

Concepts

The next level moves from the realm of fact into that of concepts. Concepts are symbols used to describe things. The symbol is expressed as the equivalent of the thing it represents (Lastrucci, 1967:77). For example, when we talk about concepts such as anxiety, we really cannot see anxiety. We cannot verify anxiety. But we can verify that clients sway back and forth in their chairs constantly, or that they keep tapping their feet on the floor, or that they sit on the edge of their chairs and rock. This constitutes a concept. You have stated the concept that a person suffers from a great deal of anxiety and have taken that symbolic meaning and connected it with a fact, or a series of facts, that are then used to describe that concept.

Hypotheses

The third important element of a theory is a hypothesis or hypotheses. A hypothesis is the statement of relationship between concepts. One can now see how facts, concepts, and hypotheses are interrelated. We can say that a man's mother died when he was three years of age, that he was shifted from foster home to foster home, that this has left him with a great deal of instability and insecurity, and that this seems to be generating a great deal of his current anxiety about raising his own children. In this hypothesis we have attempted to connect the idea of anxiety and early childhood experiences. We have formulated a hypothesis that these two things in fact are related. We are still left with the possibility that they may not be related. In the practice situation we need to test this hypothesis by helping the man to see this connection and to overcome it. His anxiety should decrease if the hypothesis is valid.

The concepts themselves do not become facts. They are still concepts. Concepts and facts taken alone are generally of little value. It is only when you make the connection between Concept A and Concept B that they have any use. This is the practical explanation of theory in supervisory practice.

Unfortunately, most of the time supervisors will teach theory by saying, for example, "This is psychoanalysis, which was founded by Sigmund Freud. He came up with concepts such as the unconscious, the preconscious, the conscious, the ego, the id, the superego, transference, countertransference, and insight. If people gain insight, they get better." Rarely do we ever connect those concepts with what goes on with clients. For example, when we apply those concepts in the case of the man mentioned above, we have half of the equation: we have anxiety. The supervisor will say that what we need to do is give this man insight, and that might be. But many times one of the problems with teaching from a purely theoretical approach is that we lack knowledge of how to give rise to insight. How *do* you do it? How can one relate what is going on unconsciously with this person to his anxiety? In terms of how we teach theory and its utilization for practice, we often fail to connect the concepts with the behavior, or even make the distinction between what are the facts in the case, what are the concepts, and what are the hypotheses.

The problem is that many times when we have a hypothesis, we do something, find there is no support for the hypothesis, and yet we keep on doing it anyway. We will keep testing the same hypothesis over, maybe getting a little different result, but nothing that ever confirms the hypothesis. This is the point at which we stray from the theory we use in practice; we fail to adhere to the idea of what the facts, concepts, and hypotheses are and how they work in relation to theory. If we did, our practices would be a lot better than they really are. All hypotheses are predictions, and the outcomes of the hypotheses should be held up to the theory in the supervision to keep the practice focused.

Another way to think of a hypothesis, rather than as the interrelationship between concepts, is that a hypothesis is always: if A, then B. The connection could be causation or association. Clearly, most of the time in the behavioral sciences we do not operate on the basis of causation. We have limited knowledge of what causes most of the behavior that we work with—although it is interesting that we do know quite a bit about what causes things to go away, that given certain conditions, B will cease. For example, if the client is psychotic, and if we give this person human contact and concern and care, he or she may get back in touch with reality. In many instances, if you take psychotic persons who are severely withdrawn and just flood them with contact—touching, holding—within two or three days they will come out of it. They will come back into reality. We do not know what caused the psychosis to subside, and we do not know that they will never go back into psychosis again, but this hypothesis has been tested time after time, and it works. We cannot go to the other side and say that if concern and touching and human contact cause psychosis to go away, lack of human care, concern, and touching must cause psychosis. We cannot make that kind of connection. We do not have enough information to make the causative statement, but based on the testing of the connection between A and B, we can act on the association between the two concepts.

Another way of approaching hypothesis testing in practice and supervision is for the supervisor to use the idea of *paired concepts* or *dual concepts*. What I mean by this is that the supervisor should prevent the supervisee from discussing one concept singly. For example, the supervisee who spends much time discussing the symptoms and behaviors that describe a male client's depression is dealing with a single concept. (This occurs frequently in the supervisee reaction of persistent diagnosis described in Chapter 5.) Two concepts should normally be the basis of discussion, so that when a man's depression is under exploration, so should be at least one other concept. The second concept could be self-esteem at a given time in relation to his children, to his wife, to his employer, to his parents. Depression might occur in cycles and be associated with any of the factors mentioned above. Depression might be associated with the loss of a significant relationship. It could be due to life-stage changes and a loss of meaning and goals. The point is that in the diagnostic phase or the treatment phase discussion of a single concept is of limited value; it is only when one concept is explored in relation to another that supervision can give meaning, direction, and focus to the supervisee's treatment effort. Several decades ago Karen Horney commented on this process in treatment: "The chain of associations that reveals a connection need not be a long one. Sometimes a sequence of only two remarks opens up a path for understanding . . ." (1942:121). This is a very simple way to approach concepts, but it is a down-to-earth description of hypothesis testing. Also, observation and content analysis of supervisory sessions reveal that much time is wasted engaging in single-concept approaches rather than dual-concept approaches. Dual-concept case exploration produces more positive supervisory interaction and higher levels of accomplishment and satisfaction than single-concept discussion.

FUNCTIONS OF THEORY

What can we use theory for in supervisory practice? There are primarily three ways we can use it: to organize, to explain, and to predict.

Organization Function

First, theory can be used to organize what we do. If we think about this in terms of the theories we use, the daily practice activity that we go through, this occurs initially in the area of gathering the social history. When the practitioner gathers social history information, unless there is some way to organize it, some theoretical basis for deriving it, it can be very confusing. Theory helps to decrease the confusion and will determine the approach to that particular case. The practitioner's orientation will affect the kind of information he or she gets from the client, and the theory used in part determines how the information is presented to the practitioner.

For instance, in many psychoanalytic agencies emphasis is placed on finding out the relationship that clients had or have with their father or mother, and what relationship their father and mother had with *their* father and mother, as this is considered to be important to the person's current difficulty. If the practitioner uses Gestalt theory, more emphasis is placed on what is going on in the client's present environment.

Even when clients make a simple statement about not getting along well with their mother, the theory will determine, in many instances, how you respond. According to some theories you would say, "And how does that make you feel?" According to others you would say, "Is there anybody else in your environment who reminds you of your mother?" Therefore, the theories do determine where you focus the interaction. There is nothing wrong with that. That is the major function of theory, and it helps us organize and gives us a perspective so that we know where we are going.

If we say we use a theory, we should then ask the questions that take us in the direction of testing the hypotheses and formulating the concepts and gathering the facts that fit the theory. If not, there is no reason for using the theory.

Situational theoretical orientations in supervision promote more analysis of the interactional process in treatment. The use of intrapsychic theory leads more to discussion of affect in the treatment. The same is true of systems-oriented supervision, which promotes focus on interaction and psychodynamic orientations that encourage expression of affect. The supervisor must recognize this difference and use different theoretical orientations depending on the practice needs of the supervisee.

In the diagnostic phase, we tend to assume that problems are manifested as feelings and that feelings and problems are the same things. For example, a practitioner begins an initial interview by stating to the client, "What feelings brought you here in relation to your marriage?" The assumption the practitioner has made, and the perception the client might well develop, is that the feelings about the marriage problems are more significant than the marital events that are conflictual and give rise to certain feelings. Separating problems from feelings about problems helps to sort out the complexity of the diagnostic phase. Later, the practitioner can relate the two areas.

Explanation Function

The second function of theory is that it explains behavior. This is a very simple, but valuable, point. The more behavior the theory explains, the better it is. Some theories do this better than others.

Theory is something that has always been used by interventionist professions to organize explanations of how they intervene. In many respects, theory has been independent of practice. For sociologists a much different framework exists in that practice for them is dependent upon the theory because theory has been so basic to the discipline. Sociological knowledge has always been organized around theories and their subsequent concepts, whereas social work knowledge has been, and continues to be, organized around behavior and action (Gordon, 1981; Reid, 1981). The unit of analysis has presented problems for both professions. The failure of both groups to recognize the origins of their orientations and the impact of orientations on outcomes has prevented creative problem-solving efforts from emerging. In social work, the mixing of theoretical orientations with action orientations has resulted, at best, in confusion. The intermingling of psychological and sociological theories and action (character structure, role, and social structure) has been unwittingly described by Chescheir. She concludes:

> As social workers, we need a number of different theories of personality and social systems to understand all the different events, behaviors, and conditions that we encounter in practice. Sorting through this wealth of theories, methods, and techniques can be a confusing process for the practitioner and this difficulty remains a principal concern of the profession. (1979:94)

Prediction Function

The third function of theory is that it must predict what the outcome will be. As was pointed out earlier, we cannot be very clear about the level of predictability, but the theory itself should predict some outcome. For example, systems theory predicts that if you change one part of the system, all the other parts will also be affected and will change. That is one level of prediction, and probably it is true. What happens so many times is that we say that this is going to have an effect on the system without explaining what the effects will be. Prediction at this level of abstraction is of limited value. It must be reduced to the level of specific behavior to be of any value in supervising practice. For instance, in a case where a practitioner is working with the family of a retarded child and they are trying to decide if they should institutionalize the child, the supervisee will mention the impacts on the family. What impacts? There could be negative impacts; there could be positive impacts. Do the positive impacts outweigh the negative impacts? You will probably have both. That is where the predictability comes in. You have to know much about other parts of the system before you can define the level of predictability. If you go back to the basic tenet from systems theory, it is still true: if you change one part of the system, the other parts will also change. But what becomes important in supervision is how will they change.

COMPONENTS OF THEORY

Organize, explain, predict—these are the three main functions of theory. You have to be able to use it to organize what you do, to explain what happens, and to predict what could happen or might happen. In addition, good theory has four other components.

First, it has to have *utility*. Often we forget about this. You have to be able to use it in your work and in the supervision.

Second, it has to be *verifiable*. That is, you have to be able to verify that the things that the theory says in fact exist or do happen. This is one area in which psychoanalytic theory has been accused of being weak. Many times practitioners who are not even closely associated with psychoanalytic theory will use the unconscious as a way to avoid verifying conclusions they have drawn. Current psychoanalytic writers are trying to move from the exclusively unconscious model to an interactional model. They are attempting to make elements of the theory more verifiable (Langs, 1979; Schafer, 1976). There is no necessary connection between utility and verifiability. For example, many of the concepts of existential theory are highly abstract. They do not have a lot of verifiability, but they do have a lot of utility. Any theory that has both utility and verifiability is more useful.

Third, it has to be *comprehensive*. How much of the behavior shown in the treatment situation is the theory able to explain? Psychoanalytic theory is strong in this component. It is a very comprehensive theory, which in turn gives it much utility, although its limited verifiability weakens it. Perhaps this weakness will be overcome as current and future writers and researchers report their findings. It appears there is going to be more and more empirical verification of psychoanalytic theory.

Part of the problem historically has been that Freud used the inductive method, and most people who do academic research have used the deductive method. Almost all of our practice theories have come from the inductive method. The inductive method involves going out into the world and gathering evidence, and from that evidence drawing conclusions upon which to formulate concepts and theories. The deductive method remains abstract: one states certain hunches, or formulates certain hypotheses, and then goes out into the world and sees if reality conforms to one's conception of it.

There are some who do not think that the inductive method is as acceptable as a scientific method. To be scientific, they believe one has to use the deductive method. The theories of practice we possess have been formulated mainly through the inductive method. However, future verification of these theories will come more from the use of the deductive method.

The fourth component is *simplicity* — not that the theory is simple, but that it explains a lot of information in a very concise, understandable way. In descriptions of great artists in any field, their ability to create simplicity out of complex material is portrayed as the essence of their creativity and greatness. No less is true of the good supervisor who is able to discover simplicity in complexity, allowing information to be communicated and understood by the supervisee.

The basic discussion of theory has been stated in simple form, and much detail has been left out because the objective has been to describe theory in terms that the supervisor can readily use in the supervisory process. The aim has been that, using this material, the supervisor can quickly and easily promote learning through the ideas of fact, concept, hypothesis, organizing, explanation, prediction, utility, verifiability, comprehensiveness, and simplicity. Generally, the first six components can be used to guide the supervisory interaction, and the last four can be helpful in selecting established theories to apply in supervision.

THEORETICAL SPECULATION

There is great variation in the ability of practitioners to apply theory to their practice. Some practitioners have difficulty boiling theoretical water, while others can apply theory to practice with much effort. Rarely will a supervisor encounter a practitioner who can apply theory with ease. In assessing the practitioner's level of theoretical knowledge and ability to apply it, the supervisor must keep in mind that using theory in supervision predominantly relates to the teaching and learning roles and has minimal relevance to the solving of immediate practice problems. We have been so indoctrinated in educational programs to the importance of espoused academic theory that we often fail to see how we use it to avoid dealing with more immediate and difficult problems that we come up against in practice. This manifests itself as theoretical speculation (discussed in Chapter 5).

Frequently practitioners will introduce theoretical speculation into supervision when they lack coping strategies to deal with practical problems. Supervisors must be aware of this and repeatedly bring the practitioner back to technical therapeutic issues. The supervisor must keep in mind the economy of supervision and its focus on aiding the supervisee in being more effective with the client. Clients do not care about theory and its relationship to the problem. This is illustrated in a study of family therapy outcome done in England in which the families made it clear they did not care about systems theory — they just wanted to be viewed as individuals in a family with problems (Howe, 1989). From this perspective, the supervision should focus on what to say or what to do next in the treatment. Any use of theory should be based on the practical aspects of the case. If theory can be used to predict an outcome or can guide the sorting out of problem areas, its use is warranted. The supervisor needs to monitor the supervision interaction constantly to ensure that theoretical speculation is being used to enhance the treatment rather than to resist confronting sensitive problems or concerns.

TIMING

The use of theory for long-range learning purposes must be reserved for less immediate points in the supervision. Cases used to teach theory need to be carefully selected. When the supervisor feels that the supervisee needs to develop more theoretical knowledge, timing is important. Cases cannot always be dealt with on a crisis basis. This is an important point because practitioners who resist learning theory show a tendency to present cases on a crisis basis and will jump from case to case in supervision. This must be guarded against, and the supervisor will need to control the rapidity and fragmentation of case presentation. In such situations, the supervisor must keep in mind his or her guidance role. The teaching of theory can leave the practitioner with the impression that theory is the important factor in supervision, and logically lead him or her into using theoretical speculation at times when a crisis or difficulty occurs.

THEORY AND TECHNIQUE

A basic question facing us is: Can one learn techniques of intervention that have been found effective without presuming such techniques can be directly related to a body of theory? The answer to this question is yes, but at the same time, this does not imply that theory is unimportant to practice and supervision.Theory is important, especially in helping practitioners develop self-confidence in their orientation to treatment and in articulating and communicating that orientation to colleagues, supervisors, and clients.

Use of theory is usually only indirectly apparent within the treatment process, but is directly applicable to consideration of the treatment process outside the actual treatment situation. One chief, underutilized vehicle for improving our treatment skills is increased articulation outside of treatment of what we do in treatment. One reason we have failed at this is that students of therapy have frequently failed to provide adequate, consistent models and theories to use in organizing explanation of their therapy. For example, some teachers and supervisors place heavy emphasis on the concept of equifinality from systems theory to argue that regardless of the theory used, the outcome is very often the same. This brings the use of theory into serious question, but at the same time, people who hold this view have students survey many theories and master none. This approach is confusing to learners and gives them little around which to organize their orientations and descriptions of practice.

Supervisors should avoid expecting supervisees to apply specific theoretical material when supervisees lack adequate knowledge of the theory or sufficient practice experience. A good rule to follow is exploration with supervisees of their own practice theory before progressing to exploration of an espoused academic theory.

Supervisors should avoid attempting to apply theories with which they lack thorough familiarity. One of the worst things supervisors can do to practitioners is to pass on to them a heritage of defective theoretical knowledge. Supervisors who get caught doing this run the risk of losing their supervisees' trust and respect. This problem is epitomized by one supervisee's comment that "my supervisor has not read anything in 10 years, but she is constantly telling me to become more familiar with the literature."

Learning theory necessitates a delicate balance that avoids confronting the supervisee with too large or too small increments of information. If the increments of learning are too large, confusion results, and if the increments are too small, frustration arises. There is no specific formula for the correct size increments because they must be based on an assessment of the knowledge, skill, and ability of each supervisee.

I prefer solid grounding in one theory and applying it to practice before moving to comparing and contrasting it with competing theories. In articulating what has taken place or will take place in the treatment situation in a theoretical context, rather than insisting that the theory be used directly in the actual treatment session to determine the course of the therapeutic interaction, some of the pressure is taken off the learning practitioner. This is not a rigid rule, but a guiding principle. It is based on the repeated discovery in research that it is the wisdom and experience of the practitioner, and the nature of the relationship he or she has with the client, that are the crucial variables related to outcome, rather than the theories or techniques used. A major point in this context that the supervisor must remember is: *Supervisors must help practitioners set up a theoretical hook on which to hang their practice hat.*

THEORY ABANDONMENT

One strategy for being more specific, and therefore more helpful in supervision, is to ask the practitioner to abandon conceptual thinking temporarily and to focus exclusively on treatment interaction. Conceptual and theoretical thinking require a gestalt thought process in the generic sense of the term. Gestalt thinking requires understanding the whole to understand the parts. This process is too complex for most practitioners and their therapy at certain stages. Nonconceptual thinking moves from the parts to understanding the whole. Theory and concepts can be applied later.

An example of this occurred when a practitioner was having difficulty understanding a client's pattern of behavior. The supervisor asked him to move to simply describing what events were apparent. He described the client as going to college, then dropping out. Soon after, she met and married an older man. Two years later the marriage was dissolved. Shortly after the end of the marriage she returned to school, and soon after completing her education, she became anxious and doubtful. Soon after graduation, she remarried. The woman sought treatment as this second marriage was collapsing, and she was contemplating returning to school to pursue a master's degree. This pattern of events was brought to light through a set of careful questions by the supervisor. Only after this pattern was identified could the supervisor help the practitioner see the relationship between marriage and education in providing structure to this woman's life.

Even though this person was a good practitioner, he failed to see the conceptual connection until he was required to identify the empirical events in sequence without reference to any pattern. He felt much better about the case after the supervisory session, and returned to the therapy situation with renewed confidence of having a grip on a major dynamic that occurs in many cases. Follow-up revealed that this material resulted in a breakthrough in the treatment and opened up identification of related patterns of functioning.

An example of abandoning theory can illustrate the relationship between theoretical argument and technical strategy. A supervisor and beginning practitioner sought consultation on a case that involved the involuntary court order that a child-abusing family receive treatment at a mental health center. During an initial interview the family members appeared quite nervous, especially the father. The worker sought supervisory assistance with this specific manifestation because he had encountered similar problems of nervousness in cases of this nature in the past, and he had had difficulty dealing with the material. In other words, the practitioner had identified a specific problem area in his practice and was requesting help in developing a technical strategy. Usually, when such material is presented for consultation, there is also some component of the supervision that has become problematic in addition to the case material that is presented, and the consultant should approach the situation in a way that will promote direct or indirect identification of possible supervision obstacles.

The consultant began by asking if this problem had come up in supervision before, and the reply was that it had. The supervisor indicated that he had focused on how the worker felt about the client's nervousness. The worker, with some difficulty, admitted that seeing agitation in clients, especially a family, made him nervous. The supervisor then pursued what made the worker nervous. The supervisor's approach was based on his stated orientation as a Gestalt theorist that the practitioner needed to deal with his "here and now" feelings and what was making him nervous. This approach simply made the worker more nervous. The consultant asked the supervisor and worker to abandon this theoretical orientation, which had resulted in a dead end and, in fact, was making the situation worse. Instead, the focus was placed on the treatment interaction and establishing goals for the treatment, as well as how the worker could keep the interaction focused on the family and its problems. It came out that the worker was not clear about how to proceed with certain content, especially sexual content. Once the worker learned some specific strategies for focusing on the family and handling its nervousness, his tension subsided, and his confidence as a practitioner grew.

In this example, theory-based exploration was a block to learning and needed to be abandoned to promote growth. Supervisors need to be alert to such situations to avoid allowing theory to block growth. Supervision should be guided by theory, but the discussion does not always have to be in theoretical or conceptual terms. One purpose of theory is to provide a frame of reference or a focus. It is necessary to return to the theory only periodically to ensure that the discussion is within the theoretical framework. Some theories focus on internal dynamics, others focus on environment influences, and others focus on a combination of the two. If the theory is used as a checkpoint for the discussion, it can be a valuable aid in keeping the supervision focused and consistent.

How theory can inadvertently lead to a block in the discussion of case material is illustrated by a supervisee's observations of a component of her group supervision:

> Larry, one of the other interns, is caught up in this struggle with the supervisor over theory and who knows the most about it. They'll get into a debate over some little point from the theory. The supervisor will give Larry some readings, and Larry doesn't read them but he will still argue about the points. It's an ongoing thing. The rest of us get tired of this and feel we aren't getting what we should out of the group. Sometimes the supervisor is accommodating toward Larry and concedes points rather than address the real issue.

This supervisor is caught in the trap of theoretical speculation and does not know how to cope with it. If the supervisor in this example does not get help, he will eventually lose the respect of the entire group, and perpetual frustration will be the result. In this situation, neither the interns nor the clients are getting what they deserve from supervision. The technique of theory abandonment would help this supervisor. The real issue of authority, power, and knowledge could be better dealt with by putting theory aside and focusing on the case dynamics.

CREATIVITY AND THEORY

Creativity and use of theory in practice are antithetical. Theories place boundaries on what we do. Theorists consistently hold us to established concepts, especially in deductive theory, while inductive theory forces us constantly to be guided by a search for patterns. Creative artists, on the other hand, cherish the freedom to go wherever their art takes them. Boundaries are not the companion of the artist. This does not mean that the artist works unfettered. Artists must master their craft. For the artist, method and technique are the means to creation and producing original outcomes. For the clinician, theory predicts the outcome. To the extent that creativity is possible in practice, it is limited to the confines of the theory, whereas for the artist, theory and technique are prerequisites to creating new forms.

This basic inconsistency of theory and art in psychotherapy has never been resolved. Some practitioners have urged us to abandon theory; others consider it folly to do so and believe such a strategy invites chaos, inconsistency, and incompetence. This issue should be explored more and could help us advance our knowledge. If we are to abandon theory, how would this contribute to our art? What are the foundation techniques to be mastered that would guide our creativity? If these questions were confronted, perhaps we could become truly artistic without fear of producing merely unrestrained performances.

THEORY APPLICATION

Haley believes that supervisors tend to supervise from the same theoretical orientation that they use in therapy (1976:170). Although this may be the case, a slightly different perspectiveis required when defining good clinical supervisory practices. Supervision involves common use of techniques and strategies regardless of the supervisor's theoretical orientation. Supervision can be superimposed on any theory of practice, just as the scientific method can be applied to any research topic. Some content and the focus of supervision may vary according to the theory, but how the supervisor asks questions, makes comments, and offers interpretations should remain consistent. This provides the supervisee with a systematic, consistent way of approaching supervision over time, and can reinforce and solidify learning.

There has been debate recently about the role of theory in treatment. Rogers holds that attitudes and feelings of the practitioner are more important to treatment outcome than theory or technique (Stein, 1961:98). Bowen views theory as important; Whitaker believes the use of theory isolates the practitioner, dichotomizes the treatment, makes the practitioner an observer, and stifles practitioner creativity (Guerin, 1976: 154-164). There has been little systematic study of how theory is actually used in therapy and how it affects what is said and what gets done. There is little conscious use of theory in the actual practice of therapy. Beginning practitioners, who are struggling with the intensity of the treatment situation, have little energy to invest in the skilled use of theory, and the experienced practitioner focuses on the therapeutic interaction and issues to be explored without conscious consideration of the theoretical implications of this activity. This does not mean that theory is unimportant in clinical practice. What practitioners have been taught about theory does show up in their work, but this is seldom consciously recognized.

Videotapes of good practitioners at work show consistent patterns of interaction that can be traced to their theoretical training and traced to the theory in use that they claim to hold when outside of a practice situation. For purposes of supervision, this becomes an important observation. In order to give practitioners the technical skill to know how to deal with therapy content, the supervisor must have some way to organize the analysis of therapy content. Although the practitioner may not always be aware of the use of theory in the practice situation, effective supervision for practice must be theoretically based. Carl Whitaker has pointed out research that suggests that nontheoretical practitioners can be effective when given good supervision (Guerin, 1976:163). A good rule to follow is that the more nontheoretical the therapy becomes, the more important theory becomes in supervision.

THEORY AND SUPERVISION INTERACTION

The supervisor must be careful of using theory in the abstract. Abstract use of theory occurs for a number of reasons. Supervisors in some instances simply lack the skill to effectively apply theory because they have never been trained in this way. Some supervisors feel it is their responsibility to identify and explain theory, and it is up to the practitioner to make the connections to practice. There are supervisors who use theory abstraction to avoid dealing directly with difficult or unfamiliar case material. Weak supervisors use this pattern consistently, but even good supervisors will occasionally handle difficult supervisory material this way.

Supervisors find it much easier and more stimulating to talk about theory rather than cases, and supervisees respond in the same way. Supervisors focus on theory sometimes out of resistance, but more often they use it to combat boredom with clinical material. Supervisees most often use theory to resist clinical material. Where both sides have so much to gain from abstract theoretical discussion, the supervisor must constantly be alert to theory in the abstract.

If the supervisor and the supervisee work consciously to apply theory to practice, much of the boredom and resistance can be overcome. These problems emerge because the participants fail to really work at applying theory to clinical material. When I observe supervision sessions, what I see most often is that the supervisor explains theoretical concepts and then the practitioner presents a case summary, but seldom do they interrelate the two. The functions of theory are to describe, explain, and predict. These concepts should be the basis of applying theory to clinical material. The theory should be used to describe what exists, to explain what is taking place in the case, and to predict or project what interventions the practitioner must make.

Theory and practice material must be defined independently before they can be integrated. The supervisor and practitioner must develop a *joint style* of how they will segment the supervision to contain the three components of theory, clinical material, and integration. Some like to lay out the theory, then summarize the case material, and finally apply the concepts to the case. Others reverse this process, and some alternate between the two styles. There is no one best way to accomplish this, but it is a good idea for the supervisor to identify the two styles and allow the practitioner to select the style with which he or she feels most comfortable.

It is important that the supervisor and practitioner work together to select a procedural style and stay with that style until they discuss and select an alternate style. This prevents the supervision from becoming unfocused or imbalanced in favor of theory or case material. The supervisor has ultimate responsibility to ensure that the procedural style is being followed. This does not mean that all supervisory sessions will be stylistically segmented. There will be times when this format will not be appropriate to the content for certain sessions.

GUIDELINES FOR APPLYING THEORY
TO CLINICAL MATERIAL

Some guidelines for using theory in relation to clinical material are:

1. Theory as such cannot be applied to clinical material; only concepts from theories can be applied. The supervisor needs to point this out to the practitioner and structure the discussion around specific concepts in relation to specific clinical examples. The supervisor should avoid the approach, for example, "How does Bowen's theory apply to this case?" and instead, "How do Bowen's concepts of individualization and separation apply to how this couple present themselves and what is going on in their marriage?"

2. Theoretical material must be related to clinical material. A good rule for the supervisor to follow is that no theoretical concept should be presented without one or more clinical examples.

3. It is easier for practitioners to handle criticism of their work when it is presented in relation to practice theory. Also, it is easier for a practitioner to understand the implications of an action in theoretical terms rather than simply in terms of practitioner or supervisor behavior or feelings.

4. Supervisors frequently complain that it is difficult to apply theory to practice and that there are no good guidelines for doing this. It can be complex and difficult to relate theory and technique, but to get started the supervisor needs only to ask the supervisee two questions:

- What would you do in this situation?
- What are your reasons for doing it?

The first question relates to technique, and the second relates to theory.

5. Beginning practitioners frequently believe that if you summarize some concepts from a theory and present a case history, you have applied a theory to practice. This is only a beginning step. Theoretical concepts must be clearly and consistently integrated with practice material. When theory and practice are being learned simultaneously, it is the supervisor's responsibility to foster integration.

6. Supervisors tend to talk about terminology, facts, and problems much less than they discuss theories, theorists, ideas, and concepts. For example, it is common for a supervisor to say, "We mainly use Minuchin's structural model here and some of Erikson's strategic methods," without any specific explanation for the young practitioner of precisely what is meant by this. This leaves practitioners to make whatever they want of such statements, which becomes the information they pass on

when they become supervisors. When discussing a theory or a theorist, both the supervisor and practitioner must know exactly what they are talking about.

7. After discussing the theoretical implications of a case, you are still left with what to do about the case. This is like the process in research of explaining a hypothesis after having provided statistically significant support for it. Rather than theoretical discussion being the ending point in supervision, it should be the beginning.

8. Knowledge developed in supervision must be explored as both an independent and dependent variable until a logical understanding is derived. This relates to the idea of dual-concepts exploration explained earlier in this chapter. Sometimes the ordering of the concepts must be reversed to understand the correct sequence of occurrence and association.

CONCLUSION

The problem of learning to use theory in practice, or integrating thought with action, has plagued and frustrated us for a long time (Argyris & Schon, 1980:3). Theory is something that has always been used by interventionist professions to organize explanations of how they intervene as well as to disguise their failures at intervention. In social work, the mixing of theoretical orientations with action techniques has too often resulted in confusion.

The best place to begin to deal with this concern is supervision. This chapter has identified some basic coping mechanisms for supervisors and practitioners to use in this effort.

SUGGESTED READINGS

Chris Argyris and Donald A. Schon. *Theory in Practice: Increasing Professional Effectiveness*. San Francisco: Jossey-Bass, 1980.

An excellent discussion of the practical aspects of theory in use in professions. This book was the source for some of the material in this chapter. It includes discussion of the issues of theory and professional education.

Joe Bailey. *Ideas and Intervention: Social Theory for Practice*. London: Routledge and Kegan Paul, 1980.

This book is an advanced treatment of sociological theory. The discussion is somewhat abstract but stimulating. There is a chapter devoted to social work and social theory.

Raymond J. Corsini (ed.). *Current Psychotherapies*. Itasca, IL: Peacock, 1986.

An excellent coverage of 13 major theories of psychotherapy. This book will be very helpful to the supervisor who is working to help practitioners apply espoused academic theories of psychotherapy.

James K. Feibleman. *Understanding Philosophy: A Popular History of Ideas*. New York: Horizon, 1973.

A good general discussion of philosophy. Recommended to supplement the brief coverage of philosophy in this chapter.

Calvin S. Hall and Gardner Lindzey. *Theories of Personality*. New York: Wiley, 1970.

An excellent overview of 13 major theories of personality. There is an introductory chapter on the nature and utilization of theory.

David Howe. *The Consumers' View of Family Therapy*. England: Gower, 1989.

Empirical study of the outcomes of family therapy treatment in England where systems theory was used. Good ideas for conducting small scale outcome studies.

Abraham Kaplan. *The Conduct of Inquiry: Methodology for Behavioral Science*. San Francisco: Chandler, 1964.

A classic discussion of the scientific method. The explanation of "logic in use" and "reconstructed logic" has much practical relevance to the use of theory in practice. This book is basic reading for the serious student of the scientific method in the behavioral sciences.

Carlo L. Lastrucci. *The Scientific Approach: Basic Principles of the Scientific Method*. Cambridge, MA: Schenkman, 1967.

A basic and thorough introduction to the scientific method.

Fred Pine. *Drive, Ego, Object, and Self*. New York: Basic Books, 1990.

Excellent survey of the different schools of psychoanalytic theory.

Herbert S. Strean. *Psychoanalytic Theory and Social Work Practice*. New York: The Free Press, 1979.

Application of psychoanalytic theory to social work practice.

Francis J. Turner. *Social Work Treatment: Interlocking Theoretical Approaches*. New York: The Free Press, 1985.

Survey of major intervention theories applied to social work.

The study of inspired error should not
engender a homily about the sin of
pride; it should lead us to a
recognition that the capacity for great
insight and great error are opposite
sides of the same coin — and that the
currency of both is brilliance.

Stephen Jay Gould
The Panda's Thumb

Chapter 9

Evaluation of Practice

The emphasis in this chapter is on evaluation from the perspective
of enhancing learning about practice. This form of evaluation is discussed separately from evaluations done in an administrative sense
for promotions, salary increments, annual performance reviews, or
letters of reference. Practice learning evaluation is illustrated in a
simple, four-cell conception derived from a complicated research
study of therapy session outcome. The importance of and methods
for dealing with practice errors are explained in connection with
evaluation. The role of the supervisor in giving criticism and the role
of the supervisee in receiving it are explored from an educational,
evaluative perspective. Lists of specific suggestions for handling
criticism are given for both the supervisor and supervisee. A self-
assessment format is explicated that can be used to place a major
portion of the responsibility for the evaluation on the supervisee to
promote a more positive outcome. The roles of research, practice,
and note taking from an evaluative perspective are covered. Legal
liability of supervisors in connection with evaluation is documented.
The relationship between educational and administrative evaluation
is articulated. The legal and ethical responsibilities of the supervisor
in conducting and directing practice research as evaluation are explained.

INTRODUCTION

Recently a teacher of a group of preschool children asked them: "If you could ask your parents one question that you don't know the answer to, what would it be?" Ninety percent of the children said their question would be: "Do you love me?" (Wiseman, 1979). This seems quite amazing in this age of communication and expression of feelings, but it seems to be a perennial question. Forty years ago, Bertha Capen Reynolds wrote, "What are the questions that press in upon everyone who has to get used to living on this planet? Most primary of all for the young child is probably: Am I loved?" (Reynolds, 1942; 1965:14). Reynolds held that as the child grows the questions evolve to,"Am I able to do what anybody else my size can do?" and "Can I hold my own with others?"

After hearing about the teacher of preschoolers and reading Reynolds' observations, I began asking a series of supervisees: "If you could ask your supervisor one question he or she has not answered for you, what would it be?" Almost all of the supervisees were intrigued by the question and gave it a great deal of thought. The overwhelming majority of the answers were some variation on the reply, "How do you think I am doing in my work?" This surprised me as much as the answers given by the preschoolers. We all need to know if we are "holding our own."

The answer given by so many supervisees was unexpected, but apparently they are not getting this much-needed feedback from their supervisors. In questioning the supervisees further, it became clear that more attention needs to be given to evaluation and feedback in supervision. The following practitioner response summarizes the attitude of many practitioners.

> I got along with my supervisor. She is a nice person. But there was something about her I couldn't understand. We were on a different wavelength. I think she is smart and knows what she is doing, but she didn't share much of it with me. During the four months she supervised me, we had only two individual sessions together, and each session was about 20 minutes long. I feel badly about that. She really didn't teach me anything. I really regret that. I can't blame her though, she is a very busy person. The hospital expects too much of her, but I can't do anything about that.
>
> I thought we would spend more time together. Aren't you supposed to meet at least once a week? I guess part of it is my problem, though. I never brought any of this up when I met with her. Even when we had our evaluation conference at the end, I didn't say anything about my problems. You see, my evaluation wasn't too good.

I had a lot of personal problems during the past four months, and they affected my work, but I didn't share any of this with her. I never told her about it, so I guess I can't blame her. I wish we would have been able to talk about it, but it's too late now.

Your question is a hard one to answer, but if I could ask her one question it would be: What do you see as my major deficiencies?

EVALUATION OF LEARNING

In exploring evaluation in supervision, the term is being used here in a much narrower sense than is commonly thought. It is not used to mean judging the outcome or effectiveness of the treatment. Nor is the evaluation done for administrative purposes, such as promotions, annual reviews of performance, or reference letters. Evaluation as used here is related to the supervisor and practitioner jointly evaluating the practitioner's practice to enhance learning and, therefore, effectiveness in practice. The assumption is that if learning is increased, effectiveness is increased. Strange as it may seem, practitioners at times will be asked to rate their own effectiveness before the evaluation begins. Evaluation for learning must be separated from measurement of effectiveness in order to remove opportunities for defensiveness as much as possible. If either the supervisor or the practitioner becomes defensive, the learning ceases.

I have found that the best way to avoid defensiveness in supervision is to:

1. openly admit that defensiveness is waiting in the wings during all discussions and can take up center stage without much provocation;
2. agree to evaluate at any given point in the supervision that defensiveness has possibly emerged and explore ways of eliminating it; and
3. remove at the outset any potential methods that could lead to defensiveness, such as annual performance evaluations, promotion reviews, or comparison to other practitioners.

Where all external evaluation processes are removed from learning-oriented supervision (i.e., when the practitioner is required to undergo such administrative evaluation only at other times), there is a tendency to greatly decrease defensiveness. Practice at nondefensive evaluative learning can aid in developing nondefensive styles in administrative evaluation that are effectiveness oriented. I call this type of evaluation *error acceptance learning*, that is, errors in practice are expected and known to occur, and the supervision process will be a search for such errors without punitive action for the errors discovered. This is similar to the Airline Pilot Association's policy of encouraging pilots to report near misses and other pilot errors without penalty so they can be studied and ways found to remedy them. This mode of evaluation is aimed more at helping the client than it is at judging the practitioner.

SIMPLICITY

Evaluation of learning in supervision must be kept simple in order to be applied effectively. The structure for discovering errors and promoting learning is simple, but the discussion of discovered errors can be quite complex. When complicated evaluative schemes are devised, error is rarely discovered because much energy and defensiveness go into mastering the scheme, and the process becomes tedious and is often abandoned. This is why it is important to separate research studies and their instruments from evaluation instruments used in supervision.

Simple evaluative instruments and structures can be derived from sophisticated research studies. For example, a study of the therapist's experiences in psychotherapy by Orlinsky and Howard (Gurman & Razin, 1977:566-589) resulted in a number of complex variables being reported in a four-cell conception that is presented in Visual 9.1. Based on 32 therapists' own perceptions, their effectiveness and the degree of patient distress were tabulated for five sessions each (160 sessions). The questions used to measure these two variables were then scored on a scale of 0-20 and divided into low (0-10) and high (11-20). This resulted in the four cells of Type A, B, C, and D that were labeled "smooth sailing," "heavy going," "foundering," and "coasting," based on the practitioner's perception of high and low effectiveness and high and low patient distress during the session. Those interested in the details of the study can refer to the citation given above, but here we are interested in how this can be reduced to a simple instrument that can be used in supervision to structure the initiation of discussion of the practitioner's response to a given session.

Visual 9.2 is a simplification of the four-cell table. The practitioner can be shown this simple diagram and asked to identify the cell that best fits how he or she perceived the session selected for evaluation. Once a cell is selected, the supervision can be focused on identifying the ways in which the practitioner saw himself or herself as being low or high in effectiveness and on discussing patient behaviors that indicated low or high distress. After the session is discussed, supervisor input and insight gained by the practitioner can result in the cell selection being changed. Regardless of the initial cell selection, there is ample basis for discussion even if the cell selected is "smooth sailing." A "smooth sailing" selection can be used to elicit from practitioners what techniques and behaviors they see as being effective so that these behaviors and techniques can be reinforced and anchored in their practice style. This type of discussion is important because practitioners will often perceive sessions as being highly effective

VISUAL 9.1. Practitioner's Perception of Sessions

		Session in Which the Therapist Was Warmly Involved, Empathic, or Effective	
		Low (0-10)	High (11-20)
Sessions in Which the Patient Was Distressed or Anxiously Depressed	Low (0-10) (N = 127; 79.4%)	Type D: Coasting 17 (10.6%)	Type A: Smooth Sailing 110 (68.8%)
	High (11-20) (N = 33; 20.6%)	Type C: Foundering 6 (3.8%)	Type B: Heavy Going 27 (16.9%)
	Total (N = 160; 100%)	23 (14.4%)	137 (85.6%)

Source: David E. Orlinsky and Kenneth L. Howard. "The Therapist's Experience of Psychotherapy," in Alan Gurman and Andrew M. Razin (eds.), *Effective Psychotherapy: A Handbook of Research*. Pergamon Press, 1977; pp. 566-589. Reprinted by permission of Pergamon Press.

VISUAL 9.2. Practitioner Perception of a Session

Patient Distress	Practitioner Effectiveness	
	Low	High
Low	Coasting	Smooth Sailing
High	Foundering	Heavy Going

and powerfully therapeutic without giving much thought to what produced the positive outcome. If the specific effective strategies can be identified, the worker can have more control over positive experiences rather than having the sense that such sessions are arcane and rare occurrences that happen without explanation, which is the orientation many practitioners have about powerful treatment sessions.

When the practitioner selects the "heavy going" cell, the supervisor can support the worker and provide encouragement, because some practitioners have slight depressive reactions to sessions in which much effort is required. Even though they perceive themselves as effective, practitioners will frequently respond in terms of whether the effort they must make is worth the outcome.

When the categories of "coasting" and "foundering" are selected, error selection begins. The practitioner needs to focus on session activity that led to low effectiveness. It is better if workers can identify the specific actions that detracted from their being effective, and the supervisor must guide them in the search for alternative techniques and behaviors that will help them avoid these outcomes in future sessions.

The diagram can be used from session to session so that, when there are cell changes, supervision can be focused on what brought about the change. This four-cell conception is just one illustration of how supervisors can simplify conceptualizations from complicated research studies to meet their own supervisory needs. In order to do this, supervisors need to read research literature from a dual perspective. First, they need to read from the point of view of how the outcomes of the research are useful in practice. Second, they need to ask how the research methodology can be reconceptualized in a way that it can be used to promote learning in supervision.

PRACTICE ERRORS

It is helpful to orient the practitioner to the fact that we all make mistakes in treatment. Mistakes can be devastating; at best, they are hard to admit. However, mistakes do happen, and more often than we realize. Mistakes and errors in technique are important to supervision, because the more closely we scrutinize our work, the more mistakes we uncover. In orienting practitioners to identifying and rectifying mistakes and errors, it is valuable to point out that skilled practitioners make mistakes. I like to point out that even Freud was subject to errors and "blind spots." I refer to Langs' analysis of Freud's treatment of Dora. Langs' analysis, based on Freud's own writings, resulted in the conclusion that there was "misalliance with his patient and [it] contributed to the premature termination of her analysis. There was also some evidence that his modifications in the frame reflected specific countertransference difficulties in his relationship with Dora and contributed to his blind spots regarding her communications and their interaction" (Langs, 1976:393-394). For a more general discussion of Freud's errors, the reader is referred to Sartre's study of the young Sigmund Freud, "when his ideas had led him into hopeless error" (Sartre, 1976:129-132). Calling attention to errors by renowned therapists can do a great deal to relieve supervisees from self-imposed expectations that they need to be perfect in their practice.

There are a number of commercially produced videotapes[1] that show renowned practitioners at work, and, in some instances, they are not at their best therapeutically. Viewing such tapes can help practitioners to develop a positive attitude toward openness to admitting error.

Frequently, practitioners will dance around the issue of errors and they will never directly admit mistakes or confusion about how to proceed with difficult cases. In such instances, practitioners will introduce much complexity into the case and point to the client's lack of clarity and resistance, rather than focusing on how and where they, as practitioners, erred or could have been more effective. It is the supervisor's role to help the practitioner overcome their failure to see the therapeutic relationship in a realistic way. The supervisor can take some of the pressure off the worker by identifying ways they themselves would have been confused or would have made mistakes in the same aspect of the treatment had they been the practitioner. This makes it easier for supervisees to begin identifying their own weaknesses. Relating to the practitioner in this way, involving such material, is one of the situations in which it is appropriate for the supervisor to use *philosophical abstraction* related to case discussion, but it should be followed by use of *technical strategy*.

At times practitioners will perceive themselves to be making errors or not making progress in a difficult case. At such times they tend to criticize themselves and occasionally to question their own competence. The supervisor can help the practitioner by pointing out that the case is an extremely difficult one and that the difficulty does not rest with the worker's lack of skills. However, the supervisor must be prepared to pinpoint the problem areas in the case and offer the supervisee assistance in how to deal with them. This strategy can lead to difficulty when the supervisor

---

1. One series of such videotapes is available from the Boston Family Therapy Institute. This series includes Virginia Satir, Carl Whitaker, Salvador Minuchin, Daniel Rubenstein, and James Framo.

recognizes that a clinical problem does arise from a practitioner's lack of skill or knowledge, and rather than dealing directly with the supervisee's shortcomings, will attribute the difficulty to the complexity of the case. To support failures in practice in this manner is an extremely unprofessional act on the part of a supervisor and is actually a process of sanctioning poor practice. Although all supervisors will periodically make such errors, to do this as a pattern is to reward bad practice, to perpetuate incompetence, and expose clients to undue risks.

FOLLOW-UP AND EVALUATION

Follow-up and evaluation of a case are related but separate functions. Evaluation deals with the progress and effectiveness during a course of treatment; follow-up relates to gathering information about the client's functioning at a given interval or at several intervals after treatment is completed. The expectation and importance of follow-up should be made clear as a part of termination to avoid client feelings of remote dependency on the worker. Follow-up can be informal-through a telephone call or letter from the client or worker — or formal — through a brief, mailed questionnaire to the client. Regardless of the method used, the nature and form of the follow-up should be made clear at the time of termination.

CRITICISM OF CLINICAL MATERIAL

To help practitioners learn and grow, supervisors will have to be critical of their work from time to time. This is a basic, inherent part of the supervisory role. In our society we dislike criticism and having to give it or receive it. We usually avoid it if at all possible and engage in it only when the situation is desperate. We cannot afford this in supervision.

Learning to offer criticism effectively takes much practice and skill. Weisinger and Lobsenz (1981) have written a book devoted entirely to how to give criticism effectively. Some of their general principles can be adapted to supervision of clinical practice. The following points will be helpful to the supervisor in offering criticism.

1. Criticism is a tool used to promote personal growth and enhance relationships.
2. To criticize is to communicate information to practitioners in ways that enable them to use it to their advantage and benefit.
3. Criticism can be delivered in a non-negative manner.

4. To be helpful, criticism must draw a distinction between the behavior criticized and the individual involved.
5. Criticism is destructive when words and phrases are used that indicate or imply that the behavior in question was done deliberately.
6. The criticism must be specific if the practitioner is expected to act on the basis of it or change as a result of it.
7. The supervisor must ensure that the practitioner understands the criticism. This is the only way that an exchange of information and learning can result from the criticism. It helps to ask if the practitioner agrees or disagrees with the criticism.
8. Criticism offered by the supervisor should be separated from his or her personal feelings or emotional aspects of the supervisor's relationship with the practitioner. The supervisor needs to assess: Am I aware of my own feelings about the practitioner? Are my feelings positive or negative?
9. When offering criticism the supervisor should avoid the words "should" and "shouldn't."
10. Criticism must be offered at a time when the practitioner is ready to deal with it, and there should be sufficient time allowed to discuss it. State the criticism clearly and concisely, and then get feedback.
11. Criticism can be offered without threats or ultimatums.
12. Criticism can be offered without being in the context of "I told you so."
13. Criticism is most helpful when it is not stated as an accusatory question.
14. When offering criticism the supervisor should consider in advance: What behavior do I want to criticize?
15. Before offering criticism the supervisor needs to consider: Can the criticized behavior be changed?
16. The supervisor needs to consider in advance: How can the criticism help the practitioner?
17. The supervisor must consider how the criticism will generate new approaches to the issue.
18. Criticism is best focused on the positive (i.e., What can be done? rather than, What was not done?).
19. The supervisor's criticism should be offered as an opinion, not as a fact.
20. When offering criticism, the supervisor needs to consider: Am I expressing my criticism in a manner that conveys that I understand how the practitioner feels and thinks?

REACTIONS TO CRITICISM

The very nature of supervision necessitates that the supervisor evaluate the practitioner's work critically, and this evaluation must involve exploration of actual case material. We can think up many euphemisms for the word criticism in an effort to make it easier for the supervisee, but the fact remains that it is criticism, and the supervisee will perceive it as such. The supervisor can make every effort to be constructive and supportive when offering criticism. This can be accomplished without too much difficulty.

What the supervisor has no control over is the supervisee's response to criticism. When criticism is viewed negatively and is resisted, the supervision process becomes tense, anger on both sides increases, and learning ceases. Educational programs do not put emphasis on how to deal with being evaluated. Educational programs place emphasis on doing evaluation or being in the role of evaluator. Most beginning practitioners have no preparation for being evaluated. Some practitioners have a fear of any criticism of their performance.

One way to help avoid some of these problems is to explain the role of criticism in supervision at the beginning and provide the supervisee with some guidelines for constructively accepting criticism of their clinical material (Munson, 1980a). These guidelines also apply to the supervisor when the worker offers criticism, a practice that should be encouraged more by supervisors to improve their effectiveness. The following guidelines (in part adapted from Weinberg, 1978) are offered in dealing with criticism.

1. Listen to the criticism in detail. Avoid rushing to defend yourself or your position.
2. Evaluate in your own mind the validity of the criticism. If the criticism is fair, formulate ways in your own mind that you could change your performance.
3. Try to gain more understanding by asking for more detailed information about the criticism. If the criticism is very general, as it often is, ask the supervisor to be more specific. Ask how the activity could have been done differently or better.
4. Avoid implying that the supervisor has some personal motive. Keep the criticism on a professional level and always relate it to professional performance.
5. **Avoid getting angry** with the supervisor and losing self-control. This accomplishes nothing.

6. Avoid attempting to shift the responsibility to someone else.
7. Avoid attributing the criticism to personal weakness, and avoid presenting yourself as a total failure in all areas.
8. Avoid trying to shut off the criticism by saying that you cannot deal with negative comments.
9. Avoid changing the subject to avoid any direct discussion of the criticism.
10. Avoid repeatedly admitting that you were wrong, and refrain from continually questioning the supervisor as to what you can do to make up for the criticism.
11. Avoid focusing the conversation on giving justifications and excuses for what you did.
12. Refrain shifting responsibility onto the supervisor by saying that the supervisor is overreacting or is just looking for something to criticize.
13. Avoid turning the criticism into a joke or verbal one-upmanship.
14. Clarify for yourself, or ask the supervisor, how your behavior was inadequate. If the supervisor cannot offer an explanation, you must assess whether the criticism is valid.
15. Regardless of whether you accept or question the criticism, let the supervisor know that you heard and understand the criticism.
16. If you accept the criticism, acknowledge it and either offer an alternative for the future or ask your supervisor for possible alternative behavior.
17. Remember that criticism is not a threat to you personally or professionally. It is a way of gaining new information about different and perhaps better ways of performing.

This list of ways to deal with criticism should be discussed openly with the practitioner at the point of initiating the supervisory process. If the expectations are made clear, the supervisee can avoid becoming defensive when the supervisor must be critical of some aspect of the supervisee's work. The supervisor may choose to review the supervisee's work through audiotapes, videotapes, bug in the ear, process recordings, or after-the-fact discussion, but to be effective, the supervision must involve open exploration of the treatment process. When supervision has been structured on the basis of positive expectations regarding criticism, the outcome is more objective for both the supervisor and the supervisee.

EVALUATION AND SELF-ASSESSMENT

The supervisee must be an active participant in the supervision for it to be effective and internalized. One way this can be done is to have the supervisee select the treatment material that will be used in the supervision and to prepare a self-assessment of the material prior to the supervision session. I have devised and used a self-assessment form that contains the following questions.

1. How long did the interview last?
2. Do you feel the interview was too short, too long, just about right? Explain what factors contributed to the interview's being too short or too long. Who contributed most to this? What could have been done to overcome this?
3. Did the interview have a focus? If yes, what was the focus? If no, what prevented a focus from being developed? What could have been done to focus the interview more?
4. Do you feel that the client got what he or she came for? If yes, what did he or she get? If no, what prevented him or her from getting what was expected?
5. Did the session have a flow or interaction or continuity? If yes, generally describe this characteristic and how it was achieved. If no, what prevented it?
6. Describe generally how you felt prior to the session.
7. Describe generally how you felt during the session.
8. Describe generally how you felt after the session.
9. Describe your behaviors during the session about which you felt good.
10. Describe client behaviors during the session about which you felt good.
11. Describe your behaviors during the session about which you felt bad.
12. Describe client behaviors during the session about which you felt bad.
13. Are you aware of any gestures or behaviors on your part that detracted from the communication process?
14. Are you aware of any gestures or behaviors on the client's part that detracted from the communication process?
15. Are you aware of any gestures or behaviors on your part that enhanced the communication process?
16. Are you aware of any gestures or behaviors on the client's part that enhanced the communication process?

17. Are there any problems associated with this session with which you would like help?
18. Now that you have had time to think about it, what would you do differently in the interview if you could do it over?
19. Based on what you know now, what are your plans for the next interview?

These questions are presented in questionnaire format in Appendix 6, and can be reproduced for use in supervision. This form can be used routinely in educationally focused supervision, or it can be used to identify a specific problem in a specific case. Having practitioners write out the answers prior to supervision for a specific problem promotes a reflection process that leads supervisees to awareness of what the problem is before they get to supervision. It is very rewarding when this happens, because this is genuine self-teaching and learning. The self-assessment format advocated here promotes more efficient use of supervisory time, and is very helpful when time available for supervision is limited. There is a trend toward self-assessment in the literature associated with the recent emphasis on autonomous practice (Wallace, 1981).

RESEARCH AND PRACTICE

Learning in supervision has been vaguely defined in relation to evaluation of and research in practice. The research on psychotherapy can help with the distinction that needs to be made. During the 1950s and 1960s, a distinction was made between process and outcome research. Process research deals with *how* changes take place in a given interchange between client and practitioner; outcome research is concerned with *what* changes take place as a result of treatment (Hersen & Barlow, 1976:20). During the early days of such studies, there was a flight into process that led to an increase in process research. Methodological problems later led to a decline in process research. This distinction between outcome and process research led to a dichotomy between the two approaches that hampered measurement of effectiveness of psychotherapy. Although these were technical considerations in psychotherapy's pure research circles, the dichotomy has implications for learning in supervision because research attention later turned the relationship between process and outcome, and this relationship is important to learning in and evaluation of practice in supervision.

There has been much speculation about, and a limited amount of questionable empirical research on, the negative effects of psychotherapy. The major source of information about negative effects in psychotherapy has been client reports. Such reports are subject to distortions, inaccuracies, and varied perceptions. Strupp et al. (1977) argue that more reliable sources of such effects are supervisors' observations of practitioners in training. The empirical research on the "deterioration hypothesis" does not provide compelling evidence that negative effects are widespread. Even with increased, sound empirical research on psychotherapy outcome, "it is doubtful that scientific evidence alone will suffice" (Strupp et al., 1977:23). Psychotherapy is an extremely complicated process that involves many personality variables, moral and philosophical issues, and diverse perceptions. Just as it can be argued that recovery occurs spontaneously in spite of therapeutic intervention, it can be postulated that deterioration occurs in spite of therapeutic intervention. We are a long way from attributing causation of improvement or deterioration to therapeutic intervention. For the time being, we are limited to making associations between these events. It is to be hoped that we will have the courage and self-confidence to report improvement and negative effects when we observe them and that the positives will outnumber the negatives. Good supervision is the best way to ensure the integrity and accuracy of our observations. Since we operate in a world of so many unknowns, supervision can help monitor our efforts and offer assessment of what to do and what not to do in treatment.

Practitioners have little concern for or patience with sophisticated research in their practice. It is difficult enough to deal with clinical dynamics from a therapeutic standpoint without adding the complex thinking and procedures required for research, especially since most clinicians have little or no training in research skills. This scientist/researcher split is epitomized by Matarazzo, who observed:

> Even after 15 years, few of my research findings affect my practice. Psychological science per se doesn't guide me one bit. I still read avidly but this is of little direct practical help. My clinical experience is the only thing that has helped me in my practice to date . . . . (Bergin & Strupp, 1972:340)

Carl Rogers, a leading clinical researcher, "as early as the 1958 APM conference on psychotherapy noted that research had no impact on his clinical practice and by 1969 advocated abandoning formal research in psychotherapy altogether" (Bergin & Strupp, 1972:313). These views continue to prevail among a large number of psychotherapists.

The anti-research attitude does not mean that research concepts cannot be applied to clinical material, especially in supervision. For example, process material and outcome measures can be applied to specific case material. The desired outcomes in a case can be related to the therapeutic processes to be used in achieving these outcomes. The supervisor and practitioner can first identify the outcomes and the processes that have the most potential to achieve the outcomes, and the case can be monitored for progress in reaching the identified outcomes. Specific cases can become the focus in supervision with the objective that this procedure of analysis becomes a routine thought and action pattern for the practitioner in all cases.

The key to a research orientation in supervision and practice is that the research focus must remain simple, understandable, and connected to clinical material. Other evaluative tools that have a simplified research orientation are the self-assessment form I have developed (see Appendix 6) and the four-cell conception of research discussed earlier in this chapter. These formats can be used by supervisors when they encounter a problem in a case. When evaluation is approached from this perspective, practitioners are less likely to resist a research-in-practice focus when they recognize a problem in a case and perceive themselves as needing help.

NOTE TAKING

There is much controversy about note taking during treatment sessions. Generally it is viewed as a distraction for both the practitioner and the client. I believe that this is a matter of style. It is difficult to do a diagnostic interview without taking notes, especially in a complex case and when case information will be shared with colleagues. When note taking is a part of the treatment from the outset, it rarely becomes an issue. I have taken brief notes in treatment for years and have not experienced it as a distraction. Note taking helps keep me alert and focused. A train of thought can be reestablished through notes, patterns of behavior can be clearly documented, and notes can aid in preparing for future sessions. The function of treatment note taking should be explored in supervision as a style issue.

Although note taking is a matter of style in treatment, I think it is a necessity in supervision for both the practitioner and the supervisor. Notes are important to case planning and follow-up. Notes are important for the worker since much time may elapse between supervision sessions and subsequent client interviews. Notes are important in settings in which periodic evaluations of the practitioner's work are required. Where disagreements occur in supervision, notes can aid in clarifying issues and determining what position each participant held in a given case or series of cases. The best time to prepare for a supervisory session is just after the previous one. Notes can be very helpful in organizing and reflecting upon what has just taken place in a session and documenting material that should be followed-up in a subsequent session.

In brief, treatment note taking is essential since the practitioner does not have the luxury of asking the client to recall and re-present forgotten material. In addition, good notes are important to learning in treatment, and are essential to research and evaluation of treatment (Lewin, 1970:58-59).

RECORD KEEPING

To some extent, organizational procedure affects supervision directly in the learning process through record keeping procedures. The supervisor must ensure that the supervisee is keeping records that conform to agency procedures to facilitate flow of information and to meet mandatory external regulations. Record keeping has taken on increased significance because in most modern agencies record keeping is tied to funding. Much funding is dependent on providing accurate, detailed, and current records to payors. In addition, it has been estimated that approximately 30 percent of practitioner time is devoted to record keeping. The supervisor who does not assist supervisees at proficiency in this area could be neglecting an important and significant part of the practitioner's work.

It is the supervisor's function to orient the newly employed practitioner to the requirements. When the supervisor is performing an educational role exclusively, the decision must be made regarding what form of record keeping will be required for learning purposes. Some supervisors rely on the basic mandatory records as a basis for teaching and rely on discussions surrounding these basic records. Others view mandatory records as minor activities that must be dealt with and tolerated so that the larger task of teaching and learning can be pursued. Some supervisors require additional record keeping, such as process recording and process summaries, that are used exclusively for learning purposes and do not become part of the agency's formal record keeping.

Regardless of the style of record keeping required by the agency or the supervisor, the important point is that the methods and procedures should be made clear to the supervisee from the outset of supervision. Some supervisors avoid this because they view record keeping as a minor irritation with which they would rather not deal at all. The reality is that record keeping is important to the ongoing functioning of the agency as an organization, is important to sustaining a record of the client's contact with and service received from the agency over time, and is therefore an important fact of organizational life.

When the details of record keeping are not attended to, they can interfere with the teaching activity in supervision. I once worked with a psychotherapist who would not dictate for months and never encouraged his supervisees to keep up on their dictation. When recertification evaluations would be scheduled, this practitioner would have to cancel all of his therapy sessions for an entire week to bring his records up to date, resulting in a disruption of treatment to his clients and placing an additional burden upon other practitioners, who would have to assume his intake cases during the time he was literally locked in his office dictating. He also created massive problems for the medical records department, which had to locate and pull all his charts, as well as type all the dictation.

This psychotherapist also spent much time having disagreements with his supervisees about records and record keeping procedures because of his resistance to performing these tasks and discussing them in supervision. His lack of clarity in this area led to many lost hours in supervision when confrontations would occur. This was unfortunate, because this supervisor was an excellent teacher, and he failed to see that his abhorrence of this topic led to its taking up more, rather than less, time in supervision, thus distracting from what he did best — teaching psychotherapy.

Agencies have varying requirements for record keeping. Beyond the agency requirements, supervisors and practitioners should consider records from two perspectives: legal liability and personal use. These can be two separate sets of records. Such separation has professional sanction and legal recognition (Schutz, 1982:52). A good record for legal purposes should contain:

1. signed informed consents for all treatment,
2. signed informed consents for all transmission of confidential information,
3. any treatment contracts,
4. notation of all treatment contacts and significant information and actions regarding the contact (including face-to-face contacts with clients and others, and telephone contacts),
5. notations of failed or cancelled appointments,
6. notations of supervision and consultation contacts,
7. all correspondence,
8. a complete social history including past and present evaluations and treatment, a medical history, record of current physical examination,

9. a diagnostic assessment or statement; this assessment should be reviewed, revised, and noted periodically,
10. all medications the person is currently taking,
11. a record of the practitioner's basis for the assessment made and the treatment provided,
12. notations of suggestions, instructions, referrals, or directives made to the client and whether they followed through.

The practitioner's personal notes have more latitude and can include such items as:

1. speculation about client dynamics,
2. impressions about the course of treatment,
3. problems resolved,
4. problems being worked on,
5. problems to be worked on in the future,
6. projections about termination,
7. summary of perceptions of significant treatment session dynamics.

In many respects the supervisor records are integrated with the client records, and for legal purposes, significant supervisory contacts should be a part of the client record. The legal status of separate supervisor records is less clear than the requirements for client records. Also, agency requirements vary for supervisory record keeping, and individual supervisors' preferences vary. Generally, supervisory records should include at least:

1. the supervisory contract, if used or required by the agency,
2. a brief statement of supervisee experience, training, and learning needs,
3. a summary of all performance evaluations,
4. notation of all supervisory sessions,
5. cancelled or missed sessions,
6. notation of cases discussed and significant decisions,
7. significant problems encountered in the supervision and how they were resolved, or whether they remain unresolved and why.

It is important that the supervisor keep good records on each supervisee. When we begin supervising someone, we do not know where or how it is going to end. It could end on a positive note several years later with pride when the supervisee becomes a supervisor or moves to another position, or it could end in an agency or professional grievance hearing. Unfortunately, some do end this way, and the only thing more difficult for the supervisor than such an ending is not being able to document in a grievance hearing how a supervisee's performance was unsatisfactory. The supervisor's memory and speculative recounting of the problems are insufficient. Supervisors who rely on their memory are open to manipulation by difficult supervisees.

The supervisory record should be a tool for promoting ongoing growth and development of the practitioner. Under the best conditions, it aids the supervisor in fostering professional growth of the practitioner. In difficult adversary situations, the record is a documented defense against unrecognized and unaccepted practitioner failure at performance.

ADMINISTRATIVE EVALUATION

Annual performance evaluations should be taken seriously and not viewed as a routine form that is filled out hastily so that the supervisor and supervisee can get on with the work of the agency. This attitude and pattern are easy to assume in agencies that focus on doing therapy, and routine forms are viewed as a necessary evil. If the supervisor has been working regularly with the supervisee using the techniques discussed in this chapter and previous chapters, the administrative evaluation will not come as a surprise and will meet with minimal resistance.

The point of this chapter has been that a distinction has to be made between administrative evaluation and the evaluation of practice as part of the supervisory process. Clearly, the two are related, but they often involve different procedures. For example, practice evaluation can involve discussion of many minute practice actions that are changed immediately by the practitioner and reevaluated in a week, and any change is the result of the supervisor and supervisee's negotiating a shared solution. Administrative evaluation is very general and may not be reevaluated for quite some time. Practice evaluation is usually confined to the supervisory relationship. Although content of the administrative evaluation is agreed upon by the supervisor and supervisee, it can result in actions taken by others outside the supervisory relationship that can directly affect the supervisee, such as the amount of a salary increase or receiving or being denied a promotion. Thus, practice evaluation is specific, continuous, and basically self-contained, and administrative evaluation is general, periodic, and external to the supervisory relationship.

Although administratively mandated evaluations can vary greatly in their frequency, form, and content, the supervisor should work with the higher-level administration to ensure that administrative evaluation procedures are fair, objective, and open, so that this form of evaluation does not hinder the supervisory relationship. Some basic guidelines for administrative evaluation of clinicians that supervisors should strive for are listed below.

1. Administrative evaluation policy should be established at the higher level in the organization, implemented at a lower level, and reviewed at the higher level.
2. The supervisee should be informed of the format, content, and procedures of the evaluation at the beginning of the evaluation period.
3. The same evaluation instrument should be used over time. This is the only way change in performance can be detected.
4. The individuals to be evaluated who make up the organizational unit should participate in development of the evaluation instrument.
5. Evaluate the position and the performance, and avoid evaluating the person.
6. Avoid evaluating any function or task you have not been designated to evaluate.
7. Refrain from evaluating someone who performs a function you know little or nothing about.
8. Evaluation assumes that you know what the process and outcome of the performance is to be.
9. If the evaluation instrument is quantified, the person evaluated must be able to determine how the composite score was calculated.
10. Evaluation begins long before the forms are to be filled out. Evaluation is an ongoing process and the person should be aware of the policies and procedures from the beginning of the evaluation period.

PRACTICE RESEARCH AND SUPERVISION

In an early study by Rosenblatt, a sample of social workers rated supervision and consultation as significantly more helpful to them in practice than research findings (1968:55). The research failed to confirm that research was of much value to practitioners, and illustrated that research was not viewed as highly relevant to or integrated with what takes place in supervision. During that era the researcher, practitioner, and supervisor were described as separate specialists performing very different functions; the researcher was portrayed as a "threat" to the practitioner and the supervisor (Rosenblatt, 1968:58). Although there has been no replication of Rosenblatt's study in recent times, similar research has produced similar results, and a study by Kirk and Fischer suggests that social workers show a propensity to avoid using research in an objective manner when it is identified as potentially useful to them in their practice (1976:69).

There has been a recent trend toward dealing with some of the problems of research and practice by attempting to integrate the two areas. Rather than approaching integration by encouraging researchers and practitioners to join forces, the effort has focused on combining the two roles in one person by training practitioner/researchers (Grinnell, 1981; Jayaratne & Levy, 1979; Wodarski, 1981; Hudson, 1982). A major focus of this new orientation to research focuses on single-subject designs, which incorporate research procedures as an integral part of practice intervention. The emphasis of these designs is on observations and analyses of the effects of interventions on specific behaviors rather than on proof of hypotheses as is the case in group research designs (Grinnell, 1981:373-375). None of these approaches mentions the role of supervision in promoting and regulating research in practice.

There is still much debate about how best to apply research principles in practice (see Geismar & Wood, 1982; Ruckdeschel & Farris, 1982). Single-subject designs have been compared andcontrasted with good process records. The debate about and use of the two approaches will undoubtedly continue. What seems to be agreed upon by those on both sides of the debate is that any research in practice must be based on an analysis of specific interactional exchanges between client and practitioner. As long as this basic principle is adhered to by the supervisor and supervisee, the chances of error will be reduced in evaluating practice.

There has to be a rational alternative to the old model of the two person research/practice combination and the current model of a single person doing both research and practice. Although research and practice involve similar procedures, as writers on the topic have pointed out, they are not the same activity. Each has its own goals and objectives. When research is combined with practice, it must be done with caution, and the purposes must be made clear. The research must be compatible with the practice and care must be taken to avoid letting it detract from, impede, or confuse the goals of the treatment. The factors just mentioned must be monitored by the supervisor to ensure that client rights are being protected and that treatment efforts are not being superseded by research interests. If they are **going to be helpful to this new type of practitioner, supervisors** need to be trained in the research procedures being used and must be experienced at doing research.

The role of the supervisor in monitoring and evaluating the ethics of practitioner research is vague and unclear. This is in part due to the fact that government regulation of research activity did not begin in earnest until 1974, after the public disclosure of the so-called Tuskegee Study, which involved research for 40 years on over 400 black men, some of whom had syphilis (see Jones, 1981). An interesting aside about this study is that a social worker was the first person to raise questions concerning the ethics of the research, and he was responsible for setting in motion the events that halted the experiment (Jones, 1981:188-205).

Most institutions that receive government funds and do research now have institutional review boards that review research protocols in order to protect human subjects. Supervisors who work in such settings have a moral and quasi-legal responsibility to be familiar with requirements for institutional review of research conducted by their supervisees. The term quasi-legal has been used in relation to research in practice because it is unclear what the responsibility of the supervisor is in this area.

What is clear is that under the legal doctrine of *respondeat superior* (let the superior give answer), the supervisor is not absolved from responsibility for actions of supervisees. Schutz has pointed out:

> While therapists are not guarantors of cure or improvement, extensive treatment without results could legally be considered to have injured the patient; in specific, the injury would be the loss of money and time, and the preclusion of other treatments that might have been more successful. To justify a prolonged holding action at a plateau, the therapist would have to show that this was maintaining a condition against a significant and likely deterioration. (1982:47)

Under these circumstances, if research is a component of treatment in a situation in which there is no improvement, the practitioner and supervisor are open to the accusation that the treatment was only a subterfuge to carry out the research. In such cases the professionals involved will undoubtedly be required to demonstrate how the research was designed to enhance the effectiveness of the treatment and to show that the client was informed about and consented to the research procedures. In light of the recent developments in practice research discussed earlier, legal and ethical issues will continue to emerge in this area, and supervisors will need to keep abreast of developments in the judicial and professional arenas regarding research and responsibility for practice outcomes. It is possible that legal action from outside the profession will bring about practice and supervision reforms that have not taken place within the social work profession during its almost 100 years of existence.

Without regard to research in practice, legal liability of the supervisor for the actions of the practitioner is changing. In the 1950s, when the social work profession was attempting to shake off the effects of supervision in the quest for autonomy and professionalism (see Chapters 1 and 2), Fizdale viewed supervision of the established professional as "potentially detrimental." She went on to argue that the caseworker is fully and independently responsible for intake decisions, referrals, techniques used, and termination decisions (Munson, 1979a: 122-127). Scherz held a similar view by advocating that supervisors cannot make social workers competent by injecting knowledge into them (Munson, 1979a:73). From a professional point of view this trend continued to evolve in the 1950s, but from a legal perspective, in the 1980s supervisors must be aware that:

> When one undertakes to supervise the work of another practitioner, one also assumes a legal liability not only for one's own acts but for those of the supervisee. Legal liability rests on the de facto or de jure (actual or mandated by law) control the supervisor has over the therapy process to coordinate, direct, and inspect the actions of the treating practitioner. (Schutz, 1982:47)

Under current conditions the supervisor and supervisee have a mutual responsibility to make every effort to ensure that all major decisions about treatment have been reviewed in supervision (Schutz, 1982: 47-52).

SUGGESTED READINGS

Edith Freeman. "The Importance of Feedback in Clinical Supervision: Implications for Direct Practice." *The Clinical Supervisor* 3 (Spring 1985), pp. 5-26.
  Discussion of feedback as a form of evaluation.

Richard M. Grinnell, Jr. (ed.). *Social Work Research and Evaluation*. Itasca, IL: Peacock, 1981.
  A collection of 31 topical chapters that survey various types of research in social work practice including ethics, measurement, design, statistics, computers, and writing research reports.

M. Hersen and D. H. Barlow. *Single-Case Experimental Designs: Strategies for Studying Behavior Change*. New York: Pergamon, 1976.
  A sophisticated, advanced explanation of single-case designs. Recommended only for experienced supervisors and practitioners well trained in research methodology and statistics.

Walter W. Hudson. *The Clinical Measurement Package: A Field Manual.* Homewood, IL: Dorsey, 1982.

This manual describes nine measurement scales that are designed to assess the severity and magnitude of a variety of personal and social problems. The scales measure depression, self-esteem, marital discord, sexual dysfunction, discord with child, discord with mother, discord with father, peer discord, and intrafamilial stress. The scales are purchased separately from the manual.

Srinika Jayaratne and Rona L. Levy. *Empirical Clinical Practice.* New York: Columbia University Press, 1979.

A good, basic survey of the role of the clinician/researcher.

James H. Jones. *Bad Blood: The Tuskegee Syphilis Experiment.* New York: The Free Press, 1981.

This book is good, general reading to gain insight about the ethics of research. The author gives a thorough account of the 40-year history of this experiment and the role of a social worker in calling the ethics of the experiment into question.

Benjamin M. Schutz. *Legal Liability in Psychotherapy: A Practitioner's Guide to Risk Management.* San Francisco: Jossey-Bass, 1982.

This book is highly recommended for the practitioner and supervisor interested in legal liability for practice activity. There is specific discussion of situations affecting social workers.

George Weinberg. *Self-Creation.* New York: St. Martin's, 1978.

This book was used to develop the material in this chapter on how to deal with criticism. It is recommended for the supervisee who wants to develop more knowledge and ability to deal with criticism and self-development.

Hendrie Weisinger and Norman M. Lobsenz. *Nobody's Perfect: How to Give Criticism and Get Results.* Los Angeles: Stratford, 1981.

An excellent, readable guide to giving and getting criticism. This book is highly recommended and was used to develop some of the guidelines in this chapter.

Suanna J. Wilson. *Confidentiality in Social Work: Issues and Principles.* New York: The Free Press, 1978.

This book is an excellent, in-depth analysis of confidentiality, privileged communication, and legal aspects of privacy and access to information in the profession of social work. Chapter 10 is devoted to confidentiality problems faced by supervisors and administrators.

John S. Wodarski. *The Role of Research in Clinical Practice: A Practical Approach for the Human Services*. Baltimore: University Park Press, 1981.

A good, basic coverage of research and evaluation techniques necessary for the supervisor to be effective.

We social case workers are asking
why others should have too much
leisure and we too little. Are we trying
to sweep back the sea with our little
brooms, when we ought to be building
solid dikes against misery?

Bertha Capen Reynolds
Between Client and Community

Chapter 10

Stress Reactions

This chapter defines stress and identifies its manifestations as well
as its causes and cures. The research on stress among social workers is reviewed along with some of the conflicting results of the research. Supervision and stress are explored, as are demands that
can lead to this stress. The chapter includes excerpts from research
interviews with workers making observations about their own experiences with stress that illustrate the conceptual material. The supervisor's role in helping practitioners prevent and overcome stress
is explained. Some specific pointers and pitfalls of aiding workers
are covered. Special attention is given to helping beginning professionals deal with stress since the research shows that, perhaps un-
expectedly, stress is highest among this group. The points for combating stress can be applied to work with supervisees, but also can
be useful for supervisors in dealing with their own propensity to burn
out.

The content of this chapter is not intended as a substitute for medical treatment
of physical or psychological symptoms. When such symptoms occur, medical
advice should be sought.

INTRODUCTION

The idea of distress associated with the helping-oriented professions was identified almost a century ago:

> He who carries self-regard far enough to keep himself in good health and high spirits, in the first place, thereby becomes an immediate source of happiness to those around, and, in the second place, maintains the ability to increase their happiness by altruistic actions. But one whose bodily vigor and mental health are undermined by self-sacrifice carried too far, in the first place becomes to those around a cause of depression, and, in the second place, renders himself incapable, or less capable, of actively furthering their welfare. (Spencer, 1902:223)

So much for the idea that stress is a recent phenomenon. In more modern terms, Hans Selye, the famous stress researcher, stated, "My own code is based on the view that to achieve peace of mind and fulfillment through self-expression, most men need a commitment to work in the service of some cause that they can respect" (Selye, 1974:4). Before reading the vast literature that now exists on the concept of stress, supervisors and supervisees should read Selye's little book, *Stress Without Distress*. Selye is considered the earliest scientist to develop a perspective on stress from a biological point of view while taking into account its psychological ramifications. Selye's work is so important because he identifies the overall origins of stress, its manifestations, and ways of combating it in a general sense.

RESEARCH ON STRESS AMONG SOCIAL WORKERS

The empirical research on distress among social workers is in the early stages of development. The few data-based studies have produced interesting, but sometimes confusing, results. Reiter (1980), in a study of clinical social workers, found that 46 percent would not choose social work as a career if they had it to do over. This is interesting in light of the view that jobs and professions in our society have always been sex-typed and since social work has traditionally been considered a woman's profession (82 percent of the respondents in Reiter's study were women). Since socialization processes prepare people for these roles in conscious and unconscious ways (Pogrebin, 1980:535), the consciousness raising of the feminist movement could be the source of this regretted career choice, or it could be the result of unfulfilled expectations and job-related distress.

Further research should provide answers to such questions. Regardless of these issues, Reiter raises an important question that is significant for supervision and practice distress:

> The data strongly suggest . . . that an impressive number of social workers who have responsibility for overseeing the training of other workers are regretful of their own career choice. Whether or not that regret translates into negative feelings of professional identity that are transmitted to the supervisee is a matter for speculation. It does not seem unreasonable . . . to assume that these feelings might emerge in ways that could hinder not only the supervisory process but the professional identity of the less experienced worker. (1980:204)

Reiter did not study distress among practitioners directly, but a study by Bissell and colleagues (1980) did. Data were collected from 50 alcoholic social workers who had been free of alcohol abuse for at least a year. The researchers reported that in spite of a combined incidence of 63 arrests, 120 inpatient admissions, 13 suicide attempts, and reported addiction to alcohol and other drugs, colleagues, supervisors, and therapists who treated them were "extremely reluctant to confront the alcoholism directly." Some participants reported that they did not approach their supervisors because the supervisor was denying that a problem existed. The social workers reported suicide attempts at twice the rate that physicians did, but at slightly lower than the rate reported by nurses. This could be a reflection of the gender difference in the professions and the fact that in the total population more females attempt suicide than males (although males are three times more successful at it) (Pogrebin, 1980:75).

What is startling about this study is the failure of the supervisors and colleagues to assist these professionals who were giving clear indications that they needed help. Perhaps these people represent the hardest ones to reach, but we do need to discuss more openly how to address these serious forms of impaired functioning when they become apparent. Supervisors cannot afford to overlook such serious problems.

The question remains: How widespread are these serious problems of distress in the profession? Two recent studies offer some perspective on this. Streepy (1981) surveyed 108 practitioners in 12 family service agencies. Over 75 percent of the respondents found job satisfactions greater than the frustrations, and very few workers were considering a job change. Stress as manifested through physical and psychological symptoms was at a very low level. The findings revealed that stress was higher when family income was low, education level was low, attitudes toward the profession were low, and work experience was low. Stress showed no correlation with type of experience, sex, or job satisfaction. It was the inexperienced, poorly trained workers who experienced the highest levels of distress, but overall, stress was not widespread among these workers.

A study of 180 practitioners and supervisors in a public welfare setting (Munson, 1982) revealed that 72 percent reported having experienced stress, and almost all reported going through cycles of stress. Physical symptoms such as headaches, persistent colds, and gastrointestinal upsets were reported by 43 percent of the group, and 37 percent reported psychological symptoms such as anxiety, depression, and inability to sleep. Even though these high levels of cycles of stress were reported, 86 percent of the participants stated that they were satisfied with their jobs and the agency. That money is not the total solution to stress is reflected in the fact that the overwhelming majority of people who leave high-risk, successful careers do so to enter low-paying service occupations. A commitment to help others and to make a contribution to society is an important factor in life satisfaction that rarely gets discussed openly. It could be that such psychological needs account for the fact that many people have high levels of distress in their jobs, but at the same time feel their agency is all in all a pretty good place to work. Writers have pointed out that child welfare service workers and supervisors are highly stressed (Daley, 1979; Harrison, 1980; Zischka, 1981). My research showed child welfare workers did not show any significantly higher levels of stress than other service areas. (See summary of this study in Chapter 1.)

STUDENTS AND STRESS

Stress among professional social workers has been a focus of increased concern during the past several years, but there has been no parallel study of stress among graduate social work students. In one of the first attempts to study stress among students, I administered a 75-item questionnaire to a random sample of 82 first- and second-year graduate students in a large, urban university (Munson, Study E). The variables under study were clustered in areas of demographics, physical symptoms, psychological symptoms, field-placement satisfaction, and supervisory satisfaction.

The findings revealed that physical and psychological stress were at very low levels for the total group. Respondents did identify that they experienced more physical and psychological stress associated with classroom work than with field work. No major differences were found in stress symptoms for men and women, for first- and second-year students, or on the basis of marital status. In general, satisfaction with supervision did not produce any significant correlations with physical or psychological stress, but specific supervisory interaction variables (friendliness, openness, and putting the student at ease) did produce moderately significant correlations with certain physical symptoms (frequency of colds, headaches, and GI upset). Number of years social work experience prior to entering graduate school showed no significant correlations with physical symptoms. In general, the respondents were satisfied with their supervision and their agency placements. These supervisory and agency satisfaction levels appear to contribute to low levels of stress among students and to help prevent depersonalization of clients. The study lends support to the notion that supervision is important to preventing burnout.

As this brief survey of the research reveals, there are many unanswered questions and mixed findings about practitioner distress. The supervisor's responsibility is to know the manifestations, help workers recognize their reactions, and support them in dealing with them. Although the research findings vary regarding the extent of distress, the supervisor must look upon each practitioner as unique and be ready to assist him or her at the earliest signs of stress.

SUPERVISION AND STRESS

As with many things, supervision can work for or against practitioners in dealing with stress. Many workers identify supervisors as offering little help for distress, and in many cases supervisors contribute to intensifying it (Edelwich & Brodsky, 1980). At the same time, workers involved in my research have identified good, supportive supervisors as the main source of help in dealing with stress. Given this information, it is surprising how little most supervisors know about distress, its causes, its manifestations, its cures. Without serious study of distress, supervisors become instant experts with instant advice, and when such quickly devised, simplistic solutions do not work, workers can become more distressed. In the worst possible situation, the worker can be assigned a formerly distressed worker as a supervisor.

Distress or burnout is not always a gradual, downhill process. My research showed that burnout occurred in cyclical patterns in the majority of workers. Little is known about how these cycles occur, their duration, or what causes them to subside. Also, the research demonstrated that practitioners experience distress differently. Some complain almost exclusively of physical symptoms, others experience mainly psychological reactions, and still others undergo a combination of the two.

We do not know what causes different workers to gravitate to one pattern of reaction. It could be preexisting personality or physical variables. It could be something specific to the work setting itself. For example, in medical settings some workers develop imaginary illnesses that mimic diseases treated in the setting (e.g., cancer, depression, heart disease). It could also be a reaction to comments the supervisor makes or behavior the supervisor manifests. As discussed in Chapter 5, practitioners form reactions to their supervisors, and if workers are exposed to supervisors who are manifesting distress, it is easy for the supervisees to follow the same pattern.

SUPERVISOR STRESS

Supervisors who are in distress have a responsibility to seek help for it, but they should avoid seeking relief through their supervisees, and they have a responsibility to avoid exposing supervisees to their own burnout. Just as practitioners should not seek solace from their clients, supervisors should not seek solace from their supervisees. Just as supervisees can become overly involved with their clients, supervisors can become overly involved with their supervisees. Supervisors can become too close personally and socially with their supervisees, so that their authority and competence are eroded. Supervisors can become overly involved professionally with their supervisees and overly directive of their cases to the point that they are perceived as meddling, which results in conflict and frustration. The supervisor must be alert to the potential for such overinvolvement, and this is most likely to occur where the supervisor has no equal or consultant with whom to share supervisory concerns. The supervisor should recognize that supervisees need some differential role model to whom to relate. The supervisor is best perceived as a more experienced, more skilled, more knowledgeable source of assistance.

Only recently has concern emerged over the importance of providing support groups for supervisors (Hamlin & Timberlake, 1982). As practice becomes more sophisticated and practice demands become more complex, more consideration will have to be given to providing such supports for supervisors. Supervisors will need to be alert to their own potential for distress if they are to be effective in assisting the practitioners they supervise. Supervisors are often placed in the same bind with supervisees as the **supervisees are with their clients. The supervisor is often called upon to** take unpopular stands with their supervisees in order to help them. For example, Wolman has pointed out:

Quite often, younger colleagues came to me for supervisory sessions with a glowing feeling of success because their patients expressed love and admiration for them. The beginning practitioners often take the expression of transference love as a sign of therapeutic success. (1976:16)

Under these circumstances, to be helpful the supervisor must dissuade the practitioner regarding such illusions of power. This can result in the supervisor's being accused of trying to turn affection into cynicism, but in order to genuinely enhance the treatment, the supervisor must aid the supervisee in being more realistic about the therapeutic interaction. The supervisor must face this issue at the onset so the supervisee avoids being set up for frustration and a sense of failure when the client eventually becomes angry and resentful. It is difficult for the supervisor to be the carrier of such news, but it is often the basis of helpful supervision. When supervisors fail to recognize the importance of this aspect of their role, it can gradually lead to supervisor distress and alienation from supervisees.

ROLE OF SUPPORT

The mere passage of time in the same demanding practice position and a heavy workload are bound to catch up with the worker and can result in distress. Recognition of this basic combination of factors by the supervisor can be one of the chief safeguards against being overwhelmed by distress in practice. A practitioner who is struggling to combat distress can be tumbled into a full-blown episode of distress if support is unavailable. A client who commits suicide, a family that is liked by the practitioner but that angrily withdraws from treatment and blames the worker, or an alcoholic who returns to a bout of heavy drinking are examples of such distress-precipitating events. Supervisors must be alert to such events and provide a supportive environment that gives practitioners the opportunity to articulate and work through their anger, frustration, guilt, sense of failure, or other strong reactions they may have to perceived responsibility for unsuccessful outcomes.

The word burnout has gained popular usage as a catchall phrase, but it is not descriptive of what most people undergo. Burnout implies a final state, something that has been reduced to ashes, rubble. My research shows that workers' responses to pressure is cyclical. Perhaps we should ask the question: Is there life after burnout for supervisors and supervisees? I believe the answer to this question is: Yes, there is life after burnout, and often it is a more realistic and effective existence if the stress is recognized and dealt with appropriately. Therefore, the following sections can be used by both supervisors and supervisees in understanding and combating burnout.

GENERAL PRINCIPLES

Selye makes a distinction between stress and distress.[1] Stress "is the nonspecific response of the body to any demand made upon it," it can be pleasant or unpleasant, and it is not necessarily something to be avoided. Physical activity produces stress, but it is not necessarily damaging. Damaging or unpleasant stress is distress. Stress is not a unitary entity, but is made up of a set of stressors that can be of various types and various origins. When stress is cumulative or the number of stressors is too great, the result eventually is distress. When the stressors are withdrawn, the more normal biological and psychological state is reestablished.

Selye has identified a process of reacting to stress that he has labeled the general adaptation syndrome (GAS). There are three stages in this syndrome:

1. alarm reaction
2. stage of resistance
3. stage of exhaustion.

In the first stage there is recognition that something is wrong, and in the second stage, the person offers resistance to the stressor. If the stressor is continually applied and not withdrawn, the person will eventually reach a stage of exhaustion. It is this stage with which the term burnout is associated. From this it can be seen that burnout, as we normally view it, is only one part of a three-stage process. Distress is usually reflected through our weakest psychological and physiological points.

Job-related distress is considered quite common, and few workers are viewed as immune to it. There is no unified definition for "burnout" or job distress. Generally, it can be defined as "to deplete oneself, to exhaust one's physical and mental resources, to wear oneself out by excessively striving to reach some very high expectations" (Freudenberger, 1977:90).

---

1. Selye's basic formulations about stress and distress are the foundation of much of the content of this chapter.

Source of Expectations

High and unrealistic expectations of self and clients are held to be a primary source of distress. Unrealistic expectations are believed to take two forms: internal and external. According to some writers, practitioners are more susceptible to internal or self-imposed unrealistic expectations, and welfare workers are more susceptible to external-societally or bureaucratically imposed—unrealistic expectations. However, during my research with child welfare workers, it was discovered that they underwent internal forms of burnout as much as they did the external forms (Munson, Study D). Thus, it is still an open question just what form certain groups undergo or whether different practice settings produce a mixture of the two forms.

To illustrate this point, the following excerpt from an interview with a child welfare worker who experienced burnout is fairly typical:

RESEARCHER: Some of the research that has been done on burn-out identifies the sources of stress as being in some cases internal—that is, the person places too many demands on herself—as opposed to external—where not enough resources are available to complete the job. Which type of burnout do you think you predominantly had, or did you have both?

WORKER: I think I definitely predominantly had the internal form of burnout because I think I did put a lot of demands on myself, and I think that was probably my biggest problem—that I wasn't able to separate emotionally enough from my clients. I got too involved and felt responsible for their whole lives, which is impossible to do and really be effective. I think you have to be able to shut off your work life at the end of your day and go home and have something else to do. I think I really carried the burden, felt real responsible for everybody, which is really not good.

RESEARCHER: Do you think you have a different attitude about that now?

WORKER: I think I do. I think right now I am able to separate it more. I think it is just something you have to realize. You have to still be compassionate and get involved with the problems, but you have to know that a lot of it is dependent on the client. They are responsible for their own lives. You can only go so far.

Whether excessively high, unrealistic expectations are internal or external in origin, it is most likely that they occur as a result of values and beliefs we adopt based on a belief in hard work, doing good for others, and the importance of being dedicated to any task we take on.

Process of Stress Reactions

Because of belief systems which we adopt and which surround us, we resist admitting that we are experiencing distress. In the work setting, this would be the practical equivalent to Selye's stage of resistance (Selye, 1974). The practitioner is unable or unwilling to admit that a problem with his or her functioning exists. This is a gradual process that can come and go over a long period of time. In the first stage the person recognizes that something is wrong, but he or she does not know what it is. Selye's alarm reaction manifests itself as anxiety and depression, which is usually focused on something or someone else.

The development of distress is not always as clear as the literature would have us believe, and this gradualness of distress makes the supervisor's job more difficult. The comment of one worker illustrates this point.

> Now that I look back on it, I went through several periods of burnout, but I didn't realize it at the time. In the past 20 years, I have had three prolonged periods of burnout. At the height of each one I changed jobs. I thought at the time that I was doing it to get ahead. Now I know there were other factors of boredom involved. It took three to four years for it to develop. At times I would tell myself that it was nothing. It was a natural reaction. I was just a little depressed. I can't tell you any point . . . where it started or when it first began to show. I just know that the result was that I was miserable for a long time, and I thought it was something that somebody was doing to me.
>
> The breakthrough came when I realized I was doing it to myself. I did all the other things you are supposed to do — jogging, diet, attitude change, etc. — until I came to the realization that I could control this, and I was not being controlled by others. To explain what I have been through and to explain the solution to someone else is very, very difficult to do.

Selye's third stage is exhaustion. In this stage the practitioner continues to function, but coping mechanisms are depleted. The person undergoes disorganization to the point that even though he or she might work harder, the person actually accomplishes less. There is no sense of reward from work, and cynicism toward clients is common. The worker can become immobilized and develop disillusionment to the point that he or she feels the whole world is dysfunctional. The worker goes through the motions of working with clients without any commitment to the belief that intervention will do any good. This attitude becomes self-defeating and self-fulfilling because clients can sense the practitioner's sense of hopelessness. A research interview with a former child welfare worker illustrates this point.

RESEARCHER: How did you know you were burned out?

WORKER: I think that probably it was just the feeling of being emotionally exhausted and actually not wanting to see the problems rather than delving into them and looking for them, wanting to gloss over things. Actually, just feeling exhausted, feeling like you have given all of your emotions up, and drained.

RESEARCHER: So when you would come home from work at the end of the day, how would you feel?

WORKER: I think child welfare really messes up your private life. I think your whole life becomes child welfare, or it did for me anyway, for a while. You sort of lose your perspective on things, like that is your whole world. You come home, and you're exhausted, and you don't have a lot to give other people, friends, and family.

RESEARCHER: How about in other workers? Could you see burnout in them?

WORKER: I think people that I saw generally became cynical, and I think it is just from the pressures of the job, of seeing so much, and feeling also inadequate to deal with a lot of it. You could see the problems, but you didn't know how to help them. A lot of times it was impossible to really make any changes, and so I think it varies from person to person because I think there are ways of dealing with it, and I even think there are probably some people that go through periods of burnout and then maybe are effective again.

I don't think it is necessarily a continuous thing, but I would think that after a couple of years that that is when most people start to burn out. I think people come in, and they are very idealistic, and they **really feel good** about their job, and they feel they are doing things, and gradually they see that a lot of their clients just don't cooperate. I think they start feeling like maybe they aren't making as many changes as they thought they would. They sort of lose their positiveness about the job, and that is when they start burning out; just maybe doing enough to get by.

And, also, I don't know if it is really all the clients, but a lot of it, I think, is administrative problems within the agency, since it is such a large organization. A lot of it does depend on the supervisor. But one supervisor in particular that I had, her whole attitude was, "If you don't like it, get out," which doesn't create real positive feelings, doesn't make you feel real good about how worthwhile you are, how good the job is, when, if you have a problem you can't discuss it, you are just told if you don't like it, leave. And that was just her general attitude with everyone.

Behavioral Indicators

The supervisor must recognize that each practitioner will have a unique way of dealing with stress. In assessing burnout the behavior gauge should not be comparing a given practitioner to other practitioners, but comparing the worker to his or her own past performance record. Since distress is a result of stages, the worker's previous performance will be the best indicator of changes in functioning. To compare the worker to others can increase the worker's distress.

Behavioral indicators usually take three forms: interactional, psychological, and physical.

Interactional. The earliest signs occur in relation to clients but are not easily observable by the supervisor because the supervisor has little contact with the practitioner in this area. This is one of the reasons it is so important that the supervisor observe and participate in the worker's practice periodically.

When dealing with clients, the worker's interactional indicators are loss of interest, inattentiveness, forgetfulness, cutting off exploration with clients, and cutting sessions short. There is a tendency to become impatient with clients and to become angry when they do not respond in ways the practitioner desires.

The more apparent interactional elements occur in relation to coworkers, supervisors, and administrators. A normally pleasant, sociable worker becomes withdrawn. Phone messages, messages, and memos are not responded to. The quiet, retiring practitioner can become argumentative and obstinate. The worker avoids the supervisor or is constantly challenging the supervisor's authority and actions. When such changes in the practitioner's relationship with others occur, the supervisor has a key indicator that a stress reaction is taking place. Coworkers will often comment to the supervisor about changes in the practitioner.

The worker's interaction with others outside the work setting is usually altered. Friends and relatives detect changes, but the supervisor is not usually aware of these changes. Marital problems can develop, and some have attributed divorce to work-related stress, but this is speculation since there is no reliable information available to determine whether, in fact, the divorce rate is higher in the helping professions than it is in the population as a whole.

Psychological. Depression and anger are common reactions. Such work-related psychological changes are very hard to distinguish from reactions originating from personal problems. General depression can be confused with work distress (Bramhall & Ezell, 1981a:23). When depression is a factor in the practitioner's functioning, the supervisor must explore the origins with the person. The worker can develop cynical attitudes toward clients and become callous about clients and their motivations. Supervision can come to be viewed as harassment rather than a source of help. Negative attitudes toward administrators emerge.

Some workers manifest rapid mood changes. Suspiciousness and feelings of isolation are accompanied by a loss of sense of humor. The practitioner questions his or her ability to help others and talks of regret about his or her career choice. There is a tendency to lose interest in others and to express a sense of uncaring attitudes on the part of others. There can be a decrease in willingness to assume new roles and expressions of hopelessness and futility about agency functioning.

Physical. Physical symptoms can be quite diverse and are caused by various factors. As with psychological symptoms, the supervisor and the practitioner should be very cautious about attributing physical symptoms to job-related stress. Where physical symptoms that are due to organic causes are blamed on job stress, the person might be engaging in denial that could result in serious damage to physical health. When the practitioner raises the issue of physical symptoms in supervision, the supervisor should encourage the person to see a physician.

While almost all writers on stress provide long lists of physical symptoms that can be associated with job stress, studies I have carried out in several settings reveal that fairly low levels of physical symptoms were reported overall, and there was a low incidence rate attributing these symptoms to job-related stress (Munson, Study D).

Given these findings, it is suggested that the supervisor consider the interactional patterns and psychological reactions primarily in assessing the worker's behavior and performance over time to detect reactions to job stress. While physical symptoms might be identified, the supervisor's role should be limited to suggesting medical evaluation. In reviewing worker behavior, the supervisor should remember that individuals will respond differently to the same amount of stress. Burnout can be manifested in a variety of forms. Each individual needs to identify the ways in which he or she reacts to stress. Also, if a person has just a few of these reactions, but the reactions are exaggerated and affect functioning, an assessment should be done to determine if the worker is experiencing distress. Once stress reactions are identified, one can begin to deal with them.

Another excerpt from the interview with the former child welfare worker will illustrate some of the points that have just been made:

RESEARCHER: How did you actually behave in relation to burning out? What were the kinds of things you felt, the kind of things that actually happened to you behaviorally?

WORKER: On the job or personally?

RESEARCHER: Both, because I don't think we can separate the two, can we?

WORKER: Well, I know I felt burned out. I think I just really wasn't as effective. I think I did what I had to to get by, and just really didn't feel good about the job I was doing—about myself, maybe.

RESEARCHER: How did you feel when you came home at the end of the day?

WORKER: Pretty exhausted. I think most of the time I was pretty exhausted, maybe even more so in the beginning, because I was more involved with my clients, and so when you came home, you were just exhausted and felt your whole life was your work, and towards the end maybe I was putting less into it, so in some ways my personal life improved, but my professional life wasn't real good. [Pause.]

I think there is a real high divorce rate. All the people I knew, most of them were single, a lot of them were divorced. I think that is a real hazard of the occupation.

RESEARCHER: How about drinking? I think a lot of people turn to alcohol or drugs.

WORKER: Definitely there is an active happy hour group—every agency that I worked in.

RESEARCHER: But yet that didn't seem to relieve the tension even though it was maybe designed for that?

WORKER: Actually in some ways I am sure it did relieve it because we were able to sit and complain about things and work out some feelings—but that only goes so far. I think there are a lot of other things that attribute to your feelings of stress, and I think a lot of it is probably, or some of it anyway, is the administrative attitude that—there is a general feeling sometimes—that if you stay too long in maybe any agency in one position, you're probably not an effective person, that you've stagnated, so I just think there is an overall feeling that unless you are constantly moving that you're not really a great worker, and you start taking some of those feelings in about yourself and your job, and you lose some of your effectiveness.

CONTRIBUTING FACTORS

The interview segments illustrate that burnout is a reaction to job related stress that can result in high rates of turnover and decreased effectiveness. Job-related stress is not caused by a simple, single stimulus, but rather by objects, emotions, and personal interactions that make up a series of contributing factors. Daley (1979) has identified four sources of stress that can be contributing factors to distress: barriers to achieving goals, poor and uncomfortable working conditions, incompatible demands, and ambiguous role expectations. For example, those seeking social work careers place value on working with people. However, Daley reports that workers in protective services spend as little as 25 percent of their time in direct contact with clients. Time is spent instead transporting clients, completing forms, keeping case records, and attending staff meetings (Daley, 1979:377). Other contributing factors are large caseloads, arbitrary deadlines, and workers being prevented from seeing a case through to completion.

In many settings the worker is attacked by the community whether he or she does or does not take action. Workers are frequently not given support by supervisors and administrators for decisions the workers make. Practitioners are often criticized by their own clients if they side with certain family members on an issue, while at the same time if they refuse to take a stand, they are criticized for being unconcerned and uncaring. Even the professional literature is contradictory about what to do in many of these situations. Practitioners frequently see their own behavior patterns reflected in clients. Many clients present problems for which there are no clear intervention strategies designed to deal with them. These and other factors can mount up on the practitioner. When such frustrations accumulate, the manifestations of distress covered in a previous section can result.

DEALING WITH STRESS

Ultimately, the practitioner is the only person who can overcome stress reactions. Most of the external contributing factors mentioned above will not change. Many organizational problems and high caseload demands are persistent factors. The critical variable is how the practitioner perceives and adapts to these conditions. The following suggestions are based on the literature and practitioners' observations from my own studies on stress.

Insight. The practitioner, with support from the supervisor, must gain insight into his or her own behavior and how he or she handles stress. It is easy for the practitioner to give up on himself or herself, to say, "I'm not worthy; I can't cope; why bother to try." Until the person finds that such an attitude is unacceptable, little can be done to change the situation. The practitioner has to develop self-confidence, make a commitment to doing the best job he or she can, and accept the limitations within himself or herself, his or her clients, and the organization. Self-awareness and insight are only a beginning. The practitioner has to work hard at maintaining a positive attitude. Minor setbacks should be accepted and not allowed to trigger a pervasive fatalistic view. Workers have commented that this form of mental self-regulation is essential to combating a cycle of stress.

Exploration. The practitioner needs to discuss his or her feelings and reactions with others, especially the supervisor. Withdrawal and internalizing feelings only increase distress.

Defining the situation. Exploration with others should not be focused exclusively on complaints. The discussion needs to be aimed at how to overcome the problems or how to adjust to the situation. The problems should be viewed as situational and not ingrained in personalities. The concern should be how to alter or manipulate this situation to produce a positive outcome. It is important to recognize that practitioners need to work within the parameters of the organization. There needs to be acceptance of the givens in the situation and concentration on the factors that can be changed. Organizations cannot be expected to be rational, and the worker should not attempt to make the organization rational. Instead, there should be acceptance of responsibility for only what the practitioner can control.

The environment. The work setting in many agencies leaves much to be desired. Practitioners can take some action to create the best possible environment for themselves and their clients. The addition of plants, pictures on the wall, lamps, and small radios can improve office appearance. The worker can request that the walls be painted, and that bookshelves and rugs be added improve office appearance.

Education. The worker should seek education and training. The practitioner should identify areas of his or her work that cause the most difficulty and request training that will help him or her overcome these problems. Self-confidence can be greatly enhanced when the worker successfully helps a client using some technique or method learned in a training seminar. If the worker desires to advance in the agency, he or she should learn what education he or she needs to achieve this goal and work toward it. The worker who has long-range goals has little time to engage in self-pity and despair.

Developing outside interests. The worker needs to develop boundaries on work time and use his or her own time to develop outside interests. Work diversions such as drug use, heavy drinking, and gambling merely add to the worker's problem. Hobbies, recreation, physical exercise, and various other activities can serve as healthy outlets. Such activities do not have to be limited to nights and weekends. A lunch period can be used to pursue some interests. Vacations can be planned in advance, and the activities of planning a vacation can be a wholesome diversion from work.

Any activity that keeps the worker focused on future goals and activities decreases the opportunity to dwell on present problems and past failures. In selecting outside activities, the worker needs to be careful to avoid activities that can increase stress. For a more detailed discussion on how to select helpful activities, the reader should see the section in this chapter titled "Distress and Recreation."

Career reorientation. If the worker suffers prolonged job stress, and all corrective efforts fail, serious consideration should be given to a career change. Such decisions should not be made hastily, but continuation in an unrewarding career can result in long-term frustrations that can influence all aspects of a person's life.

Although it is sometimes good for some people to change careers, it is tragic when practitioners with potential leave the profession because of their association with severely distressed supervisors. One practitioner's decision is reflected in her comments:

Another major obstacle is my supervisor, who is experiencing burn-out. My supervisor has gone through all the stages of burnout, and he is stuck in the exhaustion stage. I don't know if he sees it and knows it, but I do. He is in a double bind. On one hand, he enjoys his work with the patients, but on the other hand, he is frustrated by low pay, low status, and the agency system. The result of my supervisor's negative feelings toward himself, his job, and his role as a social worker has affected the quality of my supervision and my perception of the social work profession. My desire to continue to work in the field of social work has decreased. I have accepted a job outside the field of social work. It is a job in industry doing personnel work. I decided to take this job because of the pay, learning experience, and the opportunity for growth.

THE SUPERVISOR'S ROLE

All of the self-corrective efforts for the supervisee mentioned in the previous section can be supported by the supervisor. The supervisor must work to create the conditions that facilitate the worker's efforts. If the supervisor does not assume a supportive role, he or she becomes another contributing factor to the practitioner's distress. There are some other general principles the supervisor can follow in assisting supervisees.

Facilitating insight. While the practitioner is the only person who can achieve insight into his or her burnout and its control, the supervisor can foster development of insight through encouraging discussion of the problem. This can be done in individual supervision as well as through group sessions in which feelings and attitudes are explored openly. Such discussions should not be allowed to become quasi therapy for the practitioners or mere gripe sessions, which tend to increase frustration.

The supervisor has a responsibility to keep the discussion focused on job-related issues and on defining the work situation. The supervisor should listen and make suggestions that will help practitioners to gain insight and to find their own solutions. When the supervisor gives direct advice or tells workers what to do, anger on the part of the workers is likely to result. The supervisees must be approached in a non-threatening manner to avoid alienating them or producing feelings of guilt and failure. The practice of telling supervisees how the supervisor solved his or her own burnout should be used with caution, since what worked for the supervisor may not necessarily be a solution for the worker.

The environment. The supervisor should work to create the best possible work environment for practitioners. When supervisees make requests for office equipment and decorations, the supervisor has a responsibility to support reasonable requests. When supervisors fail to take such requests seriously and fail to follow through with them, they lose credibility in the eyes of the workers. It is not valid to expect that all requests will be approved, but the supervisor has an obligation to present reasonable requests to administrators who control and plan budgets.

Education. The supervisor has a key role in promoting education and training for supervisees. The importance of education and training should not be underestimated since there is research indicating that the more highly trained the practitioner, the less likely he or she is to experience stress (Streepy, 1981). The supervisor has a responsibility to monitor training to ensure that workers are getting the type of training they need. Workers who are subjected to mandatory training or even voluntary training that does not help them cope with their work become frustrated and resentful.

An educational plan should be developed for each worker, and the supervisor should evaluate with the worker each seminar or course he or she attends. The supervisor should encourage the worker to discuss career goals and what education and training he or she needs to achieve these goals. The supervisor must survey the worker's educational needs and advocate training that meets these needs.

Role model. One of the best ways the supervisor can help supervisees deal with job distress is to serve as an effective role model. Practitioners develop many of their attitudes and behaviors from the relationship they have with their supervisors. Through positive attitudes and demonstration of effective work habits, the supervisor can indirectly convey to workers many strategies for combating stress. The practices advocated in this book are designed to foster positive performance by the supervisor.

UNANSWERED QUESTIONS

There are many unanswered issues about stress. For example, why is it a serious problem? Why was it not identified as a problem earlier? There is evidence that caseworkers at the turn of the century underwent stress, so that this is not a new phenomenon, but it is coming to our attention more and more.

What about our society generates so much stress? It could be such things as high mobility, rapid change, urbanization, affluence, increased bureaucracy, increased mechanization, and professionalization of charity. For many practitioners, burnout could be the result of stress associated with conflicting moral demands in practice rather than overwhelming work loads or inadequate resources.

Some feel that stress could be a positive indicator, reflecting the fact that society is working harder to solve its ills. The real challenge is not stress, they say, but the societal ills that promote it — poverty, crime, drug addiction, juvenile delinquency, mental illness, alcoholism, child abuse, aging, terminal illness, to mention just a few of the factors that can go to make up a long list (Chance, 1981:94-95).

Keep in mind that the best practitioners may experience stress at different times in their careers. What really counts is how we deal with it.

Distress and Recreation

It has been a common practice to encourage workers to deal with distress by engaging in recreational activities. This general advice can be counterproductive. For example, people who burn out have been identified as hard working, committed, high achievers. When such people are encouraged to take up recreational sports, they often select high activity, heavily competitive sports such as tennis, racquet ball, basketball, and handball. When people seek these activities for recreation, more distress can result as they strive to be the best. If workers select sports activities for which they are not suited, instead of becoming a source of relaxation, the activity can be the cause of additional stress. High achievers tend to turn everything into work, so that a highly stressed worker who turns to a sport and takes it too seriously could be compounding his or her problems.

Since our schools encourage and support competitive sports, people naturally turn to them when they decide to take up recreational sports. The supervisor should assist the worker with this because many workers are not aware of the harm they can do to themselves by selecting the wrong recreational activity. For example, watching television or attending movies for relaxation can in fact increase tension. Much television and film content today focuses on social commentary and social problems; even comedy and variety shows have become problem focused. Stress is even portrayed as entertainment on many television shows. Many documentary television shows highlight content that can intensify feelings of burnout. The individual is portrayed as helpless, a pawn, a victim in mass society controlled by giant, impersonal, uncontrollable institutions. Little is known about people's responses to prolonged exposure to such television content.

There is some research evidence that people do have immediate mood changes associated with watching distressing news programming (Munson, 1974), but we do not know the long-term effects of such television content. The dynamics of contagion associated with stress reactions can be identified among staff in agencies, but the contagion effect through television, movies, magazines, and books remains unexplored. Practitioners who use television, movies, or books as relaxation can be in for another barrage of the problems they see and hear about in their work all day. In many psychotherapy education programs (Fritz & Poe, 1979) and in schools of social work, cinema and literature are increasingly being used to train practitioners. This can lead the practitioner unconsciously to analyze movies and books from a professional point of view rather than seeing them as entertainment.

Leisure Activity Guidelines

Given this information, can one gain any relaxation and relief from television, movies, sports, or books? Yes, but one should answer the following questions to ensure that one is engaging in leisure activities for the purpose of leisure.

1. Am I doing this because I want to do it? For example, am I playing tennis because I want to or because it is the fad in the neighborhood? Am I going to this movie because I want to or because a friend wants to go? Am I reading this book because I want to or because I want to appear informed at the book club meeting?
2. Am I physically and psychologically suited to the leisure activity I have selected? For example, sports such as tennis and basketball require good eye/hand coordination, mental anticipation of your opponent, and physical stamina. Chess, on the other hand, requires much mental anticipation of your opponent without the physical requirements of tennis. Baseball involves one in a team effort that is much different from a single-opponent sport.
3. Does this activity truly give me pleasure while I am doing it? If you play on a baseball team for leisure, and you are constantly angered by the errors and failures of your teammates, you are probably not getting much relaxation.
4. When I complete the activity, do I feel good? If you play backgammon for leisure and you pick a partner who constantly defeats you and, after a series of games, you are planning how to get even, the goal of the leisure activity has been defeated.
5. Has the activity become a chore for me? If you find yourself relieved

because the tennis match has been cancelled because of rain, there is a good chance that your recreation has become work.

6. Am I investing too much time in one form of leisure activity? If a recreational activity is consuming too much of your time and taking away from other pursuits, it is no longer leisure. The person addicted to jogging is a current common example of this. Leisure researchers recommend that for the best results, one should engage in several leisure activities rather then focusing on one.

SUPERVISOR TRAINING

Supervisors should be well educated about stress since it has been identified as having such a high risk potential in many agencies. Training programs for supervisors should include content that assists them in identifying it and helping practitioners deal with it. When training is not provided to supervisors, they should take it upon themselves to learn about it. The suggested readings at the end of the chapter are a good starting point.

A key conceptualization the supervisor should keep in mind is that stress, practice demands, and coping strategies are interrelated. Practitioners who have a large number of coping strategies to use in relation to practice demands will experience less stress. It is the supervisor's job to help the worker develop as many coping strategies as possible and to work to keep the practice demands in reasonable relationship with the coping strategies. This is illustrated in Visual 10.1 through depiction of the desired and undesired states when considering these three factors. Most of the content of this book is designed to increase the coping strategies of both the practitioner and the supervisor.

DESPAIR AND ISOLATION

The chief function of the supervisor is to translate activity into practice, but another important function is to prevent the isolation of the practitioner. This covert function has been practiced but unrecognized for decades. To avoid being overwhelmed, becoming frustrated, undergoing moderate chronic depression, and becoming callous toward clients, the practitioner must maintain a wholesome contact with colleagues.

The demands placed on practitioners in their role with clients can be devastating and produce gradual, chronic, and sometimes permanent changes in therapeutic activity and personality of the practitioner. Practitioners themselves are usually the last to recognize or admit these

VISUAL 10.1. Coping Strategies, Practice Demands, and Stress

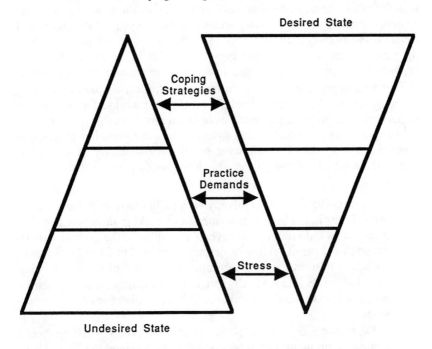

changes. The more serious the mental illnesses the practitioner treats, the greater the potential for therapeutic despair. Farber has identified this phenomenon in work with schizophrenic patients as the peculiar and painful nature of therapeutic life that produces "emptiness, meaninglessness, lack of confirmation—in short the circumstances that lead to a particular despair on the part of the therapist and that may subsequently evoke in the patient a response of pity for his doctor's plight." It is Farber's contention that this despair "is more or less intrinsic to the therapeutic life with schizophrenia and that such despair, moreover, if acknowledged rather than disowned, if contended with rather than evaded, *might* (the word is important) have a salutary effect on therapy" (Boyers, 1971:90).

Skillful recognition and articulation by the supervisor are required for such practitioner reactions to be managed positively for the benefit of the practitioner and the therapy. The supervisor must help the worker recognize what is taking place and aid in developing ways to manage and use it in the treatment. In exploring this process with practitioners, supervisors can gain insight into their own practice and use their own experience to help the practitioner. In dealing with such material, the supervisor can use a combination of the supervisory styles of *philosophical abstractions* and *technical strategies*. Philosophical abstractions are useful in identifying the process, and technical strategies are helpful in designing means of capitalizing on practitioner despair to assist in the client recovery process.

There are degrees and varying forms of practitioner despair, depending on the types of clients with whom the practitioner works. The supervisor needs to be alert to particular patterns of client problems that occur repeatedly in the worker's practice and give rise to a constellation of despair-producing symptoms. The following practitioner summary of a supervisory session illustrates the point that is being made here:

> I was doing this group therapy with eight outpatients from a state mental hospital. The group seemed to be making little progress as a group or as individuals. On several occasions in the group I experienced this wave of feeling of despair. It is hard to describe. I would withdraw into myself in the group. I was aware of what was being said, but it was like I wasn't there at the same time. It mildly scared me, and I was reluctant to talk about it with colleagues or my supervisor.
>
> On two occasions I felt like adjourning the group by telling them I couldn't help them, and it was pointless to continue meeting. These two instances occurred at times when feelings of depression were at high levels of expression in the group. During a supervisory session, my supervisor asked how the group was going. I don't know if he detected something was bothering me or not, but he commented that such groups could be demanding, and made some reference to having a similar group at one time in which he would experience feelings of being lonely without being alone. This paradox troubled him to the point that he shared it with colleagues who admitted to similar feelings. I felt relieved and shared my experiences. This became the focus of several supervisory sessions and resulted in exploration of ways I could interpret these feelings for the group as an observation of concern for the failure to make progress in the group. This helped me focus the feelings and relate them to the group task and my role as therapist. This helped me stay with the group interaction.
>
> After my interpretation to the group, they also expressed frustration about their progress and began to share problems and feelings

that provided rich therapeutic material. The group genuinely moved to a new level of therapeutic endeavor.

Supervisors must foster the kind of relationship that promotes sharing of the practitioners' deepest fears and concerns about their own feelings and attitudes that they perceive as irrational or unprofessional. Only in a trusting and accepting supervisory relationship will practitioners share these deep-seated fears. In order to deal with such content confidently, supervisors must be well prepared, experienced, and supported themselves. Wolman (1976) has argued that there are three ingredients that make a good therapist: aptitude, training, and experience. The same three ingredients are essential to good supervision. Good practitioners must function at a level different from that of their patients (Wolman, 1976:15), and good supervisors must function at a level different from that of their supervisees if they are to be helpful to them.

THE BEGINNING PROFESSIONAL

Much has been written about stress in occupations, and especially in the helping professions, but little attention has been devoted to stress that occurs before actually entering a career. There is an assumption that most burnout originates on the job. It could be that many professionals are well on the road to burnout before they enter their chosen profession. For many, this process begins during their academic training. Social work is a good example of this attempt to track the origins of stress. A key indicator is the observation of many graduate social work educators that first-year students are motivated, interested, and excited about social work, but as they progress to the second year of training, they become bitter, hostile, withdrawn, and cynical. These attitudes and behaviors are all commonly identified as being associated with stress, but ironically, when we observe such responses in graduate students, we rarely attribute them to stress.

A recent survey lends support to the notion that some students undergo high degrees of stress (Munson, Study E). In addition to the 16 hours a week spent in course work and the 20 hours a week in field placements, the survey found that 50 percent of the students spent an average of 26 hours per week employed. In addition, the majority of social work students are married women with an average of two children. With such a profile and the added hours required for study and library work, the average social work student is under a great deal of stress. Class meetings, field experience, work, and study add up to an average work week of 70 hours for many students.

Unrealistic expectations have been identified as a major factor in the process of burnout. Social work students are more fortunate than students of some other professions in that the reliance on field placements throughout undergraduate and graduate education introduces them early to some of the conditions and limitations they will face as practitioners. However, field experiences are very limited, and often students are protected from extreme cases and agency problems by their field instructors. Large numbers of students want to enter clinical practice in private settings. Their view is one of working in plush offices in the suburbs, with a psychiatrist for back-up support, with middle-class clients who have emotional and family problems. Few will enter this small, highly competitive area of social work practice. The reality for many will be large caseloads of poor, disabled clients who need services and resources that the agency is hard pressed to provide. Offices are dingy, cramped, shared with others, and poorly equipped.

During the past two decades schools have placed heavy emphasis on autonomy to promote professionalism. To some extent, such conceptions prove unrealistic as the new worker discovers that in many agencies there is little independent practice and that much of their work is controlled, evaluated, and dictated by supervisors, administrators, and community pressures.

Beginning practitioners often have little preparation for the stresses of practice. The small caseloads, frequent holidays, breaks, and supportive supervision of student training are an unrealistic preparation for long work days, heavy caseloads, and sporadic supervision in the world of full-time practice. Education programs teach little about stress, and agency orientation programs rarely mention it.

Many practitioners I interviewed in one study of stress indicated that they received no advance preparation for the demands of practice (Munson, Study D). At the same time many indicated that if they had been alerted in advance, they could have avoided many of their negative reactions, withdrawal, and persistence against overwhelming odds. These workers reported that since they were not warned in advance, there was a tendency to perceive the stress as personal and to internalize it rather than to view it as inherent in the position. Another significant finding of this study was that practitioners felt regular, supportive supervision was the most effective aid in combating stress.

SUGGESTED READINGS

Martha Bramhall and Susan Ezell. "How Burned Out Are You?"*Public Welfare* 39 (Winter 1981), pp. 23-55.
A good article on identifying distress. Includes a self-rating scale for determining the level of distress. This article is part one of a three-part series.

_____. "Working Your Way Out of Burnout." *Public Welfare* 39 (Spring 1981), pp. 32-47.
The authors offer a specific plan for overcoming stress. This article is part two of a three-part series.

_____. "How Agencies Can Prevent Burnout." *Public Welfare* 39 (Summer 1981), pp. 33-47.
Specific suggestions for administrators and supervisors on how to help prevent stress in workers. This article is part three of a three-part series.

Jerry Edelwich and Archie Brodsky. *Burnout: Stages of Disillusionment in the Helping Professions*. New York: Human Sciences, 1980.
Identifies causes, manifestations, and ways to deal with job-related distress based on interviews with distressed people in several professions.

Herbert J. Freudenberger and Geraldine Richelson. *Burn-Out: The High Cost of High Achievement*. New York: Anchor, 1980.
General discussion of distress from a personality perspective.

Walter McQuade and Ann Aikman. *Stress*. New York: Bantam, 1974.
A good general discussion of distress and methods for dealing with it.

John Murphy and John Pardeck. "The 'Burnout Syndrome' and Management Style." *The Clinical Supervisor* 4 (Winter 1986), pp. 35-44.
Burnout from a sociological perspective.

Vicky Rippere and Ruth Williams. *Wounded Healers: Mental Health Workers' Experiences of Depression*. New York: John Wiley and Sons, 1985.
Helpful in distinguishing workplace generated depression and stress reactions.

Hans Selye. *Stress Without Distress*. New York: New American Library, 1974.

This is a highly readable account of the biological and psychological basis of stress and distress. It is recommended that all supervisors read this book.

Joan Steepy. "Direct-Service Providers and Burnout." *Social Casework* 62 (June 1981), pp. 352-361.

Excellent, well-written, readable research study that can give supervisors ideas of areas on which to focus to reveal indicators of worker distress.

Jean Wallace and Merlin Brinkerhoff. "The Measurement of Burnout Revisited." *Journal of Social Service Research* 14 (Spring/Summer 1991), pp. 85-111.

A study of burnout in a public agency and how to deal with it.

Pauline C. Zischka. "The Effect of Burnout on Permanency Planning and the Middle Management Supervisor in Child Welfare Agencies." *Child Welfare* 60 (Nov. 1981), pp. 611-616.

Some general suggestions are made for supervisors in dealing with and preventing their own stress.

Obsessive personality features in top leadership
are found quite frequently. On the positive side,
the focus on orderliness, precision, clarity, and
control may foster stable delegation of authority
and clarity in the decision-making process . . . .
On the negative side, some dangers are the
leader's excessive need for order and precision,
his need to be in control, and the expression of
the sadistic components that often go with an
obsessive personality.

Otto Kernberg
"Regression in Organizational
Leadership"
in *The Irrational Executive*

Chapter 11

Administrative Activities

There are administrative tasks and functions the supervisor must attend to that go beyond the normally defined administrative duties. This chapter covers topics that the supervisor often overlooks, but which can be extremely important to the practitioner. Some of the topics covered are general record-keeping guides, legal issues in practice, duty to warn rules, ensuring practitioner safety, and credentialing requirements. The last section covers styles of administrators that can be helpful to the supervisor in dealing with their own supervisors and administrative leaders.

INTRODUCTION

It is rare that a clinical supervisor has the opportunity to exclusively do clinical supervision. It is impossible to do any clinical supervision without it having some administrative component. Most supervisors in public or private practice do administration as part of supervisory functioning. Some supervisors actually do more administration than clinical supervision. There is growing evidence that practitioners are increasingly required to do administrative tasks as a part of their clinical work. For example, there are estimates that 30 percent of clinicians' time is spent on record keeping. Others have estimated much client data is recorded as many as eight times in the record. This is indicative of the increased time the supervisor must spend doing administration and teaching supervisees about how to perform administrative functions.

Practitioner administrative tasks and supervisor tasks are often connected. For example, treatment plans must be developed in many settings, and methods for doing this must be taught by supervisors. Initial and review treatment plans done by practitioners must be reviewed and signed by supervisors. Increasingly, method of payment for services requires practitioners to complete numerous forms and submit various measures of client progress that the supervisor must approve and sign. These examples illustrate the joint nature of administrative functioning. The old view of administration in supervision as something the supervisor did to or for the supervisee has shifted, and administration is now viewed as a task the supervisor performs in conjunction with the supervisee.

RECORD KEEPING

Many times the agency accreditation can depend on the degree of completion of the complex array of forms and required documentation. A new worker, experienced or inexperienced, can be overwhelmed by the incredible detail that must be mastered to have a record be current and up to date. It is recommended that the supervisor devise a flow chart or visual of the forms that are required for each record and distribute it to supervisees. Visuals 11.1 and 11.2 illustrate the flow chart and record keeping in a typical mental health setting. No two agencies have the same record-keeping procedures, but the concepts involved are usually quite similar. The supervisor should go over these illustrations several times with new supervisees and review them with supervisees who fall behind in record keeping.

In most clinical agencies there is some requirement for an initial data

VISUAL 11.1. Typical Clinical Forms

It is helpful with beginning practitioners to provide them with a visual similar to this based on the agency's form requirements. Such visualization can decrease the time it takes to master the forms process.

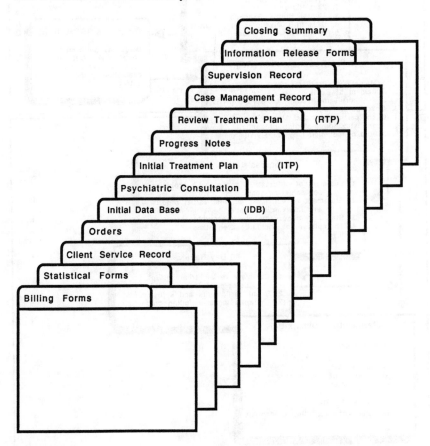

base, an initial treatment plan, progress notes done usually every 30 days (it is preferable to do a progress note for each client contact), and a review treatment plan normally required every 90 days. It is critical that the practitioner develop an understanding that clinical record keeping is a process designed to document the progress and progression of the treatment. Frequently clinicians view record keeping as an unnecessary chore that only exists for administrators to keep track of them and evaluate them. The job

VISUAL 11.2. Diagram of Typical Treatment Process

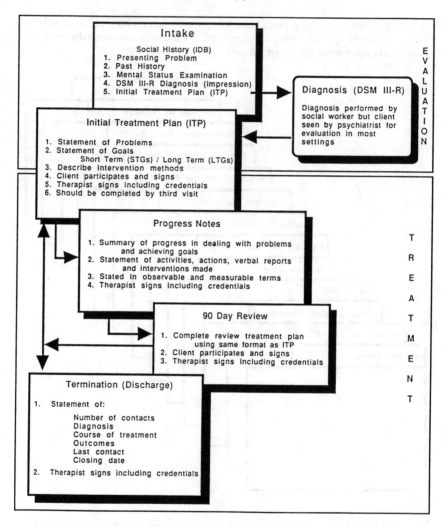

of the supervisor is not only to teach the importance of documentation and how to do it, but to also teach supervisees how to use their own documentation to benefit the client.

Documentation takes much of the practitioner's time. It is generally accepted that approximately 30 percent of clinicians' time is spent doing documentation. The supervisor has a responsibility to teach how to do this as efficiently as possible. There are several common problems that supervisors often overlook. Practitioners often have not been taught how to use dictation equipment. Frequently clinicians do not know how to summarize material or how to present the most salient features in a case or a session, and instead dictate lengthy details that give few clues to the patterns in the case. The practitioner needs to be helped in organizing time. For example, many practitioners are unaware that certain documentation can be done in treatment sessions. In fact treatment plans should be done in the session since the person is expected to be an active participant in the treatment planning, and in many settings is required to sign the treatment plan. There is limited understanding of the connection that should exist among the initial data base, the treatment plan, and the progress notes and the closing summary. These items should be an integrated whole. To develop this view takes training and practice and the supervisor plays a key role in aiding the worker in this area. Practitioners should view the dictation as a reflection of the significant activity in a case so that a person unfamiliar with the case could read the record and have a basic understanding of the case.

LEGAL ISSUES

The supervisor has an administrative responsibility to ensure that the clinician is aware of legal safeguards that must be observed in relation to clients and colleagues. The legal rights have become so complex and extensive in the past three decades that it is impossible to discuss in detail here the specific issues involved. It will be necessary instead to focus on general principles.

It has been reported that 90 percent of all malpractice suits against helping professionals have been filed in the last 30 years (Meyer et al., 1988:11). While the threat of lawsuits against mental health professions has not been extensive, most agencies and practitioners dread the thought of possible lawsuits to the extent that it impedes practice. For example, I had an office across from a colleague who would not interview a child alone. When he had a mother and daughter in the office he would not close the door and he never touched any clients. All of this was done in the belief that such actions would protect him against accusations. His actions afforded little protection, but certainly altered the nature of the treatment. Ironically, his actions even exposed him to legal liability because breach of confidence/privacy ranks fifth in liability actions (Meyer et al., 1988:21)

Some of the defensive actions agencies take are based on real threats, and some are imagined and based on erroneous beliefs about what the laws are regarding certain acts. The supervisor has a responsibility to be knowledgeable about client rights and legal developments regarding practice activity and agency obligations. This can be a significant task, but the supervisor should make a concerted effort to be aware of the legal requirements. The agency-based and private practitioner should periodically consult with a knowledgeable attorney about legal concerns. There are many excellent seminars offered by lawyers that can be helpful to the supervisor. It is important that the supervisor be able to demonstrate that reasonable steps have been taken to help people and to avoid harm.

Too often supervisors and practitioners take an absolute view of the law and feel if certain specific acts are taken, all is well. The law is not that simple. The legal system views acts as sequences and takes a more expansive view of actions. A good example of this is confidentiality. Supervisors can think that confidentiality is merely protecting the chart or not revealing information the client has shared. Confidentiality has become complex and is not a simple action. Protecting the client's confidentiality is relative and not absolute. The supervisor and practitioner must take reasonable measures to protect the client's confidentiality and privacy. The practitioners should make clear to the client the limits and exceptions to confidentiality. It is not sufficient to simply tell the client that everything they tell the therapist is absolutely confidential. The therapist must take reasonable care to guard confidentiality, but there are many situations in the modern world that make it difficult for the therapist to maintain it. One simple illustration of this is the dilemma presented by a telephone answering machine that requires leaving a recorded message for the client. The therapist has no control over who hears the message, and identifying oneself could be detrimental to the client if the message is heard by others. Society has become so complex that when a person is treated, many people can become aware of the treatment and aspects of it without the therapist sharing information. In addition to the therapist, some of the people who can be aware of the treatment are secretaries, receptionists, bookkeepers, insurance company staff, employers, custodians, other therapists, other clients, and school officials. This is a small list of the people who can come to have knowledge of treatment and illustrates that confidentiality cannot be totally guaranteed or controlled by the therapist.

DUTY TO WARN

Duty to warn, also referred to as "failure to warn" and "Tarasoff rule," is closely related to the confidentiality issues, and the concept has caused much concern and controversy in the helping professions. The arguments are lengthy and there is developing case law in this area (for a summary of this area see Meyer et al., 1988). The essence of this issue is that if a therapist learns that a client intends to do harm to others, the therapist has a duty to inform the people who have been threatened. The courts in several cases have established that therapists have a duty to warn people who have been the focus of threats made in therapy by clients, and several states have enacted duty to warn laws. In addition, the courts have held that if a client makes threats to destroy property of others, there is a duty to warn the owner of the property. For example, if a client threatens to set fire to someone's home, the therapist has a duty to warn. There is much vagueness about duty to warn regarding property, and therapists have no clear guidelines regarding to what extent the property threat extends.

The supervisor has a responsibility to ensure that practitioners understand the concept of duty to warn and offer guidelines for therapists to follow. Some states have passed laws that offer guidelines for therapist actions in such situations. The supervisor or therapist should follow the laws that govern duty to warn and should inquire of the state in which he or she practices has a law and what steps she or he must follow to meet this requirement. In the absence of a law, the supervisor and therapist should seek agency or group practice-approved procedures for duty to warn. The following general set of guidelines are merely to aid practitioners in the absence of state laws and agency policy. The guidelines should not be considered rules a for a specific situation or setting.

1. Duty to warn rests with licensed health care providers and administrators of some institutions under certain circumstances.
2. A duty to warn exists when the practitioner has direct knowledge of potential harm to an individual, group, or property. Direct knowledge consists of three elements: (a) the client's propensity to commit violence, (b) the client has the intention to inflict physical injury, and (c) the client has named a specific person or group of persons who are to be the victims.
3. Duty to warn includes reasonable and timely efforts to (a) seek commitment of the client, or (b) take treatment action designed to eliminate the carrying out of the threat, or (c) inform the police and the identified victim.
4. The warning given to the identified victim should include: (a) a description of the threat, (b) identification of the person making the threat, (c) identification of the intended victim or victims.
5. Duty to warn usually has exemption from confidentiality for the therapist. (These guidelines are in part based on a Maryland duty to warn law).

Even when the agency establishes guidelines, the practitioner will confront many situations that are ambiguous and will react to threats in different ways given the circumstances. For example, it is frequently easier for therapists to make a decision to warn when threats are made by clients with whom they have had a difficult relationship than clients with whom they have had a positive relationship. Clients the practitioner has seen for a long time will be more difficult to report about than a client one is seeing for the first time. Some therapists will deal with the duty to warn requirement by avoiding content in the treatment that could lead to threatening remarks, but this strategy does not always work since some clients will just blurt out threats.

The supervisor can help the supervisee by discussing the duty to warn requirements in detail. This includes helping the supervisee understand that a threat does not mean the therapist must immediately warn the potential victim. The practitioner can discuss the threat with the client and encourage measures to prevent the client from acting on the threat, such as encouraging the client to agree to voluntary hospitalization or seeking theclient's permission to warn the intended victim. The supervisor should be a resource for the practitioner to use in developing and considering the range of strategies to deal with the client and the threat.

VIOLENCE AND SAFETY

Social Worker Stabbed to Death in Mental Health Agency

Worker Beaten to Death with Baseball Bat During Home Visit

Workers and Patients Taken Hostage in Hospital

Worker Making Home Visit Injured When Nearby Drug Deal Goes Bad

Social Worker Shot to Death at Children's Treatment Center

Social Worker Stabbed to Death by Man Who Was Denied Service

Man Denied Services by Agency Kills Social Worker

All of these are headlines that are associated with incidents of violence against social workers. Our society is extremely violent, and there are many statistics that grimly document this. It is not clear if our society is more or less violent than has been the case in the past. What we do know is that our society is quite violent and becoming more so each year. Violence against social workers is on the increase.

There is no organization that is gathering data on violent acts against social workers. The author has been gathering data informally for the past three years. The potential headlines reported above are from seven actual cases that occurred in the last two years. In exploring these cases, some patterns occurred that are significant. First, the violence is not random. The person committing the violent act has some complaint against the agency, real or imagined, that provoked that individual. In the one case where the social worker was stabbed to death, the person was a client of the mental health center where the social worker was employed, and had recently been terminated from service because of funding cuts. Second, the precipitating incident is fairly recent and not longstanding. Third, there is often a minor incident that precedes the serious violent incident. The person gets in an argument with someone at the agency, or telephones and becomes argumentative. Fourth, the violence incident occurs when the agency does something outside the established practices of the agency. For example, in the hospital case the social worker agreed to interview the client in the waiting room when the client entered the hospital and became belligerent. This was not normally done. After the social worker was shot, the client held other people who were in the waiting room hostage for several hours. If normal procedures had been followed, it is possible the tragedy could have been avoided or the number of people involved could have been much smaller.

Supervisors and administrators frequently minimize the potential for violence in clients and inadvertently put workers at risk. One violent incident can have significant impact on staff even when no serious physical harm occurs. When staff are held hostage, they suffer psychological and emotional stress for quite some time. Some people never completely recover from witnessing or being a part of a violent incident.

The supervisor has a responsibility to prepare practitioners by orienting them to the signs of potential violence in a client. Signs of agitation, such as heavy breathing, trembling, raising of the voice, trembling in the voice, glaring at the worker, sudden use of profanity, pacing, and clenched fists are primary signs of possible impending violence (for more detail see Shea, 1988:135-177).

The supervisor has a responsibility to take precautions to protect the safety of supervisees. If the agency does not have a policy on safety, the supervisor should take the lead in organizing the staff to develop a policy. A basic safety policy should include:

1. *Office arrangement.* Offices should be arranged so that the worker is

next to the door. The workers should avoid placing the client between them and the door. All sharp objects or objects that can be easily thrown at the worker should be removed. Any object in the office that could become a potential weapon should be evaluated. For example, letter openers, glass ashtrays, lamps, etc. Where possible, the doors should have small, elongated windows installed with small blinds. The blind can be opened when the worker is interviewing a client who causes the worker to have concern about violence. The window can be a deterrent to the client taking action. Clients should never be interviewed in an office that does not contain a phone.

2. *"Buddy system."* The staff should discuss in advance a system for warning one another if they are attacked or trapped in an office by a client. There should be a general policy and an individualized policy when the worker knows in advance an interview is to be conducted with a client about whom the worker has concern. On the day that a troublesome client is to be interviewed, colleagues and supervisors should be alerted and strategies devised. The supervisor should frequently reinforce with practitioners that it is not a weakness to express concern and fears associated with interviewing certain clients. Talking in advance can offer much support and comfort to the practitioners because they can enter the session reassured and clear about what to do if the interview situation escalates.

If staff are working late at night or on weekends when there are few people in the building, they should take special care regarding an alerting system. It is not a good idea to give clients the impression you are in the building alone. Leaving buildings after dark and late at night can be hazardous. Workers should arrange to leave in groups. It is at these times that workers are most vulnerable, but the least likely to take measures to ensure safety.

3. *Warning devices.* In settings where the potential for violence is high, the staff should consider installing devices in each office that allow the practitioner to unobtrusively alert a location outside the interview room that help is needed. This can be a buzzer switch mounted on top or under the desk. If the agency will not provide an electronic system, the workers can keep whistles in desks or in clothing to use for alerting others they are experiencing difficulty.

4. *Proximity.* When clients become agitated, practitioners frequently are unsure of how to deal with the anger. This is because our society is conflicted about expressions of anger and families offer few developmental coping patterns for dealing with expressions of anger. This is the reason that we are a society that wavers between passivity and silence and explosive, violent behavior. Practitioners need to be trained in advance

how to behave when a client begins to escalate. Workers left to their own strategies will draw on the traditional ways of dealing with anger, which is to move toward the client and try to give support, often by touching. We know from experience this is most likely to increase the client's anger. The preferred strategy is for the practitioner to move slightly away from the client. Remain seated or return to your seat. Avoid the position of towering over the client that is created by the practitioner standing while the client is seated. Lower your own voice and reassure the client you heard the communication, and if possible agree with the client. It can be helpful for practitioners to role play such situations so that they have advance experience in general procedures to follow in very frightening situations. Strategies that have only been discussed in supervision can all too easily be forgotten.

5. *Restraint.* The agency should have a policy outlining conditions under which clients will be restrained and how they will be restrained. The supervisor needs to take the lead in this area if the agency has no policy. It is the supervisor's responsibility to insist that one be developed. There will be times clients have to be restrained from doing harm to themselves, others in the room, or the practitioner. When the client takes action against another person, the agency needs to have a policy and a plan for restraint. This will always require more than one staff member. The staff should receive specific training in restraining clients in a way that minimizes the possibility of hurting the client. It has been documented that untrained staff are more likely to be the victims of violence (Davis, 1991:587). If staff are not trained and injure a client in the process of restraint, the agency could be the object of legal action brought by the client. Improperly applied restraint can also increase the possibility of violence. It is under thesecircumstances that the policy and plan for restraint could be of much value to the agency in demonstrating that reasonable and prudent caution was taken. The primary reason for a restraint policy is to minimize the possibility that anyone would be physically injured in a clinical setting. In many locations the police department will offer such training for staff. There are private organizations that offer training seminars and there are continuing education seminars available. All staff should be thoroughly trained in restraint techniques.

CREDENTIALS AND EXAMINATIONS

In the past 20 years the credentialing process has ben expanding in all professions, and social work has not been an exception. Membership organizations and credentials abound today. Most states have licensing or certification at one or more levels. The National Association of Social

Workers (NASW) has the longstanding, but broadly defined ACSW (Academy of Certified Social Workers). The American Board of Examiners in Social Work (ABE) has an advanced credential, the Diplomate (BCD). The American Association of Marriage and Family Therapists (AAMFT) certifies practitioners and supervisors. There are also certification bodies for drug and alcohol counselors, and groups that certify sex counselors. The credentialing situation could become even more complex as some of these bodies are considering multiple levels of credentialing as well as specialty credentials. See Appendix 3 for a visual presentation of the array of credentialing bodies.

All of these credentials can be confusing for practitioners. The supervisor has a responsibility to be thoroughly familiar with the various credentials in social work and assist supervisees in what credentials are essential for practice, as well as what credentials may be important to career plans. For example, a practitioner in a public mental health clinic may only need a state license to practice currently, but if the person desires to develop a private practice, consideration should be given to working toward diplomate status and certification in AAMFT. We are rapidly reaching the point that career planning must include credential planning as well. The supervisor can be quite helpful to the supervisee as career planning is done in relation to credentials.

Part of credential planning and awareness must include information about how to take examinations. All credentials require some type of examination and the most common is a several hundred item, multiple-choice examination during a time-limited (usually three hours) period. There are more study guides available for preparing for the New York City sanitation workers examination than for all the social work examinations. Because of this the supervisor may be called upon to assist supervisees in how to study for the examination and how to prepare for the actual taking of the examination.

Studying for the examination and preparing for the examination are two different processes. Studying deals with reviewing content for the examination and takes place for months prior to the examination. Content review is much more difficult today because the examinations no longer deal with factual information exclusively, but consists primarily of questions that require the person to use logic and reasoning processes to arrive at an answer. Preparation deals with the way the person approaches taking the examination. This process occurs from several days before the examination to the administration of the examination. There are many hints and suggestions the supervisor can provide the supervisee that will decrease anxiety. There are manuals and workshops available for mastering content and dealing with examination anxiety. The supervisor is the best resource for the supervisee who is preparing for an examination, because the supervisor is available to the practitioner on a regular basis and can monitor and support study and preparation for the examination.

Examination anxiety is experienced by most people and can significantly influence scores. Social work schools do not rely on examinations as much as other professional educational programs, and supervisees will often have limited experience in taking examinations which can further increase examination anxiety. Office gossip about the difficulty of an examination can increase the anxiety. The supervisor who is working with practitioners preparing for a credentialing examination should devote a portion of supervisory time to the practitioner's progress and should be supportive of the worker while this difficult process of competence measurement is worked through.

DEALING WITH THE ADMINISTRATOR

The supervisor also usually has a boss. There has been little written for supervisors on how to deal with the boss. There have been several popular books written on dealing with bosses in general, but nothing that relates to the helping profession supervisor. In an effort to deal with this, the author conducted a small study of practitioners' and supervisors' perceptions of supervisors or administrators they had to deal with directly. What follows is a description of these bosses and strategies for dealing with them. The models have been tested in numerous seminars and workshops, and the responses have confirmed the accuracy of these descriptions.

Administrators have been described in stylistic categories because the theme of this book is interactional styles of supervision. By staying in this format, it will be easier for the supervisor to relate to the types that have been observed. Each type has been given an acronym to aid in identification and utilization of the types. It is recognized that there are good administrators who are effective, efficient, sensitive, open, and democratic in carrying out their duties. We can deal with good administrators and generally have little difficulty in relating to them. It is the chronically problematic administrator that supervisors struggle to find ways to deal with. Often the strategies devised by the supervisor are of limited value and make the problem worse. The purpose of devising these six categories from the research was to offer the supervisor ways to identify certain types of administrative styles and to offer some strategies for getting along better with these administrators.

The six styles that have been classified are: Benevolent, Affable Democrat (BAD); Cool, Aloof Decider (CAD); Sophisticated, Learned, Informed Commander (SLIC); Sadistic, Authoritarian Divider (SAD); Jovial, Outgoing Klutz (JOK); and Worried, Anxious Determinist (WAD). Each type is discussed in five areas, which are: communication patterns, forms of interaction, problem-solving methods, decision making, and supervisor response strategy. No administrator will conform completely to a particular categorical style, and some will manifest characteristics from all of the types. The purpose is to provide a crude classification system so that supervisors have some way to begin to organize strategies for dealing with specific actions and behaviors of administrators they perceive as problematic for them. Visual 11.3 gives details of the styles presented below.

ADMINISTRATOR STYLES

Benevolent, Affable Democrat (BAD)

Communication patterns. Communication is always pleasant, but is infrequent. In problem solving activity and communication, this type of administrator makes the same promises to different people. The motivation for most communication is to get the person initiating the communication to go away. These administrators will rarely initiate communication, and staff must approach them. When duplicate promises are discovered by the parties the promises were made to, the administrator responds by trying to get the people to share in the promises by dividing them up or working together. If this strategy does not work, the administrator will simply make a new round of promises to one of the parties involved. While these administrators makes promises, they are noncommittal regarding resources or making specific decisions.

Forms of interaction. This type of administrator will minimize and limit interaction. They detest conflict and will terminate interaction when conflict emerges. These people prefer to hear gossip and will eagerly engage in discussions about the failures, shortcomings, and problems of others if another person initiates such interaction. They will inquire about others in order to give the person an opening to discuss someone, but the administrators never initiate or share gossip.

They will avoid doing any task that has the potential for disagreement or conflict, such as doing performance evaluations or allocating salary increases. These administrators will delegate these tasks to others, and if delegation is not possible, they will not do the tasks unless forced to do

VISUAL 11.3. Administrator Styles

STYLE	COMMUNICATION	INTERACTION	PROBLEM SOLVING	DECISION MAKING	RESPONSE
Benevolent Affable Democrat	*same promises to different people *non-committal *forgets *infrequent	*avoids evaluations *enjoys gossip *hates conflict *non-confront *denies forgets	*approves requests even opposites *single-minded *forgets actions *denies forgets	*delegates freely *never Questions *avoidance / delay *non confront *questions others	*personalize *no judgments *cooperate *limit memos *socialize
Jovial Outgoing Klutz	*flood of memos *distributes everything *inconsistent	*friendly *humorous *hysterical *extensive	*impulsive *outrageous *loses focus *inconsistent	*brash *unrealistic *embarrassing blunders	*insist on rules *joke *no memos
Sophisticated Learned Informed Commander	*lengthy memos *expects loyalty *formal *regular	*brief/pointed *secret favorites *formal *pleasant gibes	*analytic *efficient *orderly *sporadic	*rational *quick *limited input *global	*be clear *be brief *be loyal *be rational
Cool Aloof Decider	*reveals when forced to *brief memos *delayed response *guarded	*pleasant when needs you *controlling *angry when challenged	*calculates *gives answers *solo *inconsistent *logical	*makes decisions does not inform *instant reactions *frequently changes	*use reason *be kind *praise *limit contact
Worried Anxious Determinist	*promise/deny *no memos *forgetful	*verbal detail *question/challenge *conceals motivation	*simplistic *secretive/solo *consult others	*contradictory *talks fast *inequitable	*limit sharing *no memos *Avoid logic
Sadistic Authoritarian Divider	*Terse demanding memos *ignores good performance *associates with weak *confrontive	*anxious *cliquish *untruthful *formal *targets people *avoids staff *masked anger	*plots *issues policies *combative *impulsive *takes all credit *denial *shallow	*solitary *sloppy *inconsistent *embarrassing blunders *covers up mistakes	*document *be silent *be calm *good reports *accept tasks *be present *be pleasant

them. When confronted with their failure to perform tasks, they will deny they forgot and blame the error on other people or events.

Problem solving methods. This type of administrator is friendly and likeable. The major problem is that they have much difficulty saying no. This leads to approve of all requests, even when the people have opposite requests. The person who benefits from this behavior is the supervisor who makes a request and who was in the administrator's office last.

The approach to problem solving is single-minded and reduced to its simplest form. In the process of defining the problem this person will take extensive notes, but it is not clear what they do with these notes, and the notes may never be seen again. In subsequent meetings where the same problems are discussed, old notes are never used, and the person continues to take new notes. The office is always neat and the desk is cleared at the end of the day. Simple problems are resolved quickly. By the end of the day, complex problems that require time to be solved are delegated to others or ignored.

Decision making. The Benevolent, Affable Democrat hates to make decisions and will go to great lengths to avoid making even the simplest ones. The strategy is avoidance and delay, which causes frustration for supervisors and staff. The delays are often so prolonged that the administrator forgets the decision that must be made, and needs to be briefed to be brought up to date. They will often respond by treating these as new problems and attempt to delay the decision again. This causes the staff to spend much time repeating explanations of problems requiring action to the point that demoralization sets in. This type of administrator will delegate decision making and likes to have subordinates who take charge and make decisions in bold and swift fashion.

Supervisor response strategy. It is good to socialize with this type of administrator. Always be pleasant and engage in small talk. If you have information about the organization and colleagues, share it with this administrator, but always be careful to avoid negative and unprofessional interaction. Offer much support and general praise, and console the administrator when he or she discusses with you how difficult it is to be an administrator. Volunteer to do projects and tasks, especially those you care about and want to see implemented. The administrator will gladly delegate them. It is unproductive to become argumentative and to avoid this type administrator. If you avoid him or her you will be on the outside and others will gain control. Avoid confronting this administrator or pushing him or her about decisions. If you must discuss problems or decisions, it is always a good idea to have a proposed solution in mind before you approach this type of administrator. Remember that instead of looking for a solution, he or she will always be looking for a way out of making a decision. This is the primary orientation of a BAD, and the supervisor can develop a strategy that will fit this style of administration.

Jovial, Outgoing Klutz (JOK)

Communication pattern. A JOK style administrator communicates everything. Every memo received by the JOK is circulated to all staff. The JOK writes frequent memos and describes items in great detail. There is much joking in memos and often the focus is lost in written communication.

Forms of interaction. This person is friendly and enjoyable to be around. They make a joke of every item or issue and they are constantly in motion. Individual sessions are brief and disorganized. Group meetings are slightly chaotic, and communication is pleasant and enjoyable, but confused.

Problem-solving methods. This administrator is the most impulsive in problem solving. Decisions are made immediately. The desk is cleared at the end of each day. If this cannot be accomplished, the briefcase goes home full and the work is finished by the next morning. In the process of problem solving, this person is so anxious to arrive at a solution that often is not even connected to the problem.

Decision making. Decisions are made in a brash, authoritative manner with an attitude that the JOK has keen insight into most situations. Announcements of decisions contain quips and quotes that are designed to bolster the effectiveness of the solution. Frequently staff have trouble making the connection between the solution and the quips. Most decisions are unrealistic and go beyond bounds of what staff can accomplish because they are so grandiose. Staff get frustrated and simply do not act on many of the decisions because they are unreasonable. JOKs become angry and depressed because they cannot comprehend why so few of their acts get implemented. When decisions are implemented, they frequently result in embarrassment for the staff and the organization. JOKs handle this by making a joke about the blunder and associate it with some philosophical comment about the ups and downs of life.

Supervisor response strategy. The supervisor in this situation should insist on following rules and procedures. This will help keep JOK in reasonable limits. Discussions should be highly structured and based on specific, written materials that require a response. Memos sent to a JOK administrator should be brief and specific. It a good approach to propose solutions to problems rather than allowing the JOK to grapple with a problem and attempt to find a solution. It is not a good idea to make jokes or quips in your communication. This should be left to the JOK to do. It could be viewed as a challenge or as sarcasm when the supervisor engages in it. When outrageous solutions are proposed by JOK, the supervisor should be prepared to indicatereasons the solution cannot be implemented, but avoid saying it will not work. This strategy avoids personalizing the efforts of the JOK.

Sophisticated, Learned, Informed Commander (SLIC)

Communication pattern. Communication is formal, but upbeat, and promotes confidence even when it is not warranted. SLIC administrators conduct lengthy planning meetings and issue memos explaining policy in great detail. These administrators expect strict compliance with rules and regulations and become upset when they discover someone has not observed the rules. They will issue memos that demand compliance with the rules. They will use the rules to avoid establishing a policy they do not like. While the SLIC sees "the big picture," most communication will focus on small increments of policies and procedures.

Forms of interaction. Interaction with SLICs is brief and to the point. They are usually preoccupied and eager to move on to the next meeting or task. Supervisors frequently feel they can never capture SLIC's attention long enough to make their point. SLICs generally have secret favorites and will use them to get information about what is taking place in the staff. These secret staff favorites receive special perks for their information and loyalty. Loyalty is a key concept for these administrators and any act of disloyalty will result in permanent banishment from significant interaction with SLIC.

Problem-solving methods. This type administrator is organized, orderly, analytic and efficient. Relational data base computer programs, automated file systems, or any system for tracking work and people are the hallmark of the SLIC administrator. The SLIC administrator will approach every problem from an analytic perspective. Unlike the CAD who appears to be burdened by administration, SLIC appears to see administration as a challenge and moves directly to deal with problems in a style like the military commander confident of impeding victory.

Decision making. This type of administrator will make decisions quickly, and will use logic and will present a rational justification for decisions. SLICs usually make comprehensive, global decisions and leave the details to subordinates to develop and implement. However, if others do not do what the SLIC thinks is effective implementation, he or she will enter the detailed decision-making process.

Supervisor response strategy. When dealing with this type of administrator, the supervisor should follow SLICs decision-making schedule and be prepared to implement decisions quickly and effectively. The supervisor should avoid having to offer justification and excuses for not having implemented a decision that SLIC has made. The best way to avoid having all control taken out of the supervisor's hands is to be on top of tasks and responsibilities as they are issued. Responses to SLIC should be brief, logical, and organized. It is best to discuss matters with SLIC and follow up with written summaries of the decisions, policies and procedures that are agreed upon in meetings.

The supervisor should seek feedback from this type of administrator. SLICs will usually be honest and direct in sharing impressions and doing evaluations. It is important to remain loyal to SLICs and use low-key strategies to express loyalty. It is good to discretely discover who the "secret favorites" are and try to have open and frequent communication with them. They will often provide clues about what SLIC is thinking or planning, or you can suggest ideas to them that they will communicate to SLIC. Do not expect to get credit for these ideas. If you are a "secret favorite," you are blessed, but you must be careful to not take advantage of this status or flaunt it with other staff. In communication with SLIC, you should be discrete and careful not to be unprofessional. SLIC will not expect this of you, but it can happen and lead to difficulty. SLIC will expect you to be logical and rational in discussions, and objectivity and factual observations should be the basis of discussions with SLIC.

Cool, Aloof Decider (CAD)

Communication patterns. Communications from this type of administrator are rare. Memos are brief and to the point. Written and verbal communication occur only when the CAD is compelled to do so. Communications that the CAD receives but decides not to act on will go unanswered. This can result in frustration for the supervisor. This type of administrator does not telephone staff, invite staff members to talk to him or her, and the CAD never just "drops in" staff offices to talk.

Forms of interaction. The CAD will interact with staff when it is necessary and the interaction is pleasant unless something is proposed with which the CAD disagrees. CADs are usually calm and soft-spoken, but will raise their voice and show slight anger or sarcasm when they do not get their way or when challenged. The CAD prefers one-on-one interaction and is quite verbal in this format. The larger the group the less the CAD will say. Interaction is always planned in the form of structured meetings, and there is no informal, spontaneous interaction. While CADs can become angered if put on the spot, they do not hold grudges, and staff are frequently relieved and amazed that they are rewarded in some way after an unpleasant exchange with a CAD administrator.

Problem-solving methods. This administrator calculates and plans most acts, and usually does so in secret. The staff only knows about actions when they are announced. Program changes, staff reorganization, and hiring of new staff are a few examples of actions that are simply announced, and no staff input is sought. The CAD sits quietly in meetings and rarely says anything. It is difficult to determine what the person is feeling or thinking. Staff are usually uncomfortable in this administrator's presence and guarded in comments, since guardedness is the style of the administrator. This is ironic since the CAD appears to use information presented in meetings to make decisions, but if the staff are reluctant to voice opinions, the administrator is denied information important to devising solutions. The CAD is generally logical in thinking, and most times attempts to be fair. The CAD approach to problems is logical, but frequently the solutions are inconsistent. When inconsistencies are glaring, the staff will fail to raise the issues because of the guardedness in relation to the CAD. The CAD gives the impression of being a lonely person and limits social contact with staff. The CAD is seen as a person who is a "solo" operator. She or he is reliable and calm most of the time, but it appears to the staff as if administration is a burden for the CAD.

Decision making. This person makes decisions in isolation and notifies staff or has others notify the staff. Some decisions are simply made and implemented without notifying staff. People find out about policies when they fail to observe them and are then told what the policy is. The CAD makes the decisions but attempts to distance from the decision if it is possible. CADs will accept responsibility for decisions if necessary, and are bold in coming to the staff with decisions when they feel the situation requires it. When a CAD administrator feels pushed, decisions are made instantly simply to get the situation resolved. Instant decisions usually occur in staff meetings, a situation the CAD generally finds uncomfortable. A CAD will frequently change decisions if he or she is not getting the desired results.

Supervisor response strategy. It is important to be pleasant toward CADs and to praise them occasionally for the good decisions they make. The supervisor should be slow to propose invitations to socialize with a **CAD administrator.** Some prefer an occasional lunch meeting, but it is best to limit such meetings unless the CAD gives indications he or she enjoys and prefers this type of contact. The more formal, regularly scheduled meeting is generally the preferred model of the CAD. The best strategy is to ask questions and develop unobtrusive methods for ensuring that you learn about policies that may have been implemented without being announced.

Efforts to change bad decisions of a CAD are best done in staff meetings where staff support can be stated, even if it is guarded support. Preparation for the attempt to change the decision can best be done by meeting with the CAD individually and casually mentioning the problem, but offering no solutions. Staff who offer solutions are viewed by CADs as trying to usurp their power, and CADs will do the opposite of what is being suggested to assert and make clear who has authority.

When new policies are implemented, it is best not to express surprise but to find out as much about the policy as possible. In other words, ask questions about the policy rather than questioning the policy. Try to base observation on logic, and focus on the organization and the meaning of the policy for clients and staff instead of attempting to personally identify the policy as coming from the administrator. Only in situations that staff members feel very strongly about should the issue of failure to get staff input before making the decision be raised with the CAD administrator. This will have to be done periodically, because CADs never change their style significantly and they will not evolve into participatory decision makers even after being repeatedly confronted about the lack of staff input.

Worried, Anxious Determinist (WAD)

Communication pattern. The WAD is friendly, but can be blunt and abrasive when working to get his or her way on an issue. These people do not send memos. They send handwritten notes. Communication is sudden, intense, and often vague and brief.

Forms of interaction. WADs are constantly in motion, they go from task to task, rarely completing a task or forgetting what task they were in the process of completing. They are quite forgetful and will deny they have forgotten. When you confront forgetfulness, they become very defensive and accuse you of having misunderstood. WADs often make promises that they forget they have made, and will deny later they made the promise. They describe everything in great detail and treat staff like children who are learning for the first time. Presentations are often confusing, and the essence of tasks get lost in the enormous detail. WADs ask many questions and challenge statements of others, but there is no logic for this and the motivation for the WADs combative stance is puzzling to the staff. WADs often complain of being overworked, and they are constantly in crises.

Problem-solving methods. This type of administrator engages in solo, secretive, and simplistic problem solving. All problems are reduced to simple black and white, right and wrong conceptions. This person will consult others by asking questions but does not reveal why the questions are being asked. Only later do staff realize the questions were used to get information to make decisions, but since the questions were not presented in this context the staff feels duped. This pattern leads eventually to the staff being guarded about any responses given to questions asked by a WAD.

Decision making. A WAD administrator makes decisions rapidly and usually before sufficient information has been gathered to make the decision. WAD decisions are frequently contradictory. There is a contagion effect among staff when a WAD feels the urgency to make a decision. The smallest of decisions often take on the quality of emergencies for the WAD. WADs consume so much energy in this process, that they will reverse themselves and say there is no hurry to complete the task. This is usually related to the fact that the WAD ran out of energy, so the problem is nolonger an emergency. In such an environment staff become distraught and withdrawn.

WADs feel they have to make decisions on everything that comes before them. If a supervisor comes in just to talk, the WAD becomes anxious early in the conversation and turns the content of the discussion into a major problem that must be solved. By the end of the conversation, the supervisor regrets having brought up the subject or even going to talk to the WAD. If the supervisor withdraws and does not come into talk, the WAD projects that into being a problem, so the supervisor has the feeling of being in a no-win situation.

Supervisor response strategy. WADs can be demanding and difficult to deal with. The supervisor must balance communication and contact with the WAD so that he or she can avoid the no-win situation described above in relation to discussing issues with the WAD. It is best to discuss with the WAD only items that you must have him or her participate in. Items that require speculation or new ideas are best explored with other staff. It is recommended that memos be sent to a WAD only when absolutely necessary. It is important to keep good notes and document discussions and phone conversations.

Trying to use logic with these administrators does not work because they will see it as a challenge and create a new logic based on their own perceptions that can be even more confusing. The better strategy is to try to determine what the WAD wants, and to ask questions that will help to make clear what he or she is trying to get. WADs are usually in a mode of trying to get something, but they will not come out and say it, so the supervisor must study the WAD's comments to determine what the exchange is actually about.

Sadistic, Authoritarian Divider (SAD)

Communication pattern. SADs communicate through terse, demanding memos. Written communication is usually issued as an order to do something or to stop doing something. SADs are not available for individual meetings with staff, and when one does get in to see them, the meetings are brief and non-committal. The key factor to remember about SADs is they desire to make decisions alone, and perceive communication to be important only in one direction—from themselves to the staff.

SADs will have staff discussions of problems, but they devalue this input and ignore it. There view is that the only requirement is that the staff be allowed to express views, but these views should not in any way influence SADs right to make decisions unilaterally.

SADs do communicate with the few people whom they take into their confidence. These people have much hidden power in that they influence decisions, and many times their recommendations are based on personal animosities.

Forms of interaction. These administrators proclaim harmony, and desire smooth operations, but they act very differently. They are constantly in conflict with staff, and they target individual staff to be recipients of punitive actions. They avoid people and communicate through memos. When confronted they become anxious and angry. They will mislead people and distort to achieve their goals. These people are unpleasant to work for and can become impossible to relate to if you become the target of punitive action. They usually only target one person at a time, and if a designated target transfers or leaves, a new target will be found. There are brief lapses between the time one person is the target and another person becomes the target. During these periods the supervisor should keep a very low profile.

Problem-solving methods. Problem solving is done in a secretive and devious manner by this type administrator. Problems are approached as a challenge that require a plot to be solved. There is a tendency to use the plot to punish and harass people. This punitive strategy usually has no behavioral basis, but seems to be part of the person's personality.

SADs solve problems alone or on the advice of one other person who has been temporarily taken into confidence. SADs constantly rely on two or three people to be their advisors. These administrators usually have much anxiety and act on impulse to solve problems. Acting on impulse, they frequently make mistakes and unjustly accuse staff of making mistakes or acting inappropriately. This leads to much conflict and frustration. When challenged, SADs become angry and upset. This occurs in private as well as group meetings. While they try to contain the anger, it is obvious to all they are irritated. After such encounters this administrator will take action that results in punitive measures for all or some staff.

Decision making. Decisions are made in solitude and occasionally after consulting a key staff person. Decisions are made hastily and frequently result in embarrassment for the administrator and the organization. Many times decisions are in direct conflict with earlier decisions this administrator has made. Logic and consistency are not important to this type administrator. Decisions that are blunders are handled by blaming staff for the failures. If decisions go well, the SAD will take personal credit and not acknowledge the work of staff.

Supervisor response strategy. The best strategy with a SAD administrator is to be laid back and do your assigned tasks. Accept requests to perform special projects and assignments without complaint. Avoid confronting SAD if your report is later distributed with SAD's name on it. To confront such issues will make you a potential target. If a targeted person has recently departed, it is best to lay low for several months and not approach SAD, because you are vulnerable during this time to becoming the new target. The supervisor should keep a low profile in relation to SAD, but be present and in frequent communication with other staff. Withdrawal is not a good strategy with SAD because this results in isolation that could make you a target. It is a good idea to befriend all staff, especially the two or three people who are the confidantes of SAD. You should share ideas you would like to see developed with these people because they will most likely share them with SAD. It is a good idea to be quiet in meetings and to retain documentation of all important actions and activities of your work. It is not a good idea to confront these administrators or send memos to them unless absolutely necessary.

SUGGESTED READINGS

Simon Davis. "Violence by Psychiatric Inpatients: A Review." *Hospital and Community Psychiatry* 42 (June 1991), pp. 585-589.
    A review of the literature on violence by patients and helpful information on violent clients.

Manfred F.R. Kets de Vries. *The Irrational Executive: Psychoanalytic Studies in Management*. Madison, WI: International Universities Press, 1984.

A conceptual discussion of leaders in organizations from a psychoanalytic perspective. Much of the information can be applied to clinical settings and associated with the styles described in this chapter.

Manfred F.R. Kets de Vries and Danny Miller. *The Neurotic Organization: Diagnosing and Revitalizing Unhealthy Companies*. New York: Harper Business, 1984.

A conceptual discussion of organizations from a management perspective. Much of the information can be applied to clinical settings.

Jonathan Kramer. *Stepping Up: How to Fight Your Boss and Win*. New York: Arbor House, 1985.

A practical guide for dealing with the type administrators described in this chapter.

Shawn Shea. *Psychiatric Interviewing: The Art of Understanding*. Philadelphia: W.B. Saunders, 1988.

Includes good information on safety issues and how to deal with potentially violent clients.

Ilga Svechs and Donald Zall. *A Curriculum Guide for the Advanced Level Review and Update Course*. National Institute for Clinical Social Work Advancement, 1989.

Study guide for preparing for clinical examinations.

"Are they going to like our film?" I ask
Ingmar. "Regard it as a surgeon's
scalpel. Not everyone will welcome it,"
he replies.

Liv Ullmann
Changing

Chapter 12

Audiovisual and Action Techniques

In this chapter audiovisual and action techniques used to promote learning in supervision are discussed. We live in a society that has experienced rapid advances in electronic technology, but very few guidelines have been developed for use of this technology in learning about practice, and most supervisors and supervisees approach this material as they approach electronic media—as entertainment. The use of television (videotape) and audiotape are explained, along with specific guidelines for sequencing and manipulating such material to enhance learning. Ethical and nonintrusive uses of electronic devices by supervisors are covered.

Role play has become a popular educational technique. Specific techniques for role play are explored along with role play procedures organized around: (1) planning, (2) monitoring, (3) evaluation, (4) debriefing, and (5) physical setting. The use of live supervision is explained. The concepts of privacy and confidentiality are discussed in relation to use of electronic devices and action techniques.

TELEVISION (VIDEOTAPE)

Most practitioners and supervisors trained in the past 30 years grew up with television as an essential and extensive component of their lives. The pervasive impact of television on practitioners, supervisors, and clients is illustrated by some powerful statistics (Finn, 1980:473-474):

1. Ninety-six percent of homes have a working television, and 25 percent have two televisions.
2. The average television is on more than six hours a day.
3. Children between 6 and 11 years of age watch television an average of 3.5 hours a day.
4. By age 18, the average person will have spent the equivalent of 2.5 years watching television — 45 percent more time than spent in classroom education.
5. By age 65, the average American will have spent nine full years watching television.

Given these statistics, it is ironic that most practitioners have not been exposed to audiovisual methods in practice and supervision. When such materials are used, there is little training for them or critical application. In this section some common techniques for using television in supervision and training are covered.

Matisse observed that invention of the camera relieved artists of the need to copy objects. In a similar sense television applied to practice is not used to permit practitioners to copy the styles of others, but is a means of enhancing the use of imagination and creativity in developing their own styles.

KNOWLEDGE GAP

The advance in audiovisual technological knowledge and mechanical application has far exceeded the development of knowledge regarding its utilization in the behavioral sciences in general, and in the field of social work in particular. There is little research or theoretical speculation available about the use of audiovisual technology in supervision.

In a study by Nelson (1978), social work trainees showed greater preference for verbal descriptions of therapy content over videotaping of treatment for use in supervision or supervisor observation than did psychiatry and psychology trainees. Although the reasons for these differences are not known, the study does illustrate that social work trainees are more likely to resist, avoid, or fear videotaping and action techniques. The supervisor needs to be aware of this reluctance and to approach the use of such techniques with sensitivity.

Nelson's findings were confirmed in my own study in which a "clinical exposure index" was developed as a special case of interaction between the practitioner and supervisor (Munson, 1975). The scale measured the extent to which workers and supervisors shared with one another their own practice methods through direct observation, videotapes, audiotapes, and process recordings. The scale ranged from 5 (none) to 20 (regularly). The mean score was 6, indicating that virtually no sharing of clinical material was taking place. Process recording accounted for most of the activity (Munson, 1975:109). Kadushin had similar findings in another study, and he concluded, "no use is made of modern technology to obtain data of on-the-job performance" (Kadushin, 1974:295).

The failure to use electronic devices to promote learning is not understandable given the current availability of videotape equipment. The most basic system for videotaping now costs less than $1,000, and even fairly sophisticated systems are availablefor under $3,000. Availability of the equipment does not seem to be the barrier because, as one study showed, almost all of the agencies reported having videotape equipment available. Perhaps other psychological resistances are at work. The material in this section is designed to help in overcoming some of these resistances.

Television as Entertainment

People have generally been oriented to watch television for entertainment. When television is used for educational purposes, the participants must develop a new perspective for viewing the material, especially clinical material. The size of the problem of overcoming television as entertainment is reflected in the estimate that the average person will spend over 16,000 hours during childhood watching television. Each visual image will last 3.5 seconds for programming and 2.5 seconds for each commercial. This adds up to 1,200 visual images per hour. People *watch* television; they do not read it, write it, and more importantly, they do not think about it or analyze it.

Television is a purely visual medium that is based on rapidity of visual images. It is not cognitively stimulating. All this must be understood in the context that the three major activities of children are sleeping, watching television, and going to school. Television is being used more and more in school, and educational viewing added to personal viewing makes television the number one educational tool in the United States.

Supervisees will comment after viewing a videotaped interview, "That was so boring; couldn't it be more lively?" Statements of this nature are an indication that the practitioners are viewing the tape from an entertainment perspective. We cannot put car chases and crashes, people falling off mountains, or scuba diving in videotapes of practitioners doing treatment. Good treatment is not always exciting or emotionally charged. Supervisees have to be prepared in advance for learning-oriented television. The supervisor must specify what to watch for, but must not pinpoint too much detail in advance.

Television as Measurement

One of the chief ways television can be used in supervision is to watch practitioners change, grow, and develop. We put much emphasis in supervision upon growth and development, but we rarely use good measures to highlight or evaluate it. Videotapes and audiotapes made of beginning students and practitioners that are preserved and reviewed a year or two later can provide valuable documentation of growth. They can be used to reinforce growth and to specify the changes that have occurred in the practitioner's style, comfort level, skill, and utilization of techniques. Practitioners and supervisors who are serious about evaluating growth will need to have such records to gauge their performance over time.

It is not sufficient to base an evaluation solely on verbally reflecting and recalling changes over time. When the verbal recall is all that is used, much of what has been learned is forgotten with time and, therefore, is not available for reinforcement at the assessment points. For the supervisee to say simply, "Well, I learned a lot this past year," is not very helpful. The verbal recall method can be manipulated by both the supervisor and supervisee to avoid dealing with sensitive, but important, issues. A comment of one supervisee illustrates this point: "I am sensitive to criticism, so I set it up that I don't get it, but when you are on tape, you can't avoid it." Also, verbal recall by the supervisor is limited even when giving the practitioner positive feedback. Another supervisee comment illustrates this: "My supervisor said, 'You really had poise in that first interview,' but I have trouble accepting his positive feedback." If the supervisee could have seen herself being poised, it might have been easier for her to accept the praise. In this case, the old saying is true—"seeing is believing."

Overwhelmingly, the use of electronic records works in favor of the supervisee. Watching a videotape of past work highlights all areas of a person's change—knowledge, skill, flexibility, confidence. It is not unusual for supervisees to say, "I forgot I did that" or "It's been a long time since I made that mistake." Such responses allow the supervisor and practitioner to get specific about the change that has taken place. Once supervisees are exposed to learning and evaluation based on electronic records, they find it stimulating and helpful.

Little information is available for the supervisor to use in deciding when, how, and where to use audio or video technology in treatment and supervision. Many questions remain unanswered, such as: When should supervisors ask practitioners to bring audiotapes of their treatment to supervision sessions? When should videotaped material be used instead of audiotaped material? When using videotape, should split screen techniques (one camera on the client and one camera on the practitioner) be used? Should the supervisory process itself be subjected to audiovisual techniques? These are just a few of the basic questions that arise regarding such techniques. The following paragraphs offer some suggestions in dealing with these basic questions as well as others.

TAPING THE THERAPY TO BE SUPERVISED

Practitioners who have not used electronic devices in their therapy generally are intimidated by such activities and usually will resist its use on the grounds that it is too threatening for the client. Repeated, unplanned, and unskillful use of electronic devices in treatment reveal that the practitioner has more difficulty in dealing with it than the client. Kagan first observed this when using videotaped material to develop the strategy of Interpersonal Process Recall (IPR) (Berger, 1978:72). Kagan found that in using videotaping for learning, the tasks had to be ordered in a progression from least threatening to most threatening. Means of accomplishing this are discussed below.

Even though most of us have been reared in an era of widespread exposure to television, we remain shy of appearing on television ourselves. This is easily observed in stores where video equipment is set up for display purposes. People will be startled at seeing themselves on the monitor. They will look at themselves briefly, quickly move out of range of the camera, and then dart back for a second, brief look. We are generally torn between wanting to see ourselves and being fearful of how we will look. The same phenomenon occurs when videotape is used in treatment. Practitioners and clients report that initially they are fearful of how they will look, and then are fearful of how they will perform and how their performance will be judged. The evaluation of the performance is more acute for the practitioner than the client. It is the practitioner who is on the spot and knows that the performance will be judged and evaluated. In dealing with such fears, familiarity breeds comfort.

It is best to introduce the practitioner to electronic devices by moving from the simple to the complex. Audiotapes of treatment sessions should be used before videotapes. The practitioner should be supported by the supervisor in advance regarding the difficulty in risking such exposure. The supervisor should explain in advance how the audiotape material will be used in supervision. The supervisor can share some of his own taped material in advance to illustrate how the practitioner's tape will be used. The supervisor should discuss with the worker procedures for getting the client's permission to do the taping.

After the initial taping, the practitioner should be encouraged to listen to the tape alone before it is used in supervision. The practitioner should be requested to make notes about the tape regarding feelings about its impact on the treatment, areas of concern to be discussed in the supervision, and plans for subsequent sessions. When the initial tape is used, the supervisor should allow the supervisee the opportunity to identify problems, blunders, unrecognized dynamics, and successful interventions before the supervisor makes any comments, interpretations, or suggestions.

When videotaping occurs, some of the most significant material regarding the participants occurs prior to the beginning of the taping and just after the conclusion of the taping. The person in charge of the taping needs to be aware of this to achieve maximum performance. The director (practitioner) of the videotaping must ensure that all participants (clients) are clear about their roles and put them at ease. At the conclusion of the taping, the participants are usually relieved, relaxed, and jovial. This is a good opportunity for the director to explore with the participants their feelings and thoughts about the session. While the material is still fresh, the participants are often quick to point out errors or what they consider as alternatives to actions they took. They frequently share what was going through their minds when they took an action or failed to do something they wanted to do.

One taping is not sufficient to develop skill in use of electronic recording. One taping session can lead to familiarity in most cases, but subsequent sessions are needed to develop comfort and skill.

The supervisor and practitioner should not be videotaped too often. The amount of videotaping will vary with the person and the circumstances, but once a month during periods of intensive learning is adequate. Workers being taped need time to apply what they learn from seeing themselves. If time to integrate visualization of self in action is not permitted, the person will become too self-conscious, and learning, as well as performance, can be hampered.

To learn from videotapes of some forms of therapy, especially family therapy, the session must be viewed twice. When viewing long tapes, the supervisor should attempt to get the practitioner to develop a comprehensive understanding of the interaction and dynamics. This can be accomplished by asking such questions as: What process is taking place? What are the unified dynamics of the session? What is the common or persistent theme? What is the thread that holds the interview together?

Videotaping the practitioner's treatment is not the exclusive means of using this medium in supervision. The supervision itself can and should be taped. Videotaping supervision sessions prevents the supervisee from developing the sense that he or she alone is being evaluated. The supervisor is subject to evaluation when supervisory sessions are videotaped, and the supervisor as well as the practitioner will be taking risks and be under scrutiny. Taping of the therapy session, and taping of the subsequent supervision of that session, can add continuity and deeper meaning to the taping.

When split screen techniques are used in individual interviews, I have found that it is easier to evaluate the interaction process when the worker and client are facing each other. When the supervisor wants to focus on the actions of the client or the practitioner exclusively, it is better to reverse the images and to have the participants appear on screen to be talking away from one another, positioned back to back. This takes some advance planning and special equipment (two cameras and a special effects generator), but it is one of the real advantages of television — reality can be manipulated for learning purposes without disturbing the actual therapy situation.

Listening to or watching portions of tapes can be helpful when specific techniques or problems are being worked on. Thematic, theoretical, or conceptual learning is more comprehensive and requires reviewing tapes of whole sessions. Portions of tapes usually are not helpful with comprehensive learning. Portions of tapes cloud the significance of prolonged silence, resistance to interventions, dissolving of resistances, dysfunctional patterns of relating, shifts in roles, interactional themes, and focusing on one person or one problem at the expense of others. A good rule to follow is to use whole session tapes with inexperienced practitioners and to use portions of tapes with more experienced practitioners. Also, it is good to begin the supervisory process with whole session tapes, and as the supervision advances, to progress to segmental tapes once the supervisor is confident that the supervisee has an appreciation for the comprehensive nature of therapy. These are general rules, and there are always exceptions. It should be remembered that whatever approach the supervisor uses should be based on an assessment of the practitioner's learning needs.

I have encountered supervisors and workers who resist videotaping because, "We only have old black-and-white equipment." This attitude is another product of advanced technology, to which we are exposed daily through commercial television. It is true that much of the equipment that is available to most practitioners and their supervisors is crude when compared to commercial television. However, research indicates that black-and-white television is better for practice training because there are fewer extraneous distractions (Berger, 1978:52). All that is needed is a good quality picture, free of distracting distortions. Only the extremes of picture quality should be avoided. Poor quality images and very high quality images are distracting. A balance between technical sophistication and simplicity must be maintained, as well as a clear and consistent focus on the treatment interaction recorded.

Rewards and Problems

It should be pointed out that television in training and therapy can be a dangerous and devastating experience for some. For the past 20 years, television has been used in treatment and has been highly acclaimed by those using it, but there has not been much independent research to document negative or positive impacts. Some practitioners have reported highly negative outcomes when videotape has been used in therapy. In one study of nine married couples, chosen by a random sampling, in a therapy setting where video feedback was used, six of the couples suffered "casualties" in the form of emotional crises, breakdowns, and suicides. At the same time, 41 other couples treated by the same practitioners without video feedback experienced only seven casualties, and none were suicides. Although the outcomes could not be directly attributed to the use of video feedback, there is sufficient reason to approach the use of television with caution and to launch more extensive research on the method (Brandt, 1980:81-82).

There are limited outcome studies of the use of television in training, and it could be some clients and practitioners in training are being put at risk without sufficient safeguards. A study by Howe (1989) found that family therapy clients resented the use of video in the therapy. This could be due to the way the video was presented and used rather than due to the technique of using video. In many training programs, students are expected to engage in video self-confrontation, to videotape family of origin groups, and to be videotaped in group supervision sessions. Many of these sessions delve into highly personal material. In some instances no supervisor is present, and no supervisor even reviews the tapes with the trainees. The unskilled trainees are expected to rummage through one another's personal thoughts and experiences in the name of personal and professional growth and development of self-awareness.

In some cases, such groups are used to give the trainees practice at developing techniques and skills in exploring feelings. It is questionable whether such exercises accomplish much of anything. Students who undergo these experiences are rarely able to connect them with learning anything tangible about the details of therapeutic technique. Some have become extremely uncomfortable in these groups and find the videotaping a source of increased discomfort. They become slightly distrustful of their fellow students and their teachers for placing them in such highly vulnerable situations, where little control is exercised over the limits of the material that becomes fair game for exploration.

These students say that they withdraw and withhold information to protect themselves. Then they are occasionally criticized by teachers, supervisors, and fellow students for being unable to be open about themselves, which calls into question their potential as practitioners. The students readily admit and understand that their learning has been limited in these situations, but attribute this to the misguided focus of the learning rather than a genuine inability to share feelings on their part. Any videotaping sessions should be well planned and supervised to guard as much as possible against negative outcomes.

AUDIOTAPING

Audiotaping has the advantage of being inexpensive, requiring little technical skill, and not being distracting in the treatment sessions. Small cassette tape recorders with built-in microphones and several tapes can be purchased for less than $50. Tapes can be easily edited for teaching purposes. As an example, audiotaping was used as part of the supervision of a young practitioner who had a tendency to use "uh-huh" to the point of distraction and to ask questions as a consistent way of responding to the client without much effect. The practitioner was asked to tape a session, and it was reviewed with her. She had some difficulty hearing the distracting speech pattern, so the tape was edited, with the client talk removed from the tape, leaving only the practitioner dialogue. When a 15-minute segment of the tape was reviewed, the practitioner said "uh-huh" 57 times and asked 24 questions. She was amazed upon hearing this pattern, and began to work on changing it. Subsequent tapes showed a change in her part of the dialogue and an improvement in the course of the treatment.

Linguistic analysis of case material is growing in importance (Grinder

& Bandler, 1976). When doing linguistic analysis of case material with a practitioner who is an active or action-oriented person and/or a client who is very verbal, it is better to use audiotaping in supervision than videotaping. It is possible to miss the linguistic elements of a videotape completely since the video aspects can be so overpowering.

AUDIO/VIDEO SEPARATION

Videotapes can be manipulated so that only the audio or video portions of the tape can be played back. Many supervisors do not realize that the audio and video elements are separate components that are merged to make a videotape and that either part can be used separately. Separation of audio and video portions of tapes in supervision can be effective in clinical interactional hypothesis testing. By listening only to the audio portion of the tape, the supervisor and practitioner can speculate about nonverbal gestures. Later the audio and video portions can be played back in unison to confirm or refute the hypotheses.

There needs to be more emphasis on coordinating use of auditory and visual material in teaching in supervision for effective learning. This is supported by research indicating people remember 15 percent of what they see, 25 percent of what they hear, but 50 percent of what they see and hear at the same time (Bagg, 1980:35).

ROLE PLAY

Role play in training, educating, and supervising social workers has increased rapidly in the past two decades, and there has been little systematic evaluation of or empirical research on its value, effectiveness, or effect on the participants. Role play is used widely in practice and supervision, and supervisors and practitioners need to learn more about its application (see Etcheverry et al., 1980). This section attempts to offer some guidelines on the use of role play for nontherapeutic purposes.

The growth of role play in education and supervision has paralleled the increased popularity of psychodrama in therapy. Also, increased use of role play paralleled the rise of anti-intellectualism of the past two decades. The search for non-traditional and nonacademic modes of learning in part gave rise to the development of role play, and for some, led toplaying at learning rather than traditional academic effort.

Role play is of limited value in education and supervision. Role play should be used as a last resort, and only after other techniques have been explored and found to be ineffective, not available, or not applicable. Live interviews, videotapes, films, audiotapes, and in some instances lectures and discussions are preferable.

Role play exercises limit the depth of feelings that can be expressed, especially when the participants have limited experience with the type of material under exploration. In training programs, this can result in students' being deluded into believing that therapy is mainly information gathering, and that complex and sensitive material is easier to deal with than it is in reality. When student practitioners are required to role play material related to serious illness, death, depression, divorce, etc., of which they have had little direct experience or knowledge, it can result in distorted views of the therapeutic skills and techniques required to deal with such material.

Videotaping or role play of therapy should not be required of student practitioners before they have been given some other form of training in how to handle the material being explored. To videotape and role play with the objective that the learning will emerge from this activity itself sets students up to fail, puts them in a vulnerable position, and can give rise to anxiety that inhibits learning. In formal courses and training programs, videotaping of sessions and role plays should take place near the end of the course or the training program. In addition, role play should take place only when a skilled supervisor or teacher is present, and the students playing the roles should have had some experience with the material being covered and/or thoroughly rehearsed in the material before the role play is attempted. Thus, the decision to use role play should always be linked to the purpose and process of the learning to be accomplished. Also, any decisions made in the process of the role play activity should be made in the context of what is to be taught and learned.

ROLE PLAY PROCEDURES

Most teachers or supervisors who attempt role play in the classroom do so without any formal training in the technique. At best, a teacher has read something about the procedure, has attended a demonstration, or has participated in a role play session. Such experiences usually provide little of the needed information to lead role play activities successfully. Role play demonstration or participation rarely includes instruction on techniques being used by the leader to conduct a successful role play. This can result in the potential role play leader's being deceived into thinking that successful role playing is easy. The teacher or supervisor who wants to do role play should get training in the method before attempting its use, but if training is unavailable, the following procedures should be followed.

There is a process the teacher or supervisor must go through in utilizing role play that can be understood as having four distinct, sequential components. These four components are: planning, monitoring, evaluating, and debriefing. Each component will be discussed separately.

Planning

Any role play activity should be planned in advance. The leader should know in advance what is to be illustrated, demonstrated, and acted out. The leader should know in advance exactly what is to be portrayed. Portrayal takes several forms, such as covering life experiences with which the participants are not familiar, bringing out into the open material that the practitioner is resisting, or rehearsing for dealing with a problem the practitioner has expressed inability to handle.

People with whom the leader thinks the person could best identify should be selected in advance to play roles. The leader should know or learn the capabilities of each participant to perform certain roles. Some people are actors, and some people are not. The leader should discuss the role play in advance with each participant. This can be done before the group arrives or in the presence of the group. None of the group members should be simply assigned or coaxed into doing a role play (Etcheverry et al., 1980:8-10).

When practitioners are asked to participate in a minimally specific role play, the pressure of performing can cause personal material to surface that the practitioner, under other conditions, most likely would not share. In educational settings in which the role play participants are unskilled students, such personal material is poorly handled, often unacknowledged as important and sensitive, and rarely given closure. In some educational programs, unskilled students are required to role play for videotaping when no skilled supervisor or teacher is present. Educational programs and supervisors should give serious consideration to the appropriateness of putting student practitioners in such uncontrolled situations.

A case example illustrates this point. A group of student practitioners was required to role play for videotaping without the teacher's being present. The teacher's logic for not being present was that she did not want to inhibit the students' performances, and she would view the tapes privately at a later time. Three students and a technician were present in the audiovisual laboratory for one of the taping sessions. The role play was set up to be about a woman who came to a mental health center for an initial interview because of unspecified depression. The practitioner was role played by a male student. The student playing the woman client eased into the role, and as the interview progressed, the source of the depression focused on the client's having a sister who was dying of cancer. The student practitioner, wanting to perform well, gratefully focused on the client's feelings about her sister. The role play client became more visibly upset as the interview progressed and was near tears at the conclusion of the session. When the role play was concluded, the technician asked the woman student if she in reality had a sister who was dying of cancer, and she indicated that she did. The students discussed this briefly, and the woman uncomfortably shared more information about her sister before leaving the laboratory in an agitated state.

This example illustrates how significant personal material can surface and not be given closure. The student performing the client's role was led into the personal material by accident, and feelings she had not acknowledged before were tapped. At the close of the session, she was left with the feelings, and no skilled practitioner or supervisor was present to help her understand, accept, or work through these feelings and make some recommendations for her to get help with the problem, if she desired it. In addition, the videotape was played back for the entire therapy class, causing the student to experience the feelings again and leaving her classmates to speculate about whether the situation was real.

The student's confidentiality was violated. Several students asked her about the situation, which she ultimately resented. Although she felt supported by some of her fellow students, she did not like so much attention on her, and she grew weary of explaining the situation to interested fellow students. She wanted to cut off the querying, but at the same time did not want to appear rude to her student colleagues. If the supervisor had planned sufficiently, this woman could have avoided exposure of this family trauma. If she had desired help with this, she could have been assisted privately by the supervisor.

Before starting the role play, explain each role again and take a few minutes to warm each person up to his or her role. Asking how they feel about playing the role helps to ease people into the role play. Such activity can help the leader identify aspects of the role with which the person might have difficulty getting in touch, and the leader can then directly or indirectly be of assistance.

The leader should explain to the group before beginning the role play that role play for educational purposes is similar to, but different from, role play in the therapeutic situation and that it requires a different focus and approach on the part of the leader. The role play audience should be instructed to take notes to use in the post-role play discussion. If specific points are to be observed and recorded, they should be mentioned by the leader before the role play begins. Also, the leader should mention briefly before beginning that the role play might have to be terminated if it moves away from the intended purpose.

Whenever possible, videotape or audiotape the role play. If the role play is successful, it can be used with subsequent groups with much less preparation. Consistent role plays are difficult to recreate even with the same actors. If the role play is recorded, written permission of the participants should be obtained.

Monitoring

Monitoring relates to directing and controlling the role play. It is the leader's responsibility to ensure that the role play remains focused and related to its intended purpose. There are two ways of managing control, based on the level of involvement of the leader. The first is for the leader to be one of the actors. In this method it can help if a co-leader is available as a non-actor, but this is not always possible. The second method is for the leader to direct the role play as a non-actor participant. The method used will depend on the style and preferences of the leader and the nature of the role play to be performed.

The role play should be of short duration. If it takes a great deal of time to set up the situation, you have most likely attempted to deal with too much or too complex material. The set-up time should be no more than five minutes, and the actual role play no more than 15 to 20 minutes. It is better to break complex material into two or three separate role plays and to use discussion time to integrate the material. Role play is one of many techniques the supervisor has available, and more consideration should be given to using a short role play in conjunction with such other techniques as lecture, discussion, written assignments, and audiotaped and video-taped case material.

If any or all of the actors are having difficulty getting into the roles, it is better to abandon the role play after several brief assists from the leader rather than to persist with the effort. This is an important part of the leader's monitoring role. The leader can salvage some aspects of a bad role play by discussing with the actors and the audience why the role play was difficult to enact. In some instances the barriers and blocks can be sufficiently identified to resume the role play.

In some instances it might be necessary to shift the roles of certain actors to overcome problems and resistances. Some people lack the experience, knowledge, or will to assume certain "as if" stances of particular roles. A sensitive leader will be able to identify such difficulties and make the necessary adjustments. If the role play is unsuccessful, and if the leader feels it is not a good idea to persist further with this method to deal with the material, the leader should not attempt to justify or explain away an unsuccessful role play.

I have developed the concept of *role play deviance* to describe situations in which role plays diverge in any way from the supervisor's original purpose or direction. When a supervisor makes the mistake of conducting a spontaneous role play without a specific focus, role play deviance will not occur, but this does not mean that difficulty cannot result. It only means that when difficulty does develop, the supervisor has no basis for terminating or reorienting the role play.

Role play deviance usually occurs when the interaction moves away from the intended focus or when an actor becomes upset by the content of the role play. When the interaction moves away from the intended focus, the supervisor has the responsibility to intervene and redirect the focus or terminate the session. To redirect the focus to the original purpose takes more skill than is apparent. The supervisor must follow the interaction closely and ask questions and make comments or suggestions without distracting the actors from their roles. In a real sense, the supervisor has to be there without being there. This can be accomplished by kneeling behind the actors and making comments or whispering commands to nonactive actors when the leader is not directly involved in the role play. When the leader is involved in the role play, he or she can use the role to refocus the interaction.

Evaluation

At the conclusion of the role play, the leader should discuss the content of the role play and emphasize the points that were to be illustrated as well as any material that emerged as a result of the role play. Observations of both the actors and the audience about certain points should be explored since actors and audiences frequently develop differing perspectives of the role play. The leader should attempt to integrate these differing perspectives to maximize learning. It is helpful in this regard to focus on what the audience *observed* about a certain role and to focus on what the actors *felt* as they performed these roles. The leader can relate these two perspectives to the practice setting, whereas often a person in a role does not perceive events in the same manner as those observing the role.

One problem of role play is that the leader has no control over wrong, weak, or inappropriate responses by actors during the role play. During the discussion the leader should pick up on such responses and help the group find different ways of handling the situation. This can be approached by exploring with the actors how they felt about the adequacy of their responses. Frequently actors readily recognize and admit weakness and inadequacy in their responses.

Debriefing

After evaluating and discussing the role play, the leader should debrief the actors and the audience. Actors' feelings about the roles they played should be discussed. Connections between feelings identified in the "as if" situation and real-life role should be explored. Insights that have been gained should be identified. Incongruent ideas and conflicts in feelings and thoughts that emerge should be kept open for discussion within the group, privately with the leader, or with other appropriate professional or personal contacts. Also, in the debriefing the leader should again explain that the role play techniques used by the leader will not always be obvious. In explaining techniques the leader should make a distinction between doing a role play to help professionals learn something about therapy and doing a role play to teach them how to use role play in the therapy situation.

Participants should be encouraged to incorporate material from the role play in their practice, but the leader should caution participants that there is no guarantee that components of the "as if" situation of the role play will emerge in the reality of practice.

Physical Setting

Good role play conditions require equipment. The average classroom, group therapy room, and office are not conducive to good role play. The supervisor who is serious about role play should be aware of this. Role play can best be performed where there is a stage and where lighting can be controlled. Where this is not possible, two or three floodlights or stage lights mounted on tripods will suffice. The room should be darkened as much as possible, and the spotlights should be placed between the audience and actors and focused on the actors.

This will assist greatly in preventing the actors from seeing the audience. Actors should be positioned in a way that will give the leader freedom of movement to assist in or direct the action. When the leader is a role play participant, he or she should be centrally positioned to see as much of the action as possible.

LIVE SUPERVISION

Live supervision, in which the supervisor actually participates in the treatment by being present during the treatment session or by observing the treatment through a one-way viewing mirror or on a television monitor in another room, is one of the most effective ways to do supervision. In situations in which the supervisor is not present in the therapy room, it is a common practice to use a telephone or "bug-in-the-ear" device for the supervisor to have direct contact with the practitioner.

This is a very effective method of conducting supervision, but it does have some limitations. This form of supervision is fast moving and leaves little time for integration and reflection. It is a much better method for teaching techniques and mastering process in treatment than it is for applying theory, developing a philosophical orientation, or planning a course of treatment. Live supervision can be used most effectively, and can come closer to bridging the gap between a technique orientation and theoretical abstractions, when there are follow-up sessions to the live supervision in which speculation, reflection, and contemplation are allowed. The follow-up meeting, and its relation to what took place in the treatment session, are extremely important because, in live supervision, there is a tendency on the part of both the supervisor and supervisee to let important points go unnoted, since they believe the points will be covered in the follow-up supervision. However, often the material is forgotten or left undiscussed as more pressing issues come up.

It has been argued that the concept of parallel process that has been developed in practice theory also carries over to supervision (Kahn, E. M., 1979). Thus, the parallel process that develops between practitioner and client can pass through to the relationship the practitioner has with the supervisor. In live supervision, the potential for such double-parallel process is increased because both the practitioner and supervisor are directly influenced by the client. If this is not recognized and clearly identified, it can lead to supervisory conflict—the origins of which neither the supervisor nor the supervisee will be able to identify.

Live supervision is more than supervision—it is teamwork and requires much role flexibility, role acceptance, and role confidence on the part of the supervisor. When live supervision is used, the supervisor has to be more responsible and aware than is the case in other forms of supervision. If television is being used, the supervisor must be sensitive to comfort levels of the practitioners and clients. The supervisor must be responsible for minimizing distractions, such as bright lights, movement by television technicians, and talking by the supervisors and others observing behind a one-way mirror. When the supervisor uses a telephone or bug-in-the-ear device to communicate with the practitioner, overuse can be a distraction for the practitioner and client.

When supervisors work behind a one-way mirror and other supervisees are allowed to observe, the supervisor must be careful of what is said about the supervisee doing the treatment. The simplest and most innocuous remarks can be repeated to the performing supervisee by the observing supervisees and can be misinterpreted. When members of a group of supervisees take turns at performing live supervision and observing, the sense of competition can become greatly increased if it is not defused by the supervisor. In one situation a supervisee got very upset when voices could be heard from the viewing room while she was interviewing. The supervisee became very distracted and did not perform a good interview. In the follow-up session she cried and accused her fellow trainees of trying to sabotage her treatment. The supervisor has an absolute responsibility to prevent such situations from occurring. Silence behind the mirror is the best policy. The supervisor and observer should take notes and do the talking during the follow-up session. A viewing room is for viewing. When people are talking, they are not observing, even if they are talking about the treatment session in progress. The supervisor should make these conditions clear to supervisees and colleagues when observing the live work of others.

Many problems can occur in the various forms of live supervision. The supervisor will have to make split-second decisions. In such situations the client's comfort and well-being must be the first consideration. In some situations, if a technical problem occurs, it is better to let the treatment continue and allow the live supervision to lapse. In other situations, it is better to stop the treatment if the live supervision is too distressing for the client. In order to avoid abrupt distraction of the practitioner, the supervisor should give thorough information about the live supervision and how it works in advance. Supervisees should be alerted to common problems that can occur and instructed on how to handle them in advance. It is a good idea to have practitioners observe live supervision before they participate in it. In live supervision the supervisor has a responsibility to be alert to the rights and amount of discomfort experienced by both the practitioner and the client. For this reason, in live supervision it is important to place emphasis on the evaluation of the supervision as well as evaluation of the treatment.

Live supervision done in a sensitive, positive manner is very effective in promoting confidence and eventual autonomy in the practitioner. When live supervision is applied in an authoritarian or punitive manner, it results in the practitioner's trying to copy the supervisor's therapy style in order to lessen the supervisory demands. This inhibits the practitioner from developing his or her own style and decreases the potential for confidence and creativity.

INTRUSION OF PRIVACY

It has been argued that any audiovisual devices used in the treatment or any observation of the treatment is an intrusion and affects the client-practitioner relationship, especially its confidentiality (Langs, 1979:25-26). I do not completely agree with this view. If the logic of the confidentiality argument is consistently applied, there would not be any supervision because any discussion of the therapy outside of the therapy threatens confidentiality. At least when audiovisual devices are used, the client has complete control over what is revealed or not revealed. Also, the use of audiovisual material in supervision provides assurance that the client and the problem will be presented more accurately than when the practitioner attempts to portray or explain the client to the supervisor.

In addition, much concern has been raised about the quality of psychotherapy as the number and type of psychotherapists increase. Clients have limited means of knowing whether they are receiving good or bad treatment. The more a practitioner's work is exposed to other professionals through supervision, the less the risk to the client of undergoing poor or unethical treatment. I think it is appropriate to share with the client the notion that use of audiovisual devices is designed to enhance the quality of the treatment he or she receives without destroying the client's confidence in the practitioner.

With respect to confidentiality, we must keep in mind that the supervisor operates within the same ethical standards as the practitioner. It is true that gaining benefits in any relationship involves taking some risks. Some protection is given up when audiovisual devices are introduced into the treatment, but something can also be gained in the form of new insights, more effective treatment, and more rapid resolution of problems.

RANKING OF TECHNIQUES

This chapter has covered the major audiovisual devices and action techniques used in treatment supervision. As a quick reference for the supervisor, I have ranked these devices and techniques on the basis of their effectiveness and efficiency. They are ranked from 1 to 10, with 1 being the most useful and 10 being the least useful.

1. live joint interviews
2. bug-in-the-ear devices
3. one-way mirror observation
4. videotapes (live material)
5. videotapes (commercially produced)
6. audiotapes (live material)
7. audiotapes (commercially produced)
8. process recordings
9. discussion of case material
10. role play.

In some ways, therapy itself and training to perform it have, like many aspects of our society, become a technological game, so that for many people, one-way mirrors, bug-in-the-ear devices, videotaping and audiotaping, and role play have emerged as therapeutic gimmicks that become ends rather than means. Any technological devices used in treatment or supervision must be planned and implemented as a supplement and focused on how they enhance the improvement of the client.

SUGGESTED READINGS

Milton M. Berger (ed.). *Videotape Techniques in Psychiatric Training and Treatment*. New York: Brunner/Mazel, 1978.
   This book covers the history, theory, and techniques of applying videotaping to practice and training. Some basic technological material is included that is helpful to the supervisor who wants to get started in videotaping.

Roland Etcheverry et al. "The Uses and Abuses of Role Playing." paper presented at Second Group Work Symposium, Arlington, TX (November 1980).
   This paper is an excellent discussion of the use of role play techniques and expands on many points made in this chapter regarding this topic.

J. Paul Gallant and Bruce Thyer. "The 'Bug-in-the-Ear' in Clinical Supervision: A Review." *The Clinical Supervisor* 7 (Fall/Winter 1989), pp. 43-58.

Literature review and summary of use of electronic feedback devices in practice.

Peter Utz. *Video User's Handbook*. Englewood Cliffs, NJ: Prentice-Hall, 1980.
An excellent book for the supervisor who wants to learn the basics of videotape and audiotape operation.

> In my own day-to-day attempt to
> provide a meaningful psychotherapy, I
> find myself increasingly thwarted by
> the reality outside the therapy, by the
> social and material culture of the
> patient and the therapist, the
> ambience, the setting, the milieu in
> which the therapy takes place.
>
> Fred Bloom
> *Psychotherapy and Moral Culture*

Chapter 13

Supervision in Different Settings

This chapter covers supervisory practice in different settings and unique situations. Since all the various settings in which social workers are employed cannot be covered, the chapter begins with a listing of eight characteristics that should be used to explore supervisory practice in any agency that is considered different or special. Then, issues of several different specific settings are explored. The settings discussed are medical, geriatrics and gerontology, criminal justice, and rural.

DIFFERENT SETTINGS

Historically there has been a gradual expansion of the number and type of settings in which social workers function. The proliferation of practice settings is advantageous as far as job opportunities for social work practitioners and supervisors are concerned, but makes it very difficult for an author to cover all the possibilities within the space limitations of a book chapter. Even in practice settings where "identical" services are offered in a number of agencies, each agency will have a unique set of characteristics that the practitioner and supervisor will need to take into account. In order to make such a complex topic more manageable, only general principles and more common settings and situations are covered here. The following list of general characteristics should be considered in aiding supervisees in a given setting:

1. social, economic, and cultural characteristics of clients
2. psychological characteristics of clients and their families
3. interactional patterns of clients
4. interactional patterns of staff
5. structural dynamics of the agency
6. organizational dynamics of the agency
7. geographical location of the setting (i.e., urban, suburban, rural)
8. locale of the agency (i.e., the neighborhood or medical complex of which the agency is a part).

MEDICAL SETTINGS

Knowledge Base

In medical settings the supervisor must be aware of and sensitive to several special areas. First, practitioners in medical settings and specialized medical service areas must master what often seems like a whole new knowledge base. In order to assist patients and their families, practitioners must learn the etiology of the disease being treated, the terminology associated with the disease, the process of the disease, and the problems associated with the course of treatment.

Organizational Structure

Second, the organizational structure of medical settings often is more complex and more diverse than those with which many practitioners are accustomed to dealing. The multidisciplinary setting in which teamwork is advocated, but may or may not be a reality, must be mastered and adapted to by the practitioner. The power of the medical and nursing professions in many settings must be understood, as well as understanding how to relate to less highly trained staff, who often have the most and closest contact with patients (see Krause, 1977:33-67). The supervisor has an important role to play in aiding the practitioner to adjust to and to influence these other disciplines in order to help the patients and their families. The nature of the supervisor's approach will vary according to the size and nature of the facility. The supervisor, who usually has spent years dealing with the complexities of the organization, will sometimes assume that the practitioner also possesses such knowledge and fail to spend adequate time helping the practitioner in this area.

Terminal Illness

Third, in some medical settings, dealing with death and terminal illness is a common experience. For example, in large cancer wards it is common to have an average of one or two deaths per day. Many times, when patients are discharged, the professional staff knows that death is imminent for the patient. Practitioners must be helped to deal with reactions to death and its onset. Many times the most sensitive and committed practitioners have the strongest reactions. Supervisors must be prepared to help practitioners work through such reactions.

Psychological Reactions

Fourth, upon entering certain medical practice areas, practitioners may have psychological reactions to intense exposure to some diseases. Cancer, kidney disease, and heart disease are a few examples of some of the diseases that can cause reactions in workers. Workers can develop responses that mimic the symptoms of the disease that is treated by the service. The supervisor must be alert and prepared to help practitioners with such reactions.

Practitioners may have reactions to trauma and disfigurement they witness in some medical settings. New as well as experienced workers can have reactions to such situations, and supervision is an arena for dealing with these reactions. Trauma debriefings are helpful but usually are only the beginning of the healing process. There must be follow-up to such debriefings. Debriefings are usually general and done in large groups. Such generalized debriefing can expose the practitioner to new stresses through content brought up by participants from other services that can actually add to the practitioner's stress. The supervisor must be available to deal with these secondary reactions.

Death and Dying

In dealing with dying patients the practitioner usually needs help relating to the patient, the patient's family, and other staff. Patient needs are often viewed as immediate. New practitioners have some difficulty accepting the fact that their own lives and work schedules go on when patients are near death. As one practitioner commented in her supervision, "Here I am planning to go sailing this weekend, and this patient is dying." Practitioners must come to accept that they do as much as they can for the patient, but that there must be limits.

Practitioners have reported that they "get more depressed" when their supervisor is away from the agency for vacations or other matters. Practitioners also become more depressed when a patient gets worse or deteriorates, and they are more affected when the dying patient is younger. Practitioners report frustration when patients are not able to accomplish things they wanted to before they became incapacitated. Practitioners have difficulty accepting the fact that they frequently cannot control the situation. The comments of one practitioner summarize this concern: "People go downhill so fast. People die in spite of how they feel and in spite of their feelings, and you can't control the process; nothing you do will stop it."

Interestingly, supervisees also report being more depressed immediately after supervision sessions in which difficult cases are discussed. At the same time the supervision is considered as helpful and worthwhile because supervisees are able to express and explore feelings that under other circumstances "just get bottled up," which can be more harmful than the temporary depression associated with sharing real feelings with the supervisor.

Often practitioners in such settings will talk in circles and deal with a series of related and unrelated issues that do not deal with the real issue of the patient's dying. As one supervisee said, "Hospitals are full of denial." The supervisor needs to be alert to this kind of rambling, confusing discussion and bring up the real issue of the dying patient.

In working with families of the dying patient, special problems can develop. Some families engage in massive denial and attempt to cut the patient off from needed communication. In some families relatives will refuse to visit the patient, leaving the patient with many doubts and concerns. Other families will go to great lengths to protect the patient from the knowledge of the condition. Some family members react with anger. Some patients also react with anger. They may remain angry until death and not "die in peace," which is what the practitioner would like for them. Families need help in dealing with the patient's unyielding anger. Some practitioners show a tendency to move psychologically and interactionally ahead of where the family is emotionally, and push them to deal with what it will be like after the patient dies before the family is ready to deal with this content. Some patients and their families lose time orientation in the stressful period before death, and practitioners need to be prepared to help them with this confusion.

Other staff who are less trained in human behavior can have adverse reactions to the dying patients and their families, and focus their lack of understanding on social workers as they try to intervene. Staff also frequently try to protect the patients and families from the realities of the illness. When social workers attempt to intervene and promote openness about the situation, they may be accused of meddling, interfering, and upsetting the patient. Such criticism, overt and covert, can be upsetting and disheartening to the social worker. The supervisor must be prepared to support and help the practitioner with such staff reactions.

The supervisor in geriatric and/or medical settings must be able to help supervisees deal with issues of death and dying confronted by patients and their families. In many instances supervisees will need to be sensitized to these issues, especially younger workers. Weisman (1972:157) has developed a set of seven questions the supervisor can explore with supervisees to help them become more empathic in this area.

1. If you faced death in the near future, what would matter most?
2. If you were very old, what would your most crucial problems be?
3. If death were inevitable, what circumstances would make it acceptable?
4. If you were very old, how might you live most effectively and with least damage to your ideals and standards?
5. What can anyone do to prepare for his or her own death, or for that of someone very close?
6. What conditions and events might make you feel that you were better off dead? When would you take steps to die?
7. In old age, everyone must rely upon others. When this point arrives, what kind of people would you like to deal with?

Hospice Settings

A new form of medical social work is developing in hospice settings. The concept of hospice care for the terminally ill and their families is relatively new in the United States, but is increasing rapidly. There are now more than 200 such settings, such as nursing homes, hospitals, and free-standing hospices. The hospice concept is organized around the idea of a team effort involving physician, nurse, social worker, clergy, patient care coordinator, volunteers, the client, and the family of the client (Ajemian & Mount, 1980:65-93). A hospice offering inpatient and outpatient care is usually viewed as a small agency by its staff even when it is part of a larger facility. The social work department usually consists of two or three social workers plus a supervisor.

The supervisor in a hospice has a unique responsibility because all of the supervisees are members of an interdisciplinary care team. Frequently, social workers, as well as other staff, have little experience functioning as a part of such teams. Supervision of the social worker participating in such teams requires a strong sense of professional independence and autonomy based on knowledge and skill. The supervisor's role is made more complex because, in many hospices, volunteers engage directly in bereavement counseling, which can lead to confusion about accountability, evaluation of intervention, and exercise of authority.

Team membership involves conflict, negotiation, compromise, participative decision making, and flexibility. The social worker and supervisor must be confident about the practitioner's independent professional competence, but at the same time not be threatened when concessions must be made to the team. Lack of professional competence can bring the practitioner into conflict with other team members because authority is diminished on the team. This model of team functioning promotes individual team members' giving way to enabling roles and leadership shared among team members at appropriate points in the treatment process (Rossman, 1977:107).

Because hospice care is a new form of practice, ground rules and clear procedures are missing. Participants are free to experiment with new methods and procedures, but at the same time fear of the unknown and untried strategies can promote insecurity and undue caution in practitioners. This situation creates new challenges and opportunities for the social work supervisor.

GERIATRICS AND GERONTOLOGY SETTINGS

Portions of this section are reprinted from Carlton E. Munson, "Social Work in Aging," Gerontology and Geriatrics Education, Vol. 1, No. 1 (Fall 1980), pp. 17-23; and Carlton E. Munson, "Social Work Educational Consultation in Church-Related Nursing Homes," Gerontology and Geriatrics Education, Vol. 1, No. 3 (Spring 1981), pp. 175-180. Reprinted by permission of the University of Texas Press.

Supervising the practitioner in geriatrics (diseases of aging) and gerontology (science of aging) settings can impose special problems for the supervisor. The most salient concern of the supervisor should be the negative stereotypic notions the young practitioner might have about the aged, which Butler (1969) has identified as "ageism." Research indicates that such stereotyping is a serious problem among children (Seefeldt et al., 1977) and students in training for the professions (Geiger, 1978). Social work and medical students have been found to be significantly lacking in information and knowledge about the elderly, fail to perceive accurately problems that the elderly are likely to identify, and show no preferences for working with the elderly. Practitioners in training, as well as practicing therapists, have few opportunities to work with healthy and active older people, and their work with the impaired elderly can reinforce the impression that aging is associated with impaired functioning, decreased activity, and gradual or sudden disengagement. This can result in certain assumptions in relating to the elderly person seeking treatment that can promote dependency and disengagement. Although there have been some limited attempts to sensitize professional students to the elderly (Birenbaum et al., 1979), the majority of young practitioners have limited experience with such programs, and their attitudes and behaviors need to be monitored for stereotypes that can distort treatment efforts. Although social work has been present in medical settings for most of this century, social workers are relative newcomers to geriatric settings.

Social work in aging has been focused in three major areas: curative, preventive, and enhancing (Lowy, 1979). Interventive efforts on the part of social workers have occurred through the three major practice methods of casework, group work, and community organization. Casework has centered on, but has not been limited to, the curative and enhancing functions through work with individuals and their families. Group work has centered on these same two functions in relation to small groups, while community organization has related more to the preventive function through work with large groups.

Social work education has been generally reactive to practice developments regarding social problems and groups to be served. Social work practice historically has lacked widespread application in the field of aging (Lowy, 1979). This is not to imply that there is no history of social work in aging or societal concern with the elderly.

In general, social workers have had limited desire to work in the field of aging because of societal and personal lack of interest in the elderly, because of low professional status associated with this area of practice, and because of low salaries. This has been the case in both community-based and institutional programs, but these factors have been especially important with respect to the institutionalized elderly. Ironically, the recent, rapid entry of social workers into geriatric settings has been due to federal and state regulatory mandates implemented in the nursing home field. At the same time there has been reluctance on the part of both the nursing home field and the social work profession to establish social work services for the institutionalized elderly.

Statistical information about manpower in various practice specializations is much more highly developed in other professions than in social work. The National Association of Social Workers (NASW) has no reliable statistics on its membership, which makes it difficult to speculate with any accuracy about the number or characteristics of trained social workers, historically or currently, with respect to practice activity in aging in comparison with other practice areas. Also, accurate statistics for social work education for geriatric practice are not available. Although the Council on Social Work Education (CSWE) compiles annual statistics on the total number of students, faculty, and accredited educational programs, no statistics exist for student or faculty specialization in various practice areas or for the number of programs offering degree specializations. In order for sound manpower and educational planning to occur, the practice and educational components of the profession — through the two major national organizations (NASW and CSWE) — must make a concerted effort to gather and analyze such information (Munson, 1980c: 17-18).

Motivation and learning needs of practitioners in aging have received limited attention from social work educators or supervisors. Some practitioners select aging because of an emotional experience with an elderly relative or because of the promise of good job opportunities, without having a realistic perception of the demands that can be placed on them. Many are quite young and have little understanding of or appreciation for the functioning or problems of the elderly. Supervisors need to be more alert to ways of sensitizing practitioners to the elderly. In accomplishing this, models for teachers and supervisors need to be developed that will appropriately orient practitioners to effective ways to intervene with the elderly. Currently, the literature is very limited in this area.

Long-Term Care Facilities

Work in nursing homes or long-term care facilities (LTCFs) poses unique problems for the social work supervisor, and special attention will be given to the supervisory role in such settings since they are so new. Social workers find the nursing home field alien because proprietary and nonprofit facilities operate from a free-enterprise perspective and use business management strategies. The pattern has been for most LTCFs to contract with professional social workers to serve as fee-for-service providers on a part-time basis. Such social workers are frequently, but it seems to me inappropriately, referred to as consultants. When social services are provided by outsiders, there is little motivation to develop services within the facility, and regular staff tend to shy away from direct helping activities for fear of intruding on the work of the outside service providers. This section presents a different view of the role of the social worker in LTCFs. An interpersonal role model of the social worker is presented that focuses on integrative functions as well as provision of clinical services. From this perspective the practitioner engages in enhancing the helping skills of regular staff, interpreting and integrating roles of various disciplines in relation to social services, and developing service programs.

In role theory, roles have been distinguished as conventional and interpersonal (Hewitt, 1976:144-146). Conventional roles are based on routine responses to human situations and regularized structures. Interpersonal roles develop out of unique interactive situations, and repeated interaction leads to creative role performance and expectation. When one accepts the position of practitioner in an LTCF, both the practitioner and the facility staff—and especially the administrator—draw on conventional role models. The administrator hires a social worker from the perception that the social worker will function structurally much as the physician; that is, he or she will be a part-time professional service provider who relates to residents' basic needs and addresses special problems as they arise. Social workers readily accept this model because conventionally they have been trained to work and have worked in agencies in which they provide casework and group work services directly to clients. Residents accept this model because they have rarely had any contact with social workers prior to admission, and this is a new role experience for them. When the social worker assumes this conventional role model, there is little incentive for the facility to develop a fully integrated social work program.

The social worker needs to assume an interpersonal role model in which the practitioner works directly with all staff, including the facility administrator. The focus of the supervisor should be on defining the role of **social services** in relation to other disciplines and departments. The major functions of the supervisor from this perspective are:

1. to establish a social service policy;
2. to define who will deliver the social services;
3. to develop job descriptions and guide recruitment efforts;
4. to provide in-service training for social service staff and other disciplines regarding the role of social work;
5. to establish admission procedures;
6. to develop treatment strategies, including goal-setting and recording procedures; and
7. to interpret regulations regarding social services.

The extent to which the supervisor focuses on specific functions depends on the nature of the individual facility. Some homes have MSW staff; others have full-time employees with little or no training who serve as social service designees. Some homes have thorough admissions procedures; others have none at all. Some homes have adequate recording procedures; others have haphazard and inconsistent methods. Some facilities master social service regulations without difficulty; others respond with frustration and confusion.

Role Differentiation

In LTCFs, the social worker often experiences difficulty with the administrator and nursing staff, especially the director of nursing. The supervisor must work to help differentiate the roles of social workers, nurses, and administrators. Frequently, in church-related homes, the administrator has a ministerial background. When administrators have not been trained to distinguish between the role of administrator and minister, role strain can develop. When a social worker is brought into this situation, role confusion often develops, resulting in conflict, frustration, and isolation. I have defined administrators who view their residents as a congregation to be ministered to as *all-inclusive* administrators. They run the facility much as they did their church. They handle all the administrative tasks as well as counseling residents and their families. They are used to dealing with death, grief, guilt, and tragedy, and often they prefer these challenging tasks to mundane administrative tasks, which they frequently are ill-prepared to perform. A social worker operating in the shadow of such an administrator feels discounted and becomes frustrated and isolated in the organization. It is easy for an administrator to bypass a social worker at any level of education, experience, and skill. For example, the all-inclusive administrator can admit patients without involving any other staff, can counsel a dying patient on wills and burial arrangements, or can deal directly with the family of a dying patient (Munson, 1980c).

This problem can be dealt with by the supervisor through role differentiation on a potential and actual basis by conducting joint sessions with both the administrator and social worker. These sessions should not be based on abstract explanations of organizational roles, but should instead deal with specific case material that is problem-oriented. In the process of discussing the case material, specific responsibilities should be delineated and agreed upon. Such cases should be discussed more than once, and should be followed for several months until the problems are resolved. A secondary outcome of this process is that the administrator and social worker get a perspective on what happens to residents over time. This allows them to recognize indicators of change in functioning and adjustment of residents. The ongoing sessions also reinforce the role differentiation and prevent the administrator from falling back into the all-inclusive pattern. There are occasions when it is determined that the administrator should have more, rather than less, involvement with some residents. For example, the majority of LTCF residents, and the majority of social workers, are women. Male residents often feel isolated, and where a male administrator is present, informal involvement with the male residents can be helpful.

Regulations

Social work services in LTCFs are much needed, poorly developed, and little understood. They are the least-regulated service, and the meager regulations are marginally enforced. Enforcement of state and federal regulations varies from state to state, and although federal regulations mandate minimal standards, supplemental state regulations vary substantially. In addition, the qualifications of evaluators and surveyors differ from state to state. In some states evaluation is done by nurses, physicians, or social workers. Where social workers are employed or contracted with to serve on evaluation teams, they usually have little or no experience in LTCFs. This can be problematic because the evaluators have limited understanding of the role of the social worker in LTCFs, and have even less understanding of the role of the supervisor. This is compounded when evaluators lack clarity about the regulations or how to evaluate their implementation.

Special attention is given to regulation because the supervisor is often expected to help the facility with the regulations and the regulators. It is easy for the neophyte supervisor to be overwhelmed by this staff concern and to devote a substantial portion of time to this subject. At the same time the supervisor who refuses to discuss meeting regulations with the staff, because he or she views the supervisor's role as dealing only with practice problems, will not be viewed as very helpful by the staff. Also, supervisor efforts to improve staff service delivery efforts will have marginal effectiveness in dealing with a group that works with perpetual concern for meeting regulations.

Instead of being overwhelmed by or ignoring regulations, the supervisor should use regulations as a means of focusing content about organizing and delivering services. In order to do this, the supervisor must become thoroughly familiar with federal and state regulations and guidelines used to implement the regulations. Usually, social service regulations are minimal and general enough to allow development of alternative styles of service delivery.

It is also helpful for the supervisor actually to participate in an evaluation of the facility to learn how evaluation reports are formulated and to assist staff at interpreting social services for the evaluators. The supervisor can assist survey team members to understand the role of social work in LTCFs and to evaluate the effectiveness of social work services. For example, in one survey an evaluator came to the conclusion that the social worker was not involved with the residents. When questioned about this, the surveyor admitted that the judgment was based solely on having asked several residents what the social worker's name was. It was explained by the staff that such a technique was not a very reliable measure when dealing with a population that is known to have substantial short-term memory loss for various reasons. The staff explained and documented for the evaluator the amount and variety of contact and activity engaged in with the residents. Such information, which can be provided only by social work staff, can do much to add balance to an evaluation. To achieve such interaction, the staff must be trained to be active participants in the evaluation process, rather than passive recipients of judgments made by evaluators that are based on resident records and simple, but not necessarily relevant, questions asked of residents. Surveyors usually welcome such input from the staff; they have admitted possessing little knowledge, little guidance, and few skills at implementing social service regulations (Munson, 1981b).

Regulations can be used to train staff to work with residents. For example, regulations generally deal with documentation of social history data, treatment plans, and long-term and short-term goal setting. The supervisor can use documentation in any of these areas to establish how to gather data, what data to gather, how to determine priority of needs, how to establish goals, what goals to establish, and how to interrelate long-term and short-term goals. For example, social history data about the childhood development of a 70-year-old resident is secondary to knowing what family members are available as a resource to the resident. In setting goals,workers and evaluators tend to think in global and total-recovery terms. Such thinking can divert the practitioner from understanding the real needs of old and frequently incapacitated residents. Goals need to be thought of in very basic and simple terms: getting a resident to sit up, to eat, to eat in the dining room, to talk. Regulations are geared more to *when* and *where* to document, and the role of the supervisor must be related to *what* and *how* to document. An entire training program for staff can be built around this basic premise.

Role Support

To carry out the role of the supervisor that has been defined here, the supervisor must have support at the highest level of the organization. For administrators, nurses, physicians, and other departments to cooperate, the supervisor must be perceived as understood, accepted, and supported by those who operate the facility. The supervisor must have access to the decision makers and must be viewed as working in conjunction with them. A supervisor who is expected simply to satisfy regulatory requirements has no basis on which to build an effective social work program.

The effective supervisor becomes a strong support for the social work staff as they carry out their jobs in a demanding setting. As other departments that do not have a similar type of supervisor see social workers gaining further training and education, having a forum for identifying and solving problems, and having assistance in dealing with regulations, they become envious and, at times, threatened. The social work supervisor can be of further assistance to the total functioning of the facility by advocating that others, such as nurses, administrators, physicians, and activities staff, be provided with supervisors, consultants, or parallel support systems (Munson, 1981b).

CRIMINAL JUSTICE SETTINGS

The main unique feature of criminal justice settings—for probation, parole, or incarceration—is the authority invested in the practitioner. Most young, inexperienced practitioners entering such settings have had little or no experience with the power and authority granted to courts and their representatives. Often they have not experienced court proceedings and do not understand the intricacies of our legal system. Also, practitioners are sometimes overwhelmed by the degree of pain and suffering inflicted on others by those who become their clients. Practitioners are often in the position of working with people who have radically different values from their own, and they react to these differences.

The supervisory role is similar in parole, probation, and institutional settings, especially with respect to authority issues. In institutional settings, the role of the family in relation to the adult offender should be given consideration in supervision of the practitioner. For the inmate, the role of family is sometimes forgotten, and the offender can be viewed by the staff in the context of institutional life exclusively. Tobin has pointed out that the practitioner can lose sight of the role of the inmate's family in promoting motivation for the offender to change through therapeutic intervention (Mishne, 1980:278). The supervisor should monitor the practitioner to ensure that this important aspect of the rehabilitation process is not neglected.

Group Home Settings

The role of the supervisor regarding adolescent offenders is discussed here in the context of group home settings, but the points can be applied to other criminal justice settings.

There has been a trend toward shifting rehabilitation efforts for acting-out adolescents from large institutional settings to small group homes. Such group homes employ paraprofessionals as front-line staff (Handler, 1975). There have been efforts to identify the major functions of the supervisor in these settings in relation to untrained staff. This section focuses on one aspect of that role, in which the staff and residents are viewed as a small group, and the dynamics of staff interaction are reflected in resident behavior. The staff and resident group process is analyzed by exploring:

1. achieving honest and clear communication,
2. accepting and using authority,
3. dealing with staff anxiety in threatening situations, and
4. developing appropriate levels of genuineness and self-awareness.

The discussion that follows is based on a specific model of group homes in which the following statements are true:

1. **The director of the group home functions both as an administrator and as a front-line staff member.**
2. All staff are predominantly paraprofessionals who have little formal training in therapeutic relationships.

3. There are regularly scheduled "house" meetings in which staff and residents participate.
4. There are regularly scheduled staff meetings.
5. The program is based on a therapeutic model in which the staff is engaged in change efforts.

A cohesive, unified staff built on the above model can be effective, regardless of the philosophic or theoretical basis on which the group home operates.

Before any change efforts can be effectively attempted, conditions must be created for honest and clear communication. This is basic in situations in which residents are accustomed to dealing with the world through manipulation, and staff is expected to accomplish a great deal with very little training. Decision making is the basis of much interaction between staff and residents. The staff exists as a group, and the residents exist as a group. Individual behavior by a member of either group is often interpreted in a group context rather than on an individual basis. Behavior in this context is based on what Redl and Wineman (1952:20) identified in one of the earliest group home experiments as "social reality." Often the two groups get polarized around issues and problems, which results in no resolution and continuing frustration. When staff use group manipulation to deal with perceived resident manipulation, communication breaks down. This is epitomized in one resident's comment in a house meeting, "We ain't going to play the staff's games, so we don't expect you to play ours." This comment occurred after an incident in which the staff attempted to decrease "horseplay" in the house by increasing fines for such activity and notifying residents after the fact. Staff felt a need to make some on-the-spot decision to maintain order in the house, but residents viewed this as a change in the rules without their input. The staff could have contained the horseplay more effectively by assessing repeated violations at the agreed-upon rates rather than increasing the amount for the sake of expediency. Rules are effectively applied only when they are carried out according to previously agreed-upon decisions that involved both the staff and resident groups.

Given the opportunity, residents as a *group* can develop self-regulation that takes the pressure off staff and allows them to intervene only when self-regulation fails. This allows the staff to avoid the "game-playing" stance, but it is very difficult to achieve when staff live with the constant fear that interpersonal conflict will escalate out of control. This fear is very real in an unstructured situation in which the staff group is smaller in number and often physically weaker than a resident group that has limited self-control under stress. Less control is not being recommended here, but control should be exercised as agreed upon. Residents will not adhere to rules when the staff is perceived as not observing them. It is recognized that unique situations develop that require immediate decision making. In situations of this type, it is important that the staff group subsequently communicate to the resident group why such decisions were made. When feedback is not provided, such staff decisions will be viewed by the resident group as arbitrary and punitive.

Individual residents use the group to negate individual deviance, as one resident's comment illustrates: "I was drinking in the house. So what? Everybody drinks in the house." The resident group will also focus on individual behavior to avoid group issues. This is illustrated when a group of residents dislikes a particular resident and reports him for various infractions, to which the disliked resident responds, "You just want to see me kicked out of the house." The staff must be trained to recognize this variable use of the individual and the group to avoid communication of the real issues. Both of the examples that have been given demonstrate dysfunctional behavior that must be exploited for clinical purposes through use of what has been identified as "influence and interference techniques" (Redl & Wineman, 1951:41-46).

Use of authority comes with difficulty in any circumstance, and appropriate use of authority is even more difficult to attain. Young, untrained staff recognize the need for authority, but at the same time question its use since no exercise of authority goes unchallenged by the resident group. First, variations of authority within the staff group must be identified. The individual staff member's authority varies when on duty and off duty. In small, informal group homes with a milieu orientation, staff are frequently in the house when off duty. Residents often attempt to negate the authority of staff at such times. This can be handled by making clear that staff are invested with their authority at all times.

Staff are more likely to use authority when angry. Thus, residents see them exercise authority inconsistently. Staff often knowingly, in full view of residents, overlook infractions of the rules when activity in the house is calm and on a positive note, but the same infractions can get the entire house put on restriction when matters are going badly. The supervisor must help the staff to develop skill at exercising authority when they are not angry, and to avoid using their authority excessively when angry. This balancing of power use can help the staff avoid the staff-resident standoffs that are so common in group homes. As one resident commented, after the staff had placed the entire house on warning in an angry exercise of authority, "You staff are idiots; with everybody on warning there are just going to be more fights in the house." What the resident was saying epitomizes the "standoff" situation: when staff put residents on warning in anger, the residents respond by putting staff on warning through their behavior.

There is space here to make only the generalization that authority must always be available for use, but it must be applied consistently and based on rational, rather than emotional, responses. There are many other authority issues, and the supervisor will find that the resolution of specific authority problems is endemic and must be dealt with regularly in staff meetings and house meetings.

The director exercises authority at another level. This can become problematic, conflictive, and confusing when the director also carries the role of front-line staff member because when in the directorial role, he or she can use more sweeping authority in a resident encounter than a regular staff member can. The director must be helped to recognize this difference and encouraged to use the directorial authority sparingly when functioning as a staff member. The director who does not make this distinction will become isolated from residents, their feelings, and their behavior. The director is by nature in a difficult position, and "is always the last one to know" about deviant behavior in the house. The power of the director is inherently recognized by the residents and other staff; by making the distinction just described, the difficulties of the position can be minimized but certainly not overcome completely.

The supervisor has the most dubious authority. Supervisors can exercise much authority if they allow the staff to view them as experts and become dependent on them for decisions, or they can function solely as facilitators who allow the staff to work out all problems within the staff group. The most appropriate role for the supervisor is somewhere between these two extremes. As the staff should rely on resident self-regulation as much as possible, the supervisor should rely on staff self-regulation to an even greater extent. To achieve this, the supervisor needs to meet regularly with the staff, and the focus of these meetings should be improved staff intervention through discussion of problem-solving efforts in the house. The supervisor is often the only source of support for individual staff members and the staff group. Staff have many conflicts and confrontations with residents that can be the focus of these sessions, but staff also have conflicts, disagreements, and occasional confrontations with each other that must be handled. Staff are more willing to discuss their conflicts with residents than their conflicts with one another, but staff conflict must be explored to promote more unified and healthy staff functioning. This is important because residents are keen observers of weaknesses in staff relationships, and they will manipulate staff conflict. Frequently, the supervisor will learn about staff conflict from the residents before it is even identified by the staff.

Residents have authority that often is not recognized as such by the staff. Often residents are assigned duties related to operation of the house that requires supervision of other residents. Daily cleanup details and meal preparation are examples. Staff must be careful that assignment of such authority does not put some residents in a difficult position or give residents the opportunity to take advantage of a position of power. For example, it is appropriate to put a resident in charge of a cleanup detail, but the evaluation of the cleanup should be done by a staff member. Any authority granted to residents requires supervision by a staff member to avoid abuse, as well as to prevent the resident in authority from being subjected to what Redl and Wineman have defined as "social death" within the resident group as a result of being perceived as allied with the staff (Redl & Wineman, 1952:20).

The group home situation is sufficient to create anxiety in the most skilled practitioner. From the moment residents enter the home, their symptomatic behavior overwhelms the staff with intensity and great velocity (Redl & Wineman, 1951:46). In the face of such behavior, untrained staff impose external controls rather than exploit the behavior for therapeutic purposes. This is only natural given the staff's coping mechanisms. Unfortunately, external controls do not necessarily result in therapeutic change. Anxiety emerges from insufficient techniques for dealing with behavior, and when the few techniques available to the staff do not work, anxiety becomes more intense. The main strategy for the supervisor to use in decreasing staff anxiety is to help them develop nonthreatening interventive skills. The emphasis should be on using external controls only as a last resort. Staff need to be exposed to interventive techniques that encourage residents to develop internal control mechanisms. Anxiety can be lowered by removing some interaction from the resident group.

Staff should be supported and trained in doing individual counseling with residents. Issues such as drug use, sexual activity, and school performance can produce much less anxiety for a staff member and a resident when discussed in an individual relationship. The opposite is also true. There are times when sensitive issues cannot be articulated on an individual basis, and a group approach in which no individual is singled out allows exploration without provoking severe anxiety among residents or staff.

No amount of training or support will relieve all anxiety. Staff get anxious for the same reasons residents do: lack of coping mechanisms (see Pearlin & Schooler, 1978). The more coping mechanisms the staff develop, the more coping mechanisms they can pass along to the residents. This is the essence of the therapeutic process in a group home. An anxiety-ridden staff will only increase anxiety among residents. It is in this area that the supervisor can contribute the most to the therapeutic program of the group home.

The helping professions have long been concerned with the importance of self-awareness in therapeutic relationships without much study of how much and what kind of self-awareness is appropriate. The concepts of genuineness and self-awareness are important for the staff that works in a highly unstructured environment in which roles are not well differentiated. Genuineness refers to sharing *how* one feels; self-awareness refers to knowing *what* one feels. Staff often engage in work activities, recreational activities, and leisure time directly with the residents as well as "living in" the house while on duty. Genuineness is more appropriately discussed in conjunction with staff-resident relationships, and self-awareness in connection with staff relationships. Thus, genuineness involves sharing with a resident *how* it makes you feel when a staff member is the object of a barrage of profanity, and self-awareness relates to discussing in a staff meeting why one responds personally to such an attack of profanity. In a threatening and anxiety-producing encounter with a resident, it is not always good to share fear and anxiety, but in a staff meeting this can be discussed to develop self-awareness about what in the situation was threatening and anxiety producing, and how new and alternative coping mechanisms can be developed.

Self-awareness can be used in encounters with residents just as genuineness can be discussed in staff meetings. For example, during a house meeting, after genuinely sharing some of his feelings about how he deals with anger, the director was helped by some residents and staff to develop the self-awareness that often, when he was angry, he would respond inappropriately by placing restrictions on the entire resident group. Also in a staff meeting, the staff shared their feelings that a house meeting was "lousy." With help from the supervisor, they were able to be more genuine and share that what they really felt was discomfort because the meeting involved some intense, negative exchanges between staff and residents. They went on to discover that they rated meetings on the basis of control and that they associated comfort and good meetings with controlled sessions in which little genuine feeling was shared. Staff have a propensity to be more genuine when angry or frustrated, which can result in inappropriate sharing of feelings. The supervisor must work to help staff be genuine when they are in control, rather than being genuine only when they are out of control.

As long as genuineness and self-awareness are discussed in the context of the work settings, staff can develop a great deal of cohesiveness resulting in a positive, supportive work group. The supervisor has a responsibility to prevent such sharing from becoming therapeutically oriented and focused on the personalities of the individual staff. When this type of sharing is the focus of the supervisor, the staff can become disillusioned, frustrated, and immobilized. Instead of concentrating on the motives of the staff for their behavior, the supervisor should function as a role model for positive therapeutic intervention with residents. In order to do this, the supervisor must have a well-articulated repertoire of interventive strategies and coping mechanisms, including appropriate levels of genuineness and self-awareness, specifically when working with aggressive, manipulative, and poorly socialized adolescents. The timid and insecure supervisor will quickly lose the respect of residents and staff, and will increase anxiety, especially in the staff group.

RURAL PRACTICE SETTINGS

Are rural social work practitioners different? If one reads the literature on rural practice, this question repeatedly emerges as a central theme. It is understandable that this is a common question since social work has always been and remains substantially an urban phenomenon (Munson, 1980d). Articulation of rural practice has emerged in the shadow of urban practice. Conceptualization of rural practice cannot be effectively accomplished in comparison or contrast to urban practice. Too much time and effort have been devoted to differentiations of rural and urban practice that rarely get beyond descriptions of clients, communities, and educational programs.

Supervision is an appropriate arena in which to begin to define and document rural practice. Much of our overall practice wisdom has been developed through the years around supervision, but unfortunately only small portions of that wisdom have been preserved and transmitted in our literature.

Although, as so many have pointed out, rural social work practice is generic—the rural practitioner being a generalist—we must keep in mind the fact that rural practice is still conducted in service-limited agencies (agencies that have specific services to be delivered and specific functions to be performed). Too often the terms generic and generalist have been used to perpetuate vagueness, uncertainty, and inconsistency about what we do in our rural practice. The fact remains that in rural areas, clients come to welfare departments, courts, family service agencies, nursing homes, and mental health centers for services that are specific to the agency. There are networks of agencies in rural areas that offer good, coordinated services, but just as often I have witnessed "generalist" supervisors and workers referring clients to other agencies because they have a "family problem" or an "emotional problem."

With more trained workers being employed in rural areas, supervision needs to relate more to the capabilities and limitations of the worker. Many BSW-level workers have been trained in interventive skills that go unused because they are led to rely on the generalist practice of referral and coordination of services that often exists only on paper. It is essential that the MSW-level professional reach out to the BSW worker to offer parallel services to some clients. In this context we might do well to revive a former practice of having a mental health worker, at the insistence of a supervisor, contact a BSW social worker and his or her supervisor in public welfare or corrections to coordinate service delivery. Distance and travel are frequently compounding factors in rural areas, but coordination of home visits and agency visits for this purpose can be accomplished. I have often seen welfare caseworkers or probation workers transport clients to a mental health center, sit in the waiting room during the visit, and never have any contact with the mental health staff. In rural areas, one overlooked function of the supervisor is that of helping the supervisee effectively utilize services and information provided by other professionals. The MSW worker needs to reach out to other professionals, but often this does not happen. Workers need to be assisted by supervisors in providing information and intervention when it is not requested. Passivity among timid workers contributes to ineffective practice, and is anappropriate issue for supervision.

Self-Reliance

It has been held that supervision is hard to find in rural practice (Ginsberg, 1976) and, therefore, that the worker must be self-reliant. In many instances, supervision is unsolicited rather than unavailable. Generalist workers can be subjected to the subtle suggestion that they are not being "good generalists" if they need help with cases—that they are not being self-reliant. It is easy for supervisors to convey this message to the worker unwittingly since the self-reliant worker makes few or no demands on the supervisor. If worker dependency is suspected, this can be worked out in the supervision process. When personal and professional performance intermingle in supervision, supervisors have the responsibility to ensure that they supervise the position and not the person (Munson, 1976).

Self-reliance is not synonymous with good practice. There are many self-reliant workers who are inefficient and ineffective, and their self-reliance merely allows them to escape being accountable. The only way to ensure that self-reliance is genuine and appropriate is through periodic evaluation of the worker's practice, and evaluation is best achieved within sound, sensitive supervision. Evaluation must be carried out within a larger context of supervision that is oriented to promoting growth and development of the worker. Supervision carried out exclusively for the purpose of evaluation becomes merely "checking up," and can lead to worker and supervisor resentment. Evaluation should be periodic, expected, scheduled, consistent, goal oriented, and verbal as well as written. It should provide continuity and contain input from both parties. Further, evaluation should deal only with activity of the worker of which the supervisor has direct knowledge. Evaluation based on speculation about behavior is to be avoided.

Self-reliance and autonomy are not synonymous with self-monitoring. Self-monitoring involves a deliberate process in which the worker evaluates his or her own practice and decisions made in practice. Self-reliance relates to the power to make decisions in the midst of a practice situation, since autonomy is oriented to the present. Self-monitoring involves after-the-fact evaluation of decision making. The granting of autonomy to the worker should be on the basis of trust in the worker's decision-making ability in his or her practice, and not because the supervisor has little time to deal with problems. Too often workers perceive their autonomy as deriving from supervisor default rather than from a design to promote autonomy. The case example that follows illustrates these points.

A social worker in a rural nursing home appealed to her supervisor, the facility administrator, for help with an 83-year-old man who had been a resident for a year. He was depicted as gradually getting worse. The patient was described as "depressed," "having hallucinations," and "paranoid." He reported seeing strange objects and former family members in his room at night, especially his deceased wife. The patient was nervous and confused at times, and hinted at suicide. This created mixed feelings among the staff since they were not certain whether the patient was capable of committing suicide. He would fight off staff and other residents when they attempted to get him out of his room. The facility physician recommended a psychiatric evaluation. The social worker had observed that the patient's deviant behavior followed a cyclical pattern as his medication was altered. Rather than discussing the mechanics of the referral, the administrator merely approved the referral and indicated that funds were available to pay for the psychiatric evaluation. The worker had never done a referral to a mental health center, and this is what she really was asking for help with, but the administrator was not prepared to provide supervision in this area. The worker, left on her own, made the following decisions: the patient was not told of the referral until the day of the psychiatric visit, resulting in an increase in his paranoia, hostility, and depression; an aide was assigned to transport the patient the 24 miles to the mental health center; and no list of questions, social history, or description of symptoms and behavior was prepared for the psychiatrist. This resulted in the patient's appearing normal and rational to the psychiatrist, and the written evaluation was of little value to the social worker or the nursing home staff because the report was mostly a new version of the patient's social history already in the facility's records. With social work supervision provided after-the-fact, the worker was able to see that the patient should have been prepared for the referral in advance, that the social worker should have accompanied the patient to the mental health center, that a special list of questions should have been prepared for the psychiatrist (especially questions about the role of medication and suicidal threats), and that the worker should have met with the psychiatrist to formulate recommendations and a treatment plan to be implemented with the patient in the facility. That could have been the basis for future case evaluation and planning of additional treatment goals.

This is just one small example of how self-reliance does not always result in good practice. Good supervision could have avoided this waste of time and the resulting sense that psychiatrists can be of little assistance in dealing with the institutionalized elderly. Another problem that developed from the worker's failure in this case was that the patient's family was not notified of the psychiatric evaluation. When they later learned of the referral, they demanded a meeting with the social worker to express their anger about the facility staff's seeing their relative as "crazy." The family was very concerned, and justifiably, about the intervention of a psychiatrist since no member of their family had ever been considered mentally ill.

Defining Need

The agency should make every effort to provide supervision for the worker, and the worker should actively seek supervision. When supervision is demanded and the need for it well articulated, agency administrators will normally make every effort to see that it is provided. When supervision cannot be effectively provided, an acceptable alternative is to bring a qualified consultant to the agency or to have the worker go to another agency in the community for consultation. When nonagency consultants are sought, workers must be alert that the consultation meets their specific needs and must be assertive about their needs when they are not being met. Another case example illustrates this point.

A rural welfare department hired an MSW consultant from the local mental health clinic for its protective service workers. The consultant came to the agency once a week and held individual consultation sessions with the three workers. The consultant was considered sensitive and helpful. One worker had been assigned a case in which a young couple had appeared in court several times for neglect of their four children. The father had recently been laid off from his seasonal orchard work. The family was suffering increased economic deprivation, and the worker's home visits led her to believe the youngest child was being abused. A court hearing was held, and the child was ordered removed from the home and placed in temporary foster care. The worker brought this case to the consultant for discussion, and the consultant offered advice on how to approach the family. The worker hesitated to act and continued to raise questions about the case. The consultant listened in a sensitive manner, but failed to pick up on the worker's real concern. Finally, the worker raised the issue. The worker was afraid to go to the home alone to remove the child. After the court hearing, the father told the worker that he would take whatever steps were necessary to prevent removal of the child, including violence. The father's history indicated that he was quite capable of acting on his threats, and during past visits the worker had observed several rifles in the home. The consultant supported the worker and recommended to the director of the welfare department that arrangements be made to have the state police accompany the worker to the home for the removal of the child. The director agreed to this arrangement, the child was removed without incident, and the worker was greatly relieved.

Workers in rural areas are sometimes placed in threatening situations that are not recognized or taken seriously by administrators and supervisors. Workers often report being threatened with firearms, physical assault, and attack by animals (mainly dogs). Consultants and supervisors should be sensitive to such threatening situations, and when they are not, the workers should not hesitate to share their feelings.

Use of Relationship

It has been argued that relationship is a key concept in rural social work practice (Davies, 1974). The use of relationship is not unique to rural practice and is an essential component of all forms of social work practice, regardless of where the practice is carried out. Unfortunately, the informality of relationship has been carried to the extreme in much of rural practice, as is illustrated by the extremist statement, "The most destructive professional in the rural area is the one who maintains a 'clinical' objective involvement with those he serves, this defense driving him further from rapport" (Davies, 1974:511). Such statements need qualification.

Research shows that clients relate better to workers they perceive as different from themselves (Munson & Balgopal, 1978). A client, regardless of his station in life or geographic location, desires a worker who has knowledge and is trained to perform in an objective manner. All theorists who have described the professional relationship view it as unique and requiring a delicate balance between empathic objectivity and "disciplined subjectivity" (Kadushin, 1972:58). It requires of the worker a certain degree of emotional and social distance—a greater degree of authority and control, self-awareness, and self-discipline than is expected of the client (Siporin, 1975:205). To conduct an interview, a social worker must engage in more than a "folksy" conversation with the client (Kadushin, 1972:8-11). In rural areas, "who you know is as valuable as what you know" (Davies, 1974:510), but the worker must know a substantial amount about services and practice principles to be effective.

In this area the supervisor can be especially helpful to the worker in maintaining an appropriate balance between objectivity and subjectivity in professional relationships. The concepts of primary and secondary relationships can be helpful to supervisors in practice situations. Primary relationships involve an atmosphere in which the participants exchange intimate knowledge, act and react with some degree of spontaneity, and provide realistic conceptions of themselves and what others expect of them. Secondary relationships are based on a necessity for cooperation that exists for the fulfillment of aims or goals of interaction of short duration with little emotional or personal involvement. Social workers engage in both types of relationships. Depending upon the setting and how the situation is defined, some workers engage exclusively in primary or secondary relationships, and other practitioners alternate between the two forms. A paraprofessional food-stamp interviewer in a welfare department engages exclusively in secondary relationships with clients; a practitioner in private practice is more likely to develop only primary relationships with clients. A caseworker in a welfare department or a mental health clinic uses both types, depending upon the situation.

Frequently, workers who have only brief contact with clients mistakenly minimize the importance of relationship, and those who interact with clients over long periods of time tend to overemphasize the importance of relationship. Primary social work relationships can be associated more with psychotherapeutic efforts to change personality and patterns of social relations; secondary relationships deal more with provision of concrete, tangible services. Both types involve varying emotional, temporal, and structural elements. If there is to be conscious use of relationship by the worker to promote change in the client, the worker must offer the client a differential model for identification at given points in the relationship. A young, black, BSW social worker who was the only black worker in a rural mental health clinic made the following observation, which illustrates this point.

> When I went to work here at the clinic, my supervisor decided to start me off by giving me all black clients since, as she put it, "I could identify the problems more easily and accomplish more in less time since I was black and could readily identify with black clients." I agreed and really thought it would be so easy for me, and I was relieved that I didn't have a lot of white clients to start out with. Well, it was terrible. It was a mistake. Since I was black, the clients felt they didn't have to explain anything. They would get angry because I didn't know exactly what they were talking about. I even had one client tell me I was dumb. After a while, my supervisor realized the problem and gave me a mixed caseload; but in the meantime, I was so frustrated I almost quit.

If the supervisor had recognized the importance of differentiation in relationship, a great deal of frustration on the part of the worker, clients, and the supervisor could have been avoided.

The worker should refrain from engaging in a cold, calculated objectivity that creates a distance between the worker and the client, and the practitioner should engage in a sensitive, empathic objectivity that enhances relationship and rapport, rather than decreases it. There is a tendency among rural practitioners to abandon theory and put in its place "down home" philosophy when conceptualizing practice (Munson, 1979d). This could be the reason social workers are not called upon to contribute to major efforts to confront rural problems (Coppedge & Davis, 1977).

SUGGESTED READINGS

Diane Blum and Sona Euster-Fisher. "Clinical Supervisory Practice in Oncology Settings." *The Clinical Supervisor* 1 (Spring 1983), pp. 17-27.
Survey of supervision in medical oncology settings.

Alex Gitterman. *Handbook of Social Work Practice with Vulnerable Populations*. New York: Columbia University Press, 1991.

Thomas Peake and John Ball. "Psychotherapy Training: Contextual and Developmental Influences in Settings, Stages and Mind Sets." *The Clinical Supervisor* 9 (Spring 1991), pp. 1-204.
This is a special issue of the journal that covers training for and supervision of practice in a number of settings.

Albert Roberts. *Crisis Intervention Handbook: Assessment Treatment and Research*. Belmont, CA: Wadsworth, 1990.

Roberta Sands. *Clinical Social Work Practice in Community Mental Health*. New York: Macmillan, 1991.

Harold Weissman and Irwin Epstein. *Agency-Based Social Work: Neglected Aspects of Clinical Practice*. Philadelphia: Temple University Press, 1983.

> . . . Clinical work is often more widely
> varying than our theories reflect.
>
> Fred Pine
> *Drive, Ego, Object, and Self*

Chapter 14

Supervision in Unique Situations

Supervisors encounter unique situations in supervision such as supervising pregnant practitioners, physically disabled practitioners, and practitioners who are in therapy. Other situations that are discussed are family therapy supervision, use of family of origin material in supervision, and supervising cotherapist activity. These areas were selected for discussion because they are increasingly encountered by supervisors of clinical practitioners.

INTRODUCTION

Supervisors tend to gloss over important, apparent variables that affect the treatment relationship in powerful ways. For example, a pregnant therapist or a pregnant client can arouse powerful emotions in the treatment. A handicapped therapist or client can also give rise to previously unrecognized feelings. When the practitioner and client are from different races or ethnic groups, different issues often arise. When the practitioner is much older or much younger than the client, a special set of difficulties can emerge.

A detailed discussion of each of these situations would be quite lengthy. In dealing with these unique situations, supervisors must give practitioners time to discuss their responses to what is taking place in the treatment. All of these special situations give rise to feelings that need to be explored, and in many instances practitioners block feelings, thoughts, and responses that affect the treatment and can even cause it to break down completely. Supervisors have a responsibility to assist practitioners in such difficult situations.

PRACTITIONERS WHO ARE IN THERAPY

No reliable statistics are available, but it appears that a substantial number of practitioners have been at one time or are currently in therapy themselves. In one sample of graduate students surveyed, 52 percent of the students indicated that they had received treatment in the past, and 12 percent of this group were currently receiving treatment. Also, a majority of those who had received treatment said that they decided to enter social work school because they identified with their therapist and had decided to use him or her as a role model (Munson, Study A).

The important factor to be taken into account by the supervisor is how these practitioners' experiences with their therapists affect their own work. When therapists' role models are limited, as often is the case, the only role models available are their own therapists, which can result in distortions (Blumenfield, 1982:146). Most practitioners work alone and in isolation from others. The distortions that commonly occur are that the practitioner is being effective when in fact he/she is not, or that he/she is ineffective when performance is adequate. This is important because practitioners who do not receive ample or adequate supervision are more likely to draw on their therapist as a role model. They see their therapist in action more than they see their supervisor, and practitioners will develop whatever coping mechanisms they can to deal with the complexities of practice.

It has been my experience that practitioners do not discriminate how they use styles and techniques learned from their own therapists. Such carryover works and serves practitioners adequately as long as their clients have problems similar to those they present in their own therapy. It is natural to think that if it works in your own situation, it will work satisfactorily for others you treat. However, practitioners must take into account that such techniques and strategies are appropriate quite often to the unique problems under treatment, and that to adopt these strategies in a comprehensive fashion is eventually bound to lead to failure. When practitioners have clients with backgrounds different from their own, the supervisor needs to be especially sensitive to these types of misapplication.

When a practitioner's own therapy is based on a theoretical orientation similar to the one the practitioner uses in his or her own practice, there is a natural tendency to imitate the practitioner's therapist. This can produce positive or negative results, depending on the situation. In some cases the practitioner uses a theory different from his or her own therapist's, and this most often results in clumsy performance in practice and frustration, especially at difficult points. There should be some exploration in supervision of the practitioner's therapist's styles and theoretical orientation, if the practitioner is open to it. Also, the supervisor should do direct observation of the practitioner's work to detect any changes in style that could be detracting from performance. At the same time, one's own therapy can enhance practice in a number of ways, and this needs to be reinforced by the supervisor.

Such exploration does not have to involve the content of the practitioner's personal therapy, but should focus on stylistic elements that carry over from therapy to practice. Dealing with this type of material requires much sensitivity and skill on the part of the supervisor. There must be clear boundaries about what is open to discussion and what is not. The supervisor should avoid judging or evaluating the practitioner's therapist. If the practitioner has lost confidence in the therapist and wants to talk about it, the supervisor can discuss this briefly and assist the practitioner in making a decision about how to deal with it, but the decision should be made solely by the practitioner.

FAMILY THERAPY SUPERVISION

Portions of this section are reprinted from Carlton E. Munson, "Supervising the Family Therapist," Social Casework, Vol. 61 (March 1980), pp. 131-137. Reprinted by permission of the Family Service Association of America.

Many supervisors assume that family therapy supervision is not different from individual therapy supervision. This belief usually grows out of supervisors' lack of skill in actually doing family therapy and on social work's reliance on generic skills. Agencies should not place in supervisory positions staff who do not have substantial skill in doing family therapy; theoretical grounding alone is not sufficient for effectively supervising the family therapist. Although generic skills are necessary to any practice situation, they are not sufficient. For example, because more people are involved, family therapy automatically decreases the control the practitioner is able to exercise when compared to the individual treatment situation. Visual 14.1 illustrates the increase in interactional combinations that can occur as the number of participants in the treatment group is increased. In order to make the treatment manageable, the supervisor and practitioner must make important decisions about how many family members and how many therapists to involve in the treatment. No amount of generic skills will help the therapist cope with a treatment group of unmanageable size. Bowen has theoretically conceptualized the complexity of adding participants to the treatment situation. There is an actual exponential numerical increase as participants are added to the treatment (see Visual 14.1). It is Bowen's view that when the therapist who thinks in

VISUAL 14.1. Combinations of Interactions
for Treatment Situations

Number of Clients	Number of Workers			
	One Worker		Two Workers	
	Two-Way Interaction	Three-Way Interaction	Two-Way Interaction	Three-Way Interaction
1	2	-	6	6
2	6	6	12	24
3	12	24	20	60
4	20	60	30	120
5	30	120	42	210
6	42	210	56	336
7	56	336	72	504

Source: Munson 1980a: 132.

terms of individual therapy is presented clinically with families, he or she cannot "hear family concepts" (Haley, 1971:163-171).

Within the context of other family members, each individual in treatment opens up an expanded, actual interactional system to the therapist that is not compatible with individual treatment models. Bowen identifies one difference for the practitioner as that of identifying family relationship patterns that do not emerge in individual treatment. The supervisor must be able to help the supervisee make this transition. For example, one pattern of family relationship and interactional patterns is for the family to put one member in the sick role or the patient role. In such dysfunctional systems, the person identified as sick will often eagerly fulfill this role outside and within the treatment. The unsuspecting practitioner with an individual orientation will adapt to this system and focus on treating the sick member, rather than focusing on the whole family in an attempt to break up this dysfunctional pattern. The supervisor must be alert to such manipulation of the practitioner by the family and help the therapist avoid conforming to the existing family interactional pattern.

At the other extreme, families may exclude a particular member from the interactional pattern. Family members will often subtly exclude members by trying to "rescue" them or expressing painful feelings for them (Luthman & Kirschenbaum, 1974:77). It is easy for the unskilled practitioner to fail to recognize this pattern of exclusion. The supervisor must help the practitioner identify such patterns, and must assist the practitioner in aiding the excluded member to get back into the interactional system.

Interactional Issues

Families will often avoid interactional issues, and the practitioner will fail to acknowledge this for several reasons. The supervisor must be alert to such observational and interventive gaps and be prepared to discuss them with the supervisee. The best way for the supervisor to introduce the beginning family therapist to this method is to have the worker serve as cotherapist with the supervisor in treating families. The supervisor can help the worker gain direct experience by sharing strategies of intervention, technique used, and skills employed. Very little of this type of sharing is currently taking place in supervision.

If the supervisor is unable or unwilling to share his or her own practice, an alternative is to have the worker exposed to videotapes or audiotapes of family therapy sessions. These can be tapes of sessions conducted in the agency or commercially produced tapes. The use of tapes to train family therapists must involve more than just allowing the worker to view or listen to the tapes. The supervisor must put the tapes in perspective before and after they are used. Differing styles and theoretical approaches must be explained, as must the reasons for specific interactions by the practitioner and family members. Family intervention is a process, and to observe segments of this process through tapes can be misleading. This is why actual involvement in the family therapy process is best. When tapes are used the supervisor must fill in the gaps of the intervention process that is occurring. Techniques learned out of context of the therapy process can lead the beginning therapist to develop a flippant attitude or a grab bag of techniques that can be confusing and, in some cases, detrimental to the families treated.

Audiovisual Devices

When one-way viewing mirrors and "bug-in-the-ear" devices are used, the supervisor needs to be aware of his or her own behavior and its impact on the practitioner. For example, the supervisor who is too active in using the bug-in-the-ear to talk can confuse, frustrate, and limit the ability of the practitioner to carry out the therapy. This can be avoided if the supervisor seeks feedback from the practitioner about the amount of his or her involvement in the treatment as "a once-removed therapist." This form of live supervision must involve evaluation of the supervision as well as evaluation of the family treatment.

The use of audiovisual aids in supervising family therapists is a much more involved process than most supervisors realize. Much more planning needs to go into use of such aids than is currently practiced. Careful selection of aids is important. Orientation of the clients, practitioners, and supervisors to use of such aids is essential. Putting the use of aids in perspective before, during, and after their use is basic. Evaluation of the aids is as important as the evaluation of the treatment. Instructional aids cannot be used with all cases or for all supervision. The supervisor must carefully plan the use of segmental audiovisual aids so that the maximum benefit can be gained. The supervisor must be clear in advance about what the objectives of the supervision are, what the focus in the case material that is scrutinized will be, and what procedures will be used in teaching the objectives of the supervision. The self-assessment instrument contained in Appendix 6 can be a good aid in focusing the material that will be evaluated during supervision. (See Chapter 12 for use of audiovisual techniques.)

Theory and Technique

Family therapists disagree about the use of theory versus technique in family treatment. This debate is not confined to family therapists, and has been a factor in the evolution of other forms of therapy. Bowen sees theory as important to family intervention (Haley, 1971:163); Whitaker believes the use of theory isolates the therapist, dichotomizes the treatment, makes the therapist an observer, and stifles practitioner creativity (Guerin, 1976:154-164). There has been little systematic study of how theory is actually used in family intervention and how it affects what is said and what gets done. There appears to be little conscious use of theory in the actual practice of family therapy. Beginning practitioners struggle with the intensity of the family therapy situation and have little energy to invest in the skilled use of theory; the experienced practitioner focuses on the interaction and issues to be explored without conscious consideration of the theoretical implications of his or her own activity. This does not mean that theory is not important in family intervention. What practitioners have been taught about family therapy does show up in their work, but this is seldom consciously recognized. For the purposes of supervision, this becomes an important point.

In order to give practitioners the technical skill to know how to deal with therapy content, the supervisor must have some way to organize the analysis of therapy content. Even though the practitioner may not always be aware of the use of theory in the practice situation, effective supervision for practice must be theoretically based. Whitaker, in making his arguments, points to research that suggests that nontheoretical workers can be effective when given good supervision (Guerin, 1976:163). The more nontheoretical the therapy becomes, the more important theory becomes in supervision. Opposition to the use of theory in supervision is often related to the fact that family dynamics change so much in the treatment process that it is very difficult to apply theory consistently. Because of the complexity of family interaction, it is important that theory be used to guide the supervision rather than be abandoned. Although it is hard work, consistent and clear use of theory can help to keep the treatment from becoming unfocused and nonspecific. Theory used in supervision must be related to the interaction process. Most family intervention theory has emerged from analysis of family interaction and fits the supervisory process quite well.

The supervisor must be careful of using theory in the abstract to avoid difficult or unfamiliar case material. The theoretical material must be related to clinical material. A good rule for the supervisor to follow is that no theoretical concept should be presented without the illustration of one or more clinical examples. It is easier for practitioners to handle criticism of their work when it is presented in relation to practice theory. It is easier for them to understand the implications of an action in theoretical terms, rather than simply in terms of therapist or supervisor behavior or feelings.

Theory and Diagnosis

In doing diagnosis in family therapy, theory is important. Some understanding of the theory in use must precede the diagnostic process. It is recommended that supervisors avoid teaching diagnosis before identifying the theoretical orientation of the supervisor or the agency. Diagnosis, it has been long held, must be accomplished in relation to treatment. Minuchin (1974) has pointed out that diagnosis and therapy are inseparable. When diagnosis and treatment goals are accomplished in theoretical harmony, the total treatment is more understandable and more easily adapted to by the clients, the practitioner, and the supervisor. It has been my experience that when theory is not used at all in supervision, or when theory is applied inconsistently in diagnosis and treatment phases, there is more practitioner dissatisfaction with supervision, and it is more likely that the family will drop out of treatment.

When diagnosis and initial intervention are discussed and reviewed in a supervision session that does not have a theoretical focus, it can result in the practitioner's spending too much time merely giving the family information and gathering information about family history, systems, functioning, and symptoms. This lost time in treatment is usually a carryover from individual intervention, in which information is gathered and a label applied to it. Minuchin has described the difference in approach in family therapy as follows: "a diagnosis is the working hypothesis that the therapist evolves from his experiences and observations upon joining the family" (Minuchin, 1974:129). A family diagnosis and treatment strategy emerge from the therapist's direct participation in the system. In family intervention the diagnosis-treatment process is internally formulated and applied rather than externally imposed and preexisting, as in individual treatment. This difference makes the supervisor's task more difficult but more effective and rewarding when logically and consistently applied.

Family therapy supervision is more complex and demanding than other forms of clinical supervision. There is necessarily more emphasis on live **supervision and use of audiovisual aids in supervision that requires** additional knowledge and skills on the part of the supervisor. Family therapy supervision should not be attempted by the nonpracticing supervisor.

The SEES System

Discovering the process of treatment and its relationship to technique is as important in learning family therapy as diagnosis and theory. The supervisor must find a way to integrate these concepts for the supervisee. I have worked for ten years on developing a conceptual scheme that is fairly simple to master and at the same time could convey how master family therapists integrate theory and practice. Content analysis was applied to master family therapists' (Study H) recorded videotape sessions with a focus on identifying the purpose and function of intervention strategies used. This resulted in a classification system of four activities that appeared to be core techniques in each session the therapist conducted. The activities generally occurred in a flexible sequence that constituted a repeated process the therapist used to make interventions.

In this sequence, the practitioner analyzes the family's *style* of relating in the first part of the session. The therapist then moves to adjusting or adapting their own natural style of intervention to the family style and this allows the practitioner to enter the family, join the family, or form an alliance with the family. This sets the stage for the therapist to *enable* individual family members to express themselves or to be protected from other family members or to assist the entire family to mobilize its resources to accomplish a task. Once this is done, the therapist then *encounters* the family by clarifying family patterns of relating and behaving. This is a form of confrontation without anger, and is done in a caring way. Once the encounter occurs, the practitioner then forces the family to relate in a different way. I refer to this procedure as *shifting the dysfunction.* in shifting the dysfunction the therapist goes through the steps of initiating the shift, implementing the shift, and implanting the shift. This involves setting up the situation as it would normally occur, then altering the pattern of interacting and working to make the alterations so powerful the family cannot return to the old pattern of relating. There are numerous ways of achieving a shift. It can be through the whole family participating, or one family member being encouraged to not respond in the usual pattern. This process of style, enable, encounter, and shift dysfunction occurs repeatedly in master therapists' work, and it is evident in some of the earliest tapes of sessions done by pioneering family therapists in the 1960s, as well as the latest models of family therapy. (See, for example, Brendler et al., 1991.)

The supervisor can use this system to assist beginning family therapists in their efforts to master this complex form of treatment. Visual 14.2

gives a summary of the SEES system for learning about family therapy by watching films of master therapists at work.

FAMILY OF ORIGIN MATERIAL IN SUPERVISION

The literature on family intervention is confusing for beginning therapists, and can leave them with the impression that "everything seems to work" (Kramer, C. H., 1980:281). This same confusion occurs in family therapy training programs. Supervisors need to help supervisees evaluate what works and what is ineffective. Younger practitioners are likely to have been exposed to family therapy theory and concepts as part of their professional training, but such exposure is often less than adequate and entered upon before the practitioner is skilled at performing individual or group therapy (Kramer, C. H., 1980:275-276). Supervisors should remember that the only actual experience in family functioning the beginning family therapist has experienced is their own family of origin, and this experience limits and blocks therapist appreciation of the diversity of family types and styles that exist.

There seems to be general agreement that personal therapy associated with exploration of one's own family dynamics leads to one's being a better family therapist. Practitioners are encouraged to enter therapy to enhance their professional performance, and family therapy supervisors are encouraged "openly to discuss with students their experiences in current relationships with their own families" as a model for their supervisees' own practice (Goldenberg & Goldenberg, 1980:234-235). Kramer has argued that "the family therapist who has not himself experienced therapy is at a disadvantage," and the family therapist "who has not worked on his own family relationships" is "handicapped" (Kramer, C. H., 1980:298).

Given these theoretical views, the confusion about what constitutes good treatment, and beginning practitioners' lack of adequate practice experience in doing family intervention, most inexperienced practitioners naturally have a tendency to commit to any strategy or technique that will aid them in coping with demanding and complex practice material. The use of family of origin material is one of these learning strategies. It uses exploration of personal experience as a means to learn about practice. This expectation is developed early in a therapist's career during the training stage. One report in the literature of the use of family of origin material in a social work classroom setting illustrates this (Magee, 1982). The report reflects a trend to personalize for the student various forms of course content. This is based on the notion that having the student draw on personal experience to understand conceptual material fosters integration of content, development of self-awareness, and learning. There is no empirical

VISUAL 14.2. SEES System for Analyzing Family Therapy Interactional Sequences

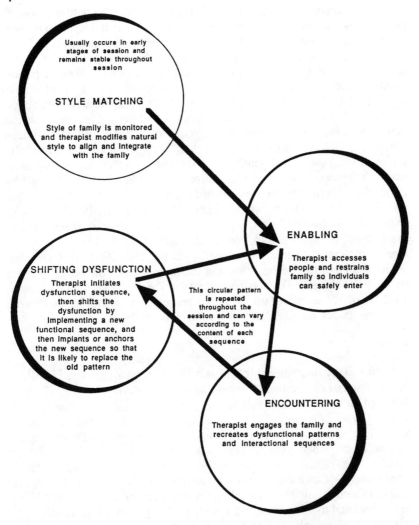

evidence to support the view that this is the most effective and efficient way to promote learning. There has not been any consideration that the use of such techniques may impede learning or, even more serious, violate students' right to privacy. Such exploration using students' personal lives to promote learning under any circumstances is unjustified. Haley has succinctly commented on such practices by observing that supervisees' personal lives are too important to be tampered with by supervisors (1976:187).

The only report on use of family of origin groups in the field component in social work education is by Thistle (1981). She holds that students believe that "unashamed inquiry in these [family] relationships is not only helpful but essential to the development of the family therapist," and asserts that "the modification of the trainee's role in his or her own family is one of the most dramatic and effective ways of teaching family therapy" (1981:248). Given these two statements, a basic contradiction emerges from the article that Thistle does not address. This contradiction is that the clients of the agency are severely mentally ill people who need inpatient psychiatric treatment, and their backgrounds are substantially different from the backgrounds of the therapist trainees. In spite of these major differences, the trainees are purported to learn about their clients by presenting "family albums and records and genograms" that make "the families come alive for group members" (Thistle, 1981:249). This type of exploration is justified on the grounds that "the individual attracted to the helping professions is often more comfortable looking at someone else's problems than his or her own" (Thistle, 1981:249). This view becomes the basis for the assertion that the main "task" of the group is for trainees "to develop skills as researchers in their own families" (Thistle, 1981:249). We are never told how this relates to or what it has to do with what the trainee does with his or her own clients.

History

Unlike many intervention techniques, the history of the use of family of origin material can be traced. It originated with Murray Bowen. The evolution of Bowen's ideas in this area is explained in his book *Family Therapy in Clinical Practice* (1978). A rather elaborate interweaving of points in the last 50 pages of the book describes this evolution. Bowen reports that he first learned to apply therapeutic dynamics to his family from a sickness perspective during his early psychoanalytic training. Later he began using his own theoretical formulations to study his own family. He worked through this by writing lengthy letters to his parents and siblings and calculated mailing them to coincide with trips to visit his family. This caused members of his family much anguish, and he reports that one brother was so angered that he threatened a libel suit (Bowen, 1978:513).

In 1967 Bowen began using his own family of origin experiences to teach psychiatric residents about treatment. These residents began using these examples with their own families, and Bowen observed that these residents appeared to be "doing better clinical work as family therapists than any previous residents'' (Bowen, 1978:531). Bowen began treating residents using this approach. He reported there was one "control" group in which he focused on extended family material, but admitted that the results were disappointing. Bowen continued to use these techniques with residents and their wives as part of his training program. Hundreds of practitioners have participated in these training seminars. Many psychotherapists from various disciplines now use family of origin groups to train other therapists. They use the same techniques with their own supervisees that Bowen demonstrated and used with them, including exploration of family of origin material and letter-writing exercises.

Case Example

There have been no empirical tests of what Bowen has produced as a participant observer in his own training seminars (Gurman, 1981:355). No specific guidelines have been developed for the use of family of origin material with therapists in training. There are no reports in the literature of positive or negative outcomes or misapplications of this approach. Although reports do occur in the literature identifying problems, there has been a tendency to overlook them and emphasize the positive assumptions of the approach (see Gurman, 1981:352-364).

One case example that illustrates the lack of differential applications of family of origin material involved a student therapist. Mary was a second-year graduate student in an outpatient mental health clinic, where her supervisor was a strong advocate of family of origin groups for practitioners. The supervisor had participated in several seminars conducted by Bowenian trainers. The supervisor urged her supervisees to participate in a family of origin group she conducted. Mary moved into one of these groups, and after several sessions was encouraged to present her family. Mary presented her father as an aloof, stern businessman who did not communicate much. When her father tried to talk with her, Mary's mother would always interfere and accuse them of "plotting against her." Mary's mother had a life-long history of mental illness and had had a series of hospitalizations. In order to avoid his wife's wrath, Mary's father was portrayed as giving up on trying to communicate with Mary, which Mary found depressing. At the same time, she felt anger at her father for not confronting his wife with her "unfounded" accusations. Mary had left home over ten years before and had visited her parents infrequently since leaving home. Mary had one younger sister, who had not attended college and had "never found her place in life." In recent years her parents, who lived over 500 miles away, were described as having settled into complacency about their life situation and acceptance of their daughter's loss of contact with them. Her parents remained reservedly proud of Mary's accomplishments. Mary desired to relate to her parents in a different way, but did not know how to achieve this.

The family of origin group convinced Mary that she was engaged in a classic triangle with her parents, and encouraged her to write a letter to her parents explaining this triangle and indicating that she wanted to break up this pattern of relating. After a holiday visit home, Mary, with much ambivalence, prepared a letter that she read to the group and subsequently mailed to her parents. The parents wrote back indicating that they did not understand Mary's comments, but that they still loved her and would like to fly in for her graduation because they were proud of her accomplishments. Mary took her parents' letter back to the family of origin group and was advised by the group to write to her parents indicating that she would refuse to see them if they came for her graduation, and that her achieving a graduate degree had been accomplished alone without help from them. It was the group's view that this would be a good way to break up the old pattern of "triangling." Mary followed through on this with another letter. The parents responded again with a long letter professing their love for her. They did not understand her position, but would honor her feelings and not attend the graduation.

The question remains whether this was the best and most appropriate way to deal with Mary's situation, but the more important question is what this had to do with Mary's own development as a family therapist. None of it was ever related by the group to her own family practice. This could be viewed as an unwarranted and unjustified intrusion into Mary's personal life.

Dynamics and Process

In groups in which family of origin material is explored extensively, it can become intertwined with group process and group dynamics that can give rise to therapeutic difficulties. Beck (1982) has reported an example of this in which a group member became reluctant to explore family of origin material, and this in turn gave rise to "considerable resentment on the part of other group members." This reaction of the group led the patient to withdraw from the group (we are not told if these patients were therapists themselves in a supervision group). The question that emerges from this case example is: What is to become of participants who exercise their right to self-determination and do not agree to such a course of treatment or supervision?

The following case report illustrates how resistance can become problematic for the therapist in supervision:

> I was only married six months when my supervisor required me to participate in a family of origin group she was conducting. I didn't know much about it, but I thought I would give it a try. My husband is very involved with his family. This didn't particularly bother me, but the group pressed me about it. I've talked to my husband about it, but without much enthusiasm. He isn't into psychology, and he discounts this stuff. I did it because the group pushed me about it. I regret having done it. I want this marriage to work. It's the second marriage for both of us. My husband doesn't understand what I'm going through. I wish I would never have brought it up. I don't think it's that important. I don't see what it has to do with learning to do good therapy. I feel comfortable with our relationship as it is. I'm being more cautious about what I reveal in the group, but I can sense some of the other members don't like the way I'm reacting.

Supervisees become frustrated and disoriented when they fail to see the connection between actions of the family of origin group and their own families. Such experiences cause the therapist in training to become resentful and to view such efforts as being involuntarily forced into personal therapy. Also, in situations like this, the therapist's learning is blocked because so much energy goes into resisting the group. When this occurs, the main objective of family of origin groups is thwarted—the supervisee ceases to learn about family therapy and how to become more skilled at doing it. Without adequate safeguards, personalizing family of origin material for the supervisee is a return to the former problematic practice of "psychologizing" the worker.

Relationship to Practice

The effect of family of origin emphasis in supervision has not been assessed from the perspective of its influence on practice activity. It has been shown that rarely is family of origin material applied in the supervision of the practitioner as it relates to the practitioner's clinical activity. When this gap exists the potential is created for practitioners to misapply this material with their cases. There must be follow-up of such learning and its application as well as clinical demonstration of its relevance to clinical situations.

Overemphasis on family of origin material in supervision can lead the practitioner to a disproportionate focus on such material in cases. Dwelling on such material can fascinate, but can lead to a narrow focus that detracts from a problem focus in the treatment. It can result in focusing on historical and inactive relationships at the expense of current relationship issues. Tangible problems and dysfunctional interactional and communication patterns in the family can be overlooked and avoided. This is especially the case in the diagnostic phase of intervention. If assessment of family functioning is inadequate or limited, the treatment will necessarily be distorted and misguided.

These issues remain unexplored in the use of family of origin material. Beck (1982) has alluded to the shortcomings of family of origin material in some situations. Supervisors who insist upon its use must be aware of these problems and develop strategies to combat them. Supervisors need to explore alternative means of promoting effective family treatment. For example, are there alternative methods of exploring family of origin material that put practitioners at less risk personally and are at the same time more practice relevant? Are other practice methods as effective, or more effective, in encouraging quality practice? Can the same ends be achieved through the use of cotherapists in family treatment? More attention needs to be given to appropriate differential application of family of origin material to practice situations.

Focus of Supervision

The amount of material that is revealed about one's family of origin should remain under the control of the supervisee and not the supervisor. To pressure supervisees to confront their own family of origin material distorts the learning process in supervision. Supervisors who press supervisees beyond the point of their comfort must ask why they are persisting in such a course of interaction. To guard against such a distortion of the supervisory learning experience, a good policy of the supervisor should be to explore family of origin material only after case material has been presented and problem areas in the case situation have been identified. The general rule being proposed here is that exploration of client dynamics should always precede exploration of therapist dynamics in the supervision. Such a policy assures that the supervision will remain learning-focused, and at any point at which therapists are reluctant to go further with personal material, they can fall back on the case material. When therapists' family of origin material is the exclusive focus of the supervision, they can feel trapped when they have reached a point beyond which they do not want to go. Dormant triangles should not be reestablished as a part of the supervisory experience. Such actions should remain in the realm of therapy. The triangles in the families being treated by the practitioner should be the focus of the supervision.

COTHERAPIST ACTIVITY

Cotherapy work can be a totally rewarding experience, a completely devastating experience, or an alternatively rewarding and devastating experience. These are generally the three categories of responses one receives when inquiring about it.

Cotherapists need some form of regular or periodic supervision. Cotherapy does not, as some believe or assume, eliminate the need for supervision. It is not a good idea to expect cotherapy to serve as a form of mutual supervision. Cotherapy often results in difficulty if one of the participants seeks such activity as a source of supervision or consultation without making this explicit. The second therapist may be incapable or unwilling to fulfill this function.

Little solid empirical outcome research exists to confirm or refute the dichotomous claims of the effectiveness and inadequacy of cotherapy. The debate about its appropriateness in family therapy epitomizes the polarities we have reached. Bowen, in describing cotherapy as a method and technique, views it as "one of the major innovations and developments in family therapy" (1978:299); Haley holds that outcome studies suggest that cotherapy is not more effective, and he believes that "the use of a cotherapist is usually for the security of the clinician and not for the value of the client" (1976:16). Rabin, in a survey of therapists, found that they preferred cotherapy but emphasized the importance of a "good" relationship between the therapists, although no clear definition of a "good" relationship was formulated (1967). Research has indicated that therapist style (Rice et al., 1972) and theoretical orientation (Gurman & Razin, 1977:212-213) affect preference for cotherapy activity. Some of this research suggests that effectiveness is associated with comfort in the cotherapy situation, and that as cotherapy activity increases, satisfaction with the method decreases. All of the research highlights the need for documenting sources and forms of conflict in cotherapy.

Currently, practitioners perceive that agencies are split evenly on whether to encourage cotherapy activity (Munson, Study F). In some agencies, acceptance of cotherapy is vague — practitioners are not encouraged to do cotherapy, but at the same time, it is not openly discouraged. Rarely do agencies have well-developed guidelines for the use of cotherapy. Generally, its use is left to practitioner interest, is undertaken at therapist initiative, and is not mandated by the agency. A strong agency expectation of cotherapy activity is usually related to a therapist training program in which a seasoned practitioner works with a student or an inexperienced practitioner.

Attitudes toward cotherapy conflict are mostly related to differences in style or theoretical orientation. Personality differences and conflicts are occasionally a factor, but are generally held to be of little significance and easily resolved. Competition is expected more where both practitioners are very inexperienced or very experienced.

Conflict

Conflict is perceived as being resolved more easily outside the treatment in meetings conducted immediately before or after the therapy sessions. Practitioners expect that they and their colleagues will make serious efforts to understand each other's style and orientation prior to entering cotherapy activity. Ironically, most practitioners do not mention supervision or consultation as an arena for dealing with cotherapy conflicts. This could be due to the current emphasis on autonomy in practice and to the increasingly vague role and purpose of supervision and consultation in agencies. Cotherapy conflict is a legitimate concern in supervision.

When supervisees are doing cotherapy, the supervisor must be alert to potential for cotherapist conflict. Cotherapy activity and compatibility should be explored periodically to allow the practitioners to express and identify problem areas. It is rare that cotherapists are able to work together smoothly and effectively from the beginning. More often the cotherapists go through a period of struggling with compatibility of styles and strategies. Some cotherapists are able to work through these problems; others struggle to no avail and eventually go their separate ways. Supervision can often speed up the achievement of compatibility or help overcome what seem to be insurmountable differences. Supervision of cotherapy efforts aids in promoting effectiveness of therapy since clients frequently pick up on cotherapist conflict and use it to subvert the therapy.

Also, cotherapists who have substantial covert conflict act this out through their interventions with clients, and use clients to vie with one another and prove their respective views. Even though such problems can develop, there is increasing belief that cotherapy benefits to the practitioners and the clients outweigh the difficulties that can emerge.

Dominant Therapist

When cotherapy is attempted, usually one of the therapists emerges as dominant, based on experience, style, and amount or type of training. It has been observed that cotherapists are rarely equals (Grotjahn, 1977:248). However, this does not have to be a permanent state of affairs. When experience or amount or type of training interferes with equality, this can be brought into the open in supervision, but minimized in the actual treatment situation. The less experienced or less trained practitioner can be encouraged to become more active, because such therapists tend to defer to the other therapist. The more experienced or more trained practitioner can be aided in monitoring interaction or interventions that promote the inequality. Dominant therapists can inadvertently reinforce the inequality in order to stay in control or enhance their status in the treatment. The therapists can be assisted in ways of interacting directly in the treatment that conveys to the clients that they are genuinely working together. For those who believe that clients do not take cotherapists' styles of being active and passive into account, a story told by Carl Whitaker, the famous family therapist, is thought provoking:

> The decision to use residents as co-therapists was also a deliberate one. I decided I could not tolerate playing games and trying to tease the residents into working with families . . . . They were free to participate or to watch. They automatically become part of the sessions, many times to their own amazement. I remember one resident who had said little or nothing for five interviews. When the . . . family came back for the sixth session, he wasn't there, having been up all night on call. They stayed for five minutes and then said, "Well, if Bill isn't going to be here, we might just as well come back next week," and walked out. This was a bit of a surprise to me, but it was a massive shock to the resident, who thought he was very unimportant. (Kopp, 1976:201)

Beginning practitioners show a tendency to need to be in control and to be overactive in the treatment. When two inexperienced practitioners do cotherapy, their combined need to be in control can lead to serious conflicts, especially when they disagree about how to direct and guide the therapy. In this situation, supervision by an experienced practitioner is important. The supervisor will need to assist such therapists more directly with their specific interventions, and will need to be more involved in focusing the patterns that emerge in the treatment process and in designing the goals of the therapy.

When style promotes inequality, it can be handled in a manner similar to that just mentioned. Stylistic inequality is also supported when one practitioner is more assertive than the other. Once this pattern is identified in supervision, techniques can be identified that will promote reversal of the styles. With practice of the techniques, equality can be accomplished.

Access to Clients

Conflict can develop when inequality grows out of one practitioner's having more access to some of the clients than the other therapist. For example, in group therapy and family intervention, one of the therapists sometimes sees certain members individually in treatment, and when the group or family meets, their therapist will have more information to use in planning and making interventions. The second therapist often becomes aware of this information after the intervention is made and must seek clarification inside or outside the treatment. The second therapist can develop feelings of isolation if this knowledge difference becomes a pattern. The supervisor can help with such conflict by discovering the origin of the knowledge difference and encouraging pre- and post-therapy session meetings in which the more involved therapist shares knowledge of the individual cases with the less involved practitioner. Also, during the treatment the more involved therapist can share the information directly, explain it briefly, and put the material directly into the group or family therapy, rather than intervening without explanation, but this strategy must be weighed against concerns about protecting the confidentiality of the individual treatment.

When students are placed in a cotherapy situation with an experienced therapist, they have no real control over their role. There is an inherent tendency to be passive and follow the lead of the experienced practitioner, rather than alternating activity levels. Only the most sensitive, experienced therapist should be asked to do cotherapy with a student. When a student is placed with a practitioner from a different discipline, special care must be taken. Not only do these students tend to be more passive, they often do not have the knowledge base to understand many of the interventions made by the other therapist. The experienced practitioner may not have the patience to explain to the student the background information essential to developing understanding. The problems of inequity and lack of knowledge are compounded when a student is placed in an existing group that the experienced practitioner has been conducting.

Decision Guidelines

Holt and Greiner (Guerin, 1976) have summarized five important questions that should be addressed before attempting cotherapy:

1. For what goals should cotherapy be used?
2. In what treatment situations should cotherapy be used?
3. With what type of clients should cotherapy be used?
4. With what type of practitioners should cotherapy be used?
5. With what theoretical orientations should cotherapy be used?

Practitioners considering this form of therapy can use and expand upon these five basic questions to avoid problems in advance. Usually, little pre-treatment planning goes into cotherapy, and the attitude seems to be that "we can deal with problems if they develop." This is unfortunate. Planning can prevent some problems from developing and lessen the shock and impact of other problems when they do occur.

There needs to be more assessment of the interactional impact of having more than one therapist. The interactional combinations increase as participants are added to the treatment (Munson, 1980a:132). The five questions listed above can be helpful in exploring the interactional impact of an additional therapist. A major question becomes: Do complexity and dynamics, based on a diagnostic assessment of the case or group, warrant inclusion of an additional therapist? A second question is: Do the concerns of a single practitioner justify adding a cotherapist, and how will this contribute to a different outcome? In some situations, it is better to initiate single-therapist treatment and regulate the therapy process by increasing supervision. This approach can prevent the situation that frequently develops in which cotherapy is sought to overcome a single therapist's feelings of inadequacy.

Evaluation

To guard against conflict, there must be as much evaluation of the cotherapy activity as there is of the treatment. For this reason, supervision of the cotherapy becomes important. The supervisor must be alert to unrecognized conflict, floundering on the part of both therapists, and unstated feelings of secondary status on the part of one of the therapists. A rarely used but effective tool in dealing with this is to require each practitioner to record independently his or her feelings and thoughts about the therapy and the cotherapy work. This is referred to as self-monitoring. An excerpt from an individual supervisory session with one cotherapist illustrates this point:

> I never gave much thought to what was going on between us until you had me write down my observations and thoughts. When we started the group, the stated agreement was that we would be co-equal therapists. As I reflect on what has taken place, this has not happened. I have fallen into or have been put in the position of not being as knowledgeable or skilled as Marvin. Through writing the notes, I know now that I do much better when Marvin misses a session and I have the group to myself. I think the group members know this. When he returns, I revert to my more passive role. I don't like this pattern, but I don't know what to do about it.

With the help of the supervisor, the practitioner was able to do something about the situation. The supervisor brought the practitioners together and raised this material. The dominant therapist was also aware that this was happening, but did not know how to deal with it. The offended therapist was able to share examples of how the dominant therapist fostered the inequality interactionally. The dominant therapist was not aware of the impact of his behaviors and agreed to alter them, and the second therapist agreed to make efforts to be more active and assertive. Follow-up on this revealed that the cotherapists' relationship improved. This carried over to the therapy and resulted in more effectiveness, increased feelings of mutual support, and more compatible therapeutic efforts.

Supervision of cotherapists should be developed with the awareness that there is no supervision when authority is absent and that, therefore, self-monitoring should be emphasized whenever possible. When coequal practitioners work together, authority is absent, and a third person—a supervisor—is needed to mediate the relationship.

However, self-monitoring by each practitioner should be encouraged to help focus the potential problems in the cotherapy relationship. Each therapist should be expected to undergo a process of self-monitoring before entering a formal supervisory session. Langs (1979) refers to "self-supervision" as "silent activities" during a therapy session. It can occur before, during, or after a treatment session, but before the supervisory session. Self-monitoring can occur even during a multi-person supervisory session, and should be encouraged by the designated supervisor. Self-monitoring prior to supervision will make the designated supervision more effective and focused. In a sense, self-monitoring is rehearsal for the time when designated supervision is withdrawn or decreased. As therapist skill and experience increase, self-monitoring should also increase.

Theory and Cotherapy

There is disagreement about the importance of theory in learning and doing treatment. There has been little systematic study of how theory is actually used in therapy and how it affects what is said and done (Munson, 1980a:136). Speculative positions have been taken that theory is essential to good practice (Guerin, 1976:42); others hold that theory is of no value to practice and, in many instances, can be inhibiting (Guerin, 1976:162). Theory does play an important role in cotherapy activity, but not in the sense that we normally use it. When attempting cotherapy, it is important that the therapists develop a basic compatibility of style and that each therapist be able to understand and anticipate a sequence of interaction in which the other engages. To promote this, the practitioners must share with one another their theoretical orientations and how these orientations guide the interventions they make. Therapists do not need to adhere to the same theory, but they must discuss with one another what theory they use and how it guides what they do. This is especially important during the early stages of the cotherapy, when the therapists are least familiar with each other's interactional style. When theory is used to promote understanding of the therapists' interactional style, compatibility develops more rapidly, and when serious incompatibility exists, it becomes apparent much earlier in the treatment. As cotherapists become comfortable working together, theoretical exploration becomes less important and planning specific interventions becomes the focus.

In addition, this emphasis on theory in use is beneficial to the overall effectiveness of the treatment. It places a form of control on the interaction that helps keep the treatment focused on problems and therapeutic efforts. Practitioners who have used this approach to cotherapy have reported that they have transferred this orientation to their individual treatment cases, which has resulted in more effective interventions throughout their practice and not just in the cotherapy situation.

Joint Style

As part of the supervision of cotherapy, it is helpful to focus periodically on the joint style that emerges. Practitioner style is a neglected element in assessing treatment interventions and outcomes. Although each therapist who engages in the cotherapy has his or her own style, a unified style of working together can be identified. It is helpful to have the practitioners describe the combined style. Many times the descriptions of the unified style are very different from the styles of the individual practitioners, and the therapists may differ on what they perceive the unified style to be. Identification and discussion of the unified style can reinforce and advance the compatibility of the practitioners through the increased understanding and sense of accomplishment that results from such awareness. Striving for unity and cohesiveness of style and their articulation in supervision can be beneficial to the therapy outcome, since there are indications that therapist cohesion is correlated with a positive therapist-client relationship (Munson, Study F).

Client Perception

Clients accept cotherapy fairly readily and tend to view such efforts as being positive because more than one person is interested in their difficulties and because the agency is willing to commit adequate resources to ensure quality treatment. The view that the presence of an additional therapist gives rise to feelings within clients that their problems must be very bad is generally unfounded. However, if the clients sense conflict and animosity between the therapists, they will not commit themselves to the therapy, and may withdraw from treatment completely. This does not mean that clients should be protected from any therapist disagreement. There is a difference between specific disagreement over an interactional sequence and persistent underlying conflict. At times, it is therapeutic for the clients to hear disagreement or divergent views about the meaning of behavior or interaction. Such disagreement can help to bring out inconsistencies in the clients' actions. Where persistent unstated conflict exists, the clients are usually the first to recognize and verbalize it in the therapy. This is especially the case when cotherapy is used in group treatment. When clients broach this topic, the therapists should encourage them to express their observations so that they can gain insight into how their performance is perceived by the clients. This type of interaction can also help the practitioners validate their assessment of the clients' general ability to perceive events, interactions, and meanings of behavior accurately.

CONSULTATION

Increasingly, social workers are being called upon to provide consultation services within agencies that employ them as well as for other agencies where they serve as outside consultants. Social workers provide consultation mainly to schools, welfare agencies, law enforcement, and aging settings. These consultation services are provided primarily to other social workers, but to nurses, teachers, psychologists, doctors, clergy, lawyers, police, and judges (Kadushin, 1977). When supervisors do consultation work for diverse agencies and different professions, they are required to assume new roles and orientations quite different from their supervisory roles. The emphasis in this section will be on the practical aspects of consultation rather than on theoretical models (for theoretical orientations see O'Neill & Trickett, 1982; Gallessich, 1982).

A study by Wallace (1982) identified the demographic factors that are reportedly associated with successful consultation. Some of the factors identified by Wallace are geographic location, working in full-time private practice, sex of the consultant, and development of community contacts. The emphasis in this section will focus on the actions taken and procedures used by the consultant in order to be successful at this activity. For example, developing good community contacts is more likely to occur through developing a quality reputation by providing sound consultation rather than by having lunch frequently with various agency representatives.

Consultation is easy for an organization to arrange, but getting good consultation is much more difficult to achieve. The supervisor who is entering consultation work must recognize that consultation is different from supervision. Supervision is mandated, and the supervisor has power by virtue of agency sanction of the position. The supervisor can give directives and expect that they will be implemented. The consultant role necessitates dealing with an agency or organization that seeks guidance and direction voluntarily. The organization employing the consultant is in a position to utilize, reject, or simply ignore the advice of the consultant.

The consultant is in a position only to give advice and make recommendations. When this advice is followed, it is rewarding, but if recommendations are ignored, the consultant can become frustrated and angry, and may lose commitment to aiding the organization and its clients. This loss of commitment to promoting changes and improvements can result in demoralization by staff who participate in the consultation process, because the consultant is often perceived as an external ally who can advocate change without reservation.

The consultant must accept the advisory role and offer recommendations firmly, consistently, and continually, regardless of whether or not they are implemented. In reality, some recommendations get implemented and, for various reasons, others do not. The consultant has a responsibility to follow up on all recommendations to determine barriers to unimplemented recommendations and to seek alternative ways to deal with problems. If the majority of recommendations are not implemented, the consultant does need to raise the question of the value of continuing the consultation within the existing framework.

The consultant should be forceful and use an interventive approach, while at the same time being sensitive to the organizational complexities and the right of the organization to use the consultant's input voluntarily. As long as this basic premise regarding the difference between supervision and consultation is kept in mind, most of the principles covered in this book can be applied to clinical case consultation or programmatic-oriented consultation.

Type and Focus of Consultation

The consultant must be clear about the type of consultation that is to be provided. This is important because many organizations know that they need a consultant, but are not sure why they need a consultant or what they need a consultant to do. If the consultant can draw distinctions for the client between the different types of consultation that are available, the distinctions can be helpful to the organization in specifying the purpose of the consultation. Generally, the types of consultation are organizational consultation, program consultation, case consultation, and a combination of organizational, program, and case consultation.

Within these types of consultation, the consultant will need to give added specificity to the consultation through helping the client identify the focus. The variation in focus can take the form of *program implementation* focus. In this form the consultant focuses on what organizational participants should do and how they should do it. This model is often used when an organization is attempting to establish or to reorganize a program or a department. This model is also useful when those assigned to carry out a program have little experience or skill with the services the program is designed to deliver.

A *relationship* focus deals with improving communication within an organization or program staff. This model is most useful where there is much staff conflict or a mixture of old and new staff. In some agencies, reorganization requires staff who have been functioning independently to work more closely with others in a team effort, and they often need help in making this transition. When focusing on relationships, the consultant will need to be more concerned with how work gets done and the nature of staff interaction.

The *personal* focus occurs when the agency manager or department head is provided with personalized consultation. The consultant serves as a highly individualized resource for the manager and is in a sense a sympathetic ear for the consultee. This form of consultation can result in an intense, highly personalized relationship in which recommendations of the consultant, if implemented, can have widespread effects.

Consultation with a *clinical* focus occurs when the consultant gives advice about service delivery in specific cases. This can take the form of case presentations or actual intervention provided by the consultant through working directly with clients.

Consultation Structure

Regardless of the type or form of consultation utilized with an organization, there are five structural elements that should be part of the process.

The Contract. The consultant should have a contract with the organization and should insist on a written contract. In organizations where serious problems exist or where staff conflict is severe, the consultant can become the "scapegoat," or be caught up in the confusion and conflict. A written contract can help the consultant avoid straying or being subverted from the original purpose of the consultant role. Staff changes over time can result in confusion about the role of the consultant even in healthy organizations. A written contract can save time when new managers enter a situation where long-term consultation arrangements exist.

The written contract should include information about consultant compensation, frequency and duration of visits, time period of the contract, the individual with whom the consultant will have direct contact, requirements for written reports by the consultant, functions of the consultant, and tasks of the consultant. These are general items that should be included, and either party to the contract should be free to ask for inclusion of any items they feel important to providing clarity.

The Plan. The consultation plan should be developed early in the consultation process and after an initial assessment has been done by the consultant. Based on the contractual functions and tasks, the consultant should assess the needs of the organization. The plan should be performance-oriented and stated in terms of goals and objectives, both short-term and long-term. The consultation plan should expand on the contractual agreement. Some consultants prefer to negotiate the written contract after this assessment and plan development stage is completed.

In the stage of developing the plan, the consultant should be sensitive to the nature and culture of the organization. The nature of the organization relates to the services, programs, policies, and procedures of the organization. The consultant must develop a plan that is consistent with the nature of the organization and that can be reasonably implemented. The culture of the organization is the informal structures that exist—the unwritten rules and interactional patterns of the staff. While these elements would not necessarily be part of the written plan, they are essential to the type of plan the consultant develops. If these informal elements are not observed by the consultant in the plan development stage, they can later interfere with implementation of the formal plan.

Contact. The contract and plan should specify frequency and duration of consultant visits. The structure of consultant visits will depend on the nature of the agency and the purpose of the consultation. In some cases, it is better to plan infrequent visits for large blocks of time, while in others frequent visits for small blocks of time are preferable. As a general rule, the more serious the problems, the more frequently the visits should occur. Also, educationally oriented (clinical) consultation is more easily adapted to infrequent visits in large time blocks, while administrative (program) consultation is better suited to frequent visits in small time periods.

The timing of the visits should be established in connection with the time required to implement recommendations of the consultant. The organization must be given time to implement recommendations before being required to attempt additional changes. Change takes place slowly, and the consultant needs to provide latitude in order to avoid frustration and poor adjustment to change on the part of the staff.

The consultant needs to be clear about whom he or she will have contact with during visits. It can be cumbersome to have too many staff involved and ineffective to have too few staff involved. All staff who will be required to implement recommendations should be involved. The critical point is to plan and think through in advance what changes are to be made and where they are to be made, and then include all staff who will be essential to implementing the change.

Reporting. The consultant should provide a written report for each visit. This can aid the organization in documenting and justifying the consultation activity. The consultant can use reports to evaluate and plan the evolution of the consultation process as well as to keep track of the sequencing of the recommendations and their implementation. Written reports can provide continuity from visit to visit and help the staff understand that the consultant will follow up on actions that were discussed during visits. Written reports allow staff to refer to the consultant's suggestions between visits rather than waiting for the consultant's next visit to seek clarification. The written report should include, but not be limited to, information regarding date of visit, length of visit, names of people with whom the consultant had contact, problems discussed, accomplishments, list of recommendations, and date and time of next visit.

Evaluation. The consultation process should also be evaluated. Consultation work that is provided for one visit only should be evaluated at the conclusion of the visit. Open-ended consultation should be evaluated periodically. Evaluation should occur at least once annually. The evaluation should be written as well as verbal. It should be focused on goal attainment, and based on the contract, the plan, and the visitation reports. It is reasonable to expect that not all goals will be achieved. A primary purpose of the evaluation is to determine what has been accomplished and what remains to be done. Unmet goals might have been unrealistic, or perhaps problems were misperceived initially and need to be reconceptualized.

Resistance

Organizations seek consultation for various reasons ranging from a genuine desire to improve functioning to saving money and avoiding criticism by regulatory bodies. Consultation is frequently perceived as a refreshing, creative, innovative opportunity for change, but it can also be viewed with resistance and suspicion and as unnecessary. For consultation to have a positive outcome, it must be accepted in principle by all levels of authority in the organization, especially by the higher levels of power and authority.

Individuals within the organization will vary in their reactions to the consultant. Rarely will all elements of the organization have an equal and consistent reaction to the consultation process. Some people will resent the consultant and attempt to subvert his or her recommendations. Others will accept the consultant but show no strong commitment to the recommendations. Others will support the consultant and use advice effectively. It is not unusual for some individuals to see the consultant as a savior who will solve all the organizational ills. People with this perspective will make individual appeals to the consultant to solve various problems or to help overcome powerful or troublesome individuals in the organization. The consultant must use information obtained from such appeals in a cautious and sensitive manner. Such information should be considered only in the context of the specific role of the consultant and the specific tasks or problems that the consultant has been employed to address.

Consultants can inadvertently and inherently threaten directors, administrators, supervisors, and ineffective practitioners. Even effective practitioners can be threatened by consultants if the consultation process is not implemented openly and with a clear understanding of why consultation has been sought. The consultant should request that staff be prepared in advance, but should also begin the consultation process with an explanation of his or her own conceptions of the consultation. Administrators can imply that a consultant is being brought in "to straighten things out" and set up the consultant as a quasi manager. This is not an appropriate role for the consultant.

Rather than telling the staff what consultation is, it is better to inquire what they perceive it as being and what they expect to get from it. This approach allows the consultant to learn how consultation has been presented to staff by the administration, as well as how the staff perceive it personally. After exploring these perceptions, the consultant can correct any misperceptions the staff may have.

There are strategies that organizational occupants can consciously and unconsciously use to resist the consultant. The types and forms of resistance are as varied as the number of participants in the consultation process. Some of the more common direct reactions are such comments as, "The consultant does not understand our situation," "The consultant is not here often enough to know what is going on," or "You need to know about the history of this agency to understand why we do things the way we do." All of these responses are aimed at negating the consultant's knowledge base for intervention.

Rather than confronting such reactions or becoming defensive, the consultant should request the participant to explain the situation or to describe the history of the agency so that the consultant's knowledge gap can be overcome. The consultant should acknowledge that he or she is less knowledgeable than the staff and then focus on getting the information needed to do the consultation work.

More subtle resistances are structural and interactional. For example, some agencies will flood the consultant with nonessential issues or they will change the agenda items for each visit. It is true that in some agencies activity is crisis-oriented and changes from day to day, but the basic issues and problems remain. When these strategies are used, the consultant needs to observe the patterns and formulate ideas about the major problems and then reconceptualize the nonessential issues and specific agenda items in the context of the persistent and real issues.

GENDER AND SUPERVISION

Issues in clinical social work supervision related to the sex of the worker have received little empirical study, and there has been little theoretical writing on the subject. This neglect is ironic in that supervision is the arena in which issues regarding sex discrimination are usually encountered. For example, salary increases, performance evaluation, employment decisions, and promotions are all components of supervision that have been identified as the major sources of discrimination against women.

Discrimination in these areas is related to hierarchical organizational arrangements in which supervisors are paid more than clinicians, and administrators are paid more than supervisors. Truly, power is position. Scotch (1971) holds that unless women are free to move up in supervisory and administrative positions, the hidden inequities become exaggerated. Although sex typing of positions has diminished, the salary and promotional inequities still exist, often leading to covert resentment and in some instances to open conflict. Women have fared badly in this hierarchical process, and this has generally been attributed to processes of socialization with respect to sex roles (Williams, Ho, & Fielder, 1974).

Social work has not been as vigorous as other disciplines in investigating and documenting expectations and performance that are based on sex-role stereotypes of men and women. Most researchers have found that workers who had a male or female supervisor found no significant differences in job satisfaction, satisfaction with salary, satisfaction with supervision, or promotional opportunity (Bartol & Wortman, 1976). Changes in clinical practice and the role of women and men over the past two decades require reexamination of supervision, practice, and male/female practitioner relationships.

Background

From the beginning of the social work profession in the 1800s to the mid-1960s, most of the major works on supervision were written by women, but subsequently the reverse has been true. This has led to a male stereotype of the supervisory relationships. Psychiatry, psychology and social work (the three major professions delivering psychotherapy services) have been slow to address issues related to gender, and almost completely lacking in attention to gender and supervision issues.

Trends indicate that the pool of available professionally trained practitioners increasingly will be female. This has implications for supervision. Virtually no literature exists on the nature of supervision practice based on sex. No reliable statistics exist regarding the percentage of female practitioners and supervisors. A study conducted by the author in the mid-1970s of a random sample of social work practitioners revealed that 66 percent of the practitioners were female and 57 percent of supervisors were female (Munson, 1979a, p. 105).

Historically, there has been little exploration of the roles of males and females in supervision. In a study of males in social work, Kadushin (1976) found that only 21 percent viewed being supervised by a female as a problem, but 37 percent preferred to be supervised by a male. Kadushin considers the movement of males toward administration in part as an attempt to resolve the concerns associated with being supervised by a female. He concludes that his findings support previous speculation that males resist subordination to women. Wilensky and Lebeaux (1975) also hold this point of view, arguing that men do not remain in direct service positions, and women are seldom assigned top administrative posts because of the conflicts that are created when males are subordinate to females. They point out that strains are created for both sexes in such positions, and they attribute the stress to cultural socialization processes that are carried over to the work relationships.

In supervision it has been pointed out that helping supervisees gain knowledge involves different processes than those required to change attitudes (Pettes, 1979:5). Acquiring knowledge and changing attitudes is fundamental in dealing with gender issues in supervision. Changing attitudes in large measure is dependent on acquisition of knowledge. Through use of facts, concepts, theories and guidelines, the conditions for developing positive attitudes toward supervision based on gender can be explored.

Women and Evolution of Supervision

We have to recognize that, in the past, in the day-to-day life of agency practice the average female practitioner and supervisee lived in a traditional society where women showed deference to men and were rarely afforded the professional promotional opportunities men experienced. Women supervising women was a common occurrence but women supervising men was a unique, brief encounter in the man's rise to higher levels of administration (Reynolds, 1965:193).

Historically, the female supervisor's lot was a difficult and suppressed one. Many of the skilled, knowledgeable female supervisors and teachers had to live in the shadow of male psychiatrists even though much of what the psychiatrists had to offer was at best ineffective and at worst inappropriate in meeting practice demands (Reynolds, 1965:47-48). Many of the inroads and creative practice methods made by females relied on the influence of psychiatrists, as illustrated by the wife of Adolf Meyer, a psychiatrist, when she became the first psychiatric social worker in New York in 1907 (Munson, 1983a:43). While this model prevailed for over a century, the women's movement during the past two decades has produced many changes and demands a new perspective of supervision.

Feminist Practice

Current supervisory practice and gender issues can be portrayed as centering around the emerging literature on a feminist approach to practice. Feminist therapy has emerged from the modern women's movement which began in the early 1960s (Sturdivant, 1980). The initial rejection of psychotherapy by the general feminist movement was subsequently refocused by therapists into a specific model of feminist therapy. Sturdivant (1980) has conceptualized feminist therapy around the idea of "philosophy of treatment." The core of feminist therapy is a set of values and attitudes that get translated into practice skill. Feminist practitioners reject traditional sex roles and view societal and cultural values as necessarily making traditional therapy sexist.

Since approximately 20 percent, about 34 million Americans, hold to traditional values, the nascent practitioner subscribing to the feminist therapeutic approach can be subjected to many conflicting pressures just as the population as a whole is caught up in conflicting expectations (Yankelovich, 1981). This conflict increases the importance of the role of the supervisor. The supervisor must give the practitioner the opportunity to explore the philosophy of practice and how it is manifested in what the practitioner does with the client. Without the opportunity to explore these attitudes, values, thoughts and actions, the treatment can be misguided and confusing for the client. Symptoms, problems, roles and responsibilities take on different meanings when a feminist perspective is introduced into the professional relationship.

The literature on feminist practice does not mention supervision as a way to help one build a feminist perspective, but implies this can be done through reading, introspection, and drawing on life experiences (Gibbs, 1984:22). The literature suggests the "going it alone" approach is necessary to emulating the male-dominated professions (Robbins & Siegel, 1983:1), and others have pointed out the loneliness, doubt, and fear that can accompany the solitary approach (Milwid, 1983:68). There is a paradox here. Since feminist theory and therapy are so new, "going it alone" will only isolate the practitioner and prevent the spread of the approach. Historically, supervision has been the source of theory development and the spread of theory (application) in practice. Supervision is the place where the inexperienced practitioner grapples with theory and case material to produce a rewarding, skilled, confident practice style.

The evolution of theory is essential. For example, modern research on psychoanalytic theory is confirming some of its tenets, modifying others, and discarding some. Some feminist therapists have attempted to build the theory by countering against psychoanalytic theory. This has not helped feminist theory, nor has it greatly altered psychoanalytic practices. Both approaches have much to offer, and the focus in supervision, research, and practice should be the advancement of each theory and differential application. There have been recent efforts to reconcile feminist perspectives with traditional psychoanalytic approaches (McGoldrick, 1991). In the process of forging a place for feminist theory in conjunction with earlier theories, there has been disagreement about whether feminist approaches to therapy constitute a method, a modality, a theory, or a philosophy. Some have argued that feminist therapy is a philosophy that can be used to enhance other approaches (Porter, 1985:334). Much more research and application are needed before this process can be considered complete.

The practitioner cannot merge philosophy and practice of feminist treatment alone. Commitment to the cause is not sufficient, and the supervisor plays a crucial role in a successful outcome of a course of treatment. Intervention based solely on academic abstractions can result in loss of confidence, disillusionment, and withdrawal from a feminist or any approach. Such shifts on the part of the practitioner can result in the client becoming discouraged, lapsing back into former ineffective coping strategies, or withdrawal from treatment. It has been pointed out that the feminist practitioner must be comfortable and secure in her own role (Sturdivant, 1980:152). The practitioner who adopts this perspective out of insecurity, rather than security, can do harm within and expose the client to potential harm outside the treatment. The supervisor's role in monitoring such limitations is critical. There is evidence that supervision is essential to identifying feminist therapists' blind spots and anger they "did not hear" in treating female clients (Kaplan, Brooks, McComb, Shapiro, & Sodano, 1983:29).

Although some would disagree, generally, psychology sees trends as theory evolution and expansion, psychiatry is returning to biological explanations of deviance, and social work is moving to a diverse number of specializations. All of these trends seem somewhat removed from the situational stresses clients face in a society undergoing exponential change and poor at translating theory into practical, useful information (see Steininger, Newell, & Garcia, 1984:146). Feminist therapy holds much reality-based assistance for many clients and deserves more attention in educational programs and supervision.

Feminist Practice and Supervision

The emergence of feminist practice raises issues for supervision and practice. There is debate whether males should treat female clients, there is disagreement whether the supervisor of a feminist practitioner should necessarily be a woman, and whether men are capable of a feminist perspective. Another issue that needs exploration is the advisability of feminist therapists treating men. With so many new underlying issues, the feminist therapist should undergo adequate supervision or consultation rather than being left to resolve the issues without support.

Female practitioners are less likely to have experienced supervision by a female during training (Seiden, 1982:287), and given the high percentage of men who have moved into administrative and supervisory positions, the chances of a female practitioner having a female supervisor in many settings are limited. Male supervisors of women are most likely inadequately prepared and unsuspecting of many of the relevant practice issues because of their own lack of exposure to female supervisors or feminist issues. Some supervisees, both male and female, will not understand the value of a feminist approach with certain clients, and these supervisees offer a special challenge for the feminist supervisor.

In the situation where the male is the supervisor of a feminist practitioner, there is a high risk of surprise, confusion, frustration, and defensiveness (Keefe & Maypole, 1983:104) on the part of the supervisor who lacks insight into traditional male behavior. The female supervisee can experience the same reactions when having to deal with an insensitive male supervisor. In such a situation, it is incumbent upon the supervisor to be open, and aware, to develop understanding of the supervisee's position, and to examine his own biases about women. The same advice holds for the female supervisor who does not subscribe to the feminist philosophy. It is unrealistic to expect that because the supervisor is a woman, she will necessarily accept, understand, and advocate a feminist view. Although the effects of the women's movement on education and practice are growing, it has been pointed out that the theory of female sexuality and feminine development continues to be based on a conventional variation of the male model which could be resulting in history repeating itself (Gould, 1984).

Feminist therapists hold that more equality of power and authority between supervisor and supervisee is a basic notion just as it is in the relationship between practitioner and client (Porter, 1985). Some have pointed out that the power relationship can be effectively reversed in some situations, such as when a male supervisor can be given insight about female clients by a female supervisee (Brodsky, 1980:513). The question that remains to be addressed is: How much equality is necessary for effective feminist supervision? If there is to be total equality, it is no longer supervision.

Agency Function

Supervision of a feminist-oriented practitioner must take into account the needs of the client and the function of the agency. Although there are feminist practitioners, there are few feminist agencies per se. Where the client comes to a specific agency with a specific problem or set of problems, a feminist approach to service must be compatible with client needs and agency function. Service should be based on client problems and needs, not practitioner interest. This does not mean agency function and intervention cannot be integrated with a feminist approach. It is critical that the feminist perspective, the agency function, and the client needs be parallel. This is identified by Niles in a case example where a client had talked about her ex-husband being behind in support payments, a son's appearance in juvenile court, and a sister's illness; then the worker suggests they discuss the woman's obesity and how the woman could be attractive if she lost weight (Keefe & Maypole, 1983:104). In this example, the worker is depicted as reflecting sex bias. Exploring the client's obesity is considered valid onlyif it is introduced as a problem by the client. This would be true of genuine specific feminist issues, which could be easily related to the three issues presented by the client. Another more extreme example of this would be the battered wife whose therapist recommends marital or family intervention when the client requires shelter and protection, which is consistent with a feminist perspective. The supervisor should conceptualize treatment issues in the context of client identified problems and agency function. This should be the background consideration of any treatment issues in feminist-oriented supervision.

Supervision should focus on the interventions to be made by the practitioner. In analyzing these interventions, feminist supervision can be oriented toward: (1) the practitioner, (2) the client, or (3) the context of the treatment. In discussing feminist material in supervision, the emphasis is on the practitioner or the client. The question remains whether this is the most efficient way to learn about or supervise treatment. Some theorists have placed more emphasis on the treatment context because it is a more comprehensive approach. In this approach the focus is on exposure, interventions, and techniques (Lecker, 1976:185). Any treatment supervision that fails to integrate all components of the treatment will be necessarily limited in utility (Gurman, 1981:420-422). Haley (1967) goes so far as to say that self-expression of the client (and in the supervisory framework the **self-expression of the** supervisor) cannot be separated from the context of the treatment. For feminist material to be effective in treatment and supervision, this is a basic point that is paramount. The main consideration is that any exploration of feminist material in supervision should be case-related to avoid the supervision going astray. This approach can help promote a feminist orientation rather than detract from it. For example, Gould holds that the use of Freudian theory in practice prohibited the development of feminist psychology. This inhabiting factor was reinforced through extension of Freudian theory use in the supervisory relationship to promote self-awareness (Gould, 1984:101).

Feminist material in supervision is relevant in the context of other practice questions, such as: What are the problems that face the client? What techniques are most appropriate in relating to client problems? What are the goals of the treatment? How will outcomes be measured? How will practitioner "blind spots" be identified and overcome? Within the framework of these questions and other similar questions feminist material can ultimately benefit, help, and be useful to the practitioner and client.

Sex Bias

Sex bias in the practitioner-client relationship can be a difficult problem to deal with in supervision, whether it be a male practitioner with a female client, or a female practitioner with a male client. Sex bias has been found to be inversely correlated with self-concept and positively correlated with homophobia. One study found that homophobia was lowest among psychologists, moderate among psychiatrists, and highest among social workers (Anderson & Henderson, 1985:522). In supervision, dealing with such issues can be clarified by supervising the position, not the *person*. To avoid conflict and combativeness, the supervisor can focus on the case, tasks to be carried out, goals to be accomplished, and problems to be solved, rather than the personality, attitudes, and values of the practitioner. Awareness techniques and exercises have been developed to explore stereotypes and biases in relation to clients of the opposite sex (Brodsky, 1980:518-520). In efforts to enhance feminist practice, it has been argued that feminists who supervise can use the supervisory relationship to foster a sensitivity to feminist issues in treatment in order to promote understanding among neophyte practitioners that a problem exists (Marecek & Kravetz, 1982:302). This approach can be helpful, but if the supervisor and supervisee are not clear about the objectives of such an approach this can lead to conflict in supervision. In order to avoid supervisory conflict, any awareness-development-oriented supervision must be client-related and connected to specific case material. In some cases, avoidance of feminist issues in supervision is preferable. This is especially the case where authority is highly structured.

In highly structured organizations where authority is emphasized, the potential for supervisory conflict is increased. For example, in hospitals where authority is structurally defined and divided along lines of professional disciplines (medicine, nursing, social work, psychology, etc.), supervisees are more acutely aware of authority division, and this awareness carries over to the supervisory relationships. In the normal course of events, these relationship issues get worked out. In the case of mild problems, passage of time and the skill of the supervisor are the crucial factors.

For example, Tim, an advanced graduate student placed in a large government hospital, was required to do three rotations of four weeks each. He began his first rotation with a sense of superiority and spent much supervisory time ridiculing the bureaucracy and being sarcastic about his perceived insensitivity of the staff. He manifested a need to convince the supervisor he knew more than the regular staff, had insights into clients and the organization that others could not see, and that he had taken an existential view of the plight of the clients, the staff, and himself in the situation. The supervisor, a seasoned, feminist practitioner, allowed Tim to express these views and did not challenge his views or attempt to defend or explain the system. The supervisor used Tim's observations to help him learn about organizations, clients, and staff at a conceptual level. The supervisor managed each supervision session in a way that guided Tim to focus on, "Under these circumstances, what could be done to help the patient?" She led Tim to express his views in the context of specific cases, and what could be done to aid the patient and/or the family. By the middle of the second rotation, Tim talked less about organizational and staff issues and focused on patient dynamics and difficulties to be addressed. He began to identify skilled and committed staff who were important to learn from and observe working. By the end of the third rotation, all the "old bravado" was gone and was replaced with professional exploration of strengths, weaknesses, limitations, and problems to be managed. The supervisor's patience and skill led to overcoming the student's defensiveness and anxiety produced by an underlying sense of inadequacy. The positive outcome in this case is best described in the words of the supervisor: "I know Tim was feeling overwhelmed and needed to defend against it. I gave him the flexibility to express his views. I knew he would come around when he realized that superiority stuff would not get him very far around here." The supervisor avoided conflict by not allowing this situation to become a sex-based power struggle, and focused instead on the practice issues facing the supervisee.

Not all gender-linked supervisory authority relationships result in such positive outcomes. In cases where supervisees have more authority-related issues and the supervisor is less skilled and not open to exploring feminist issues, the conflicts can escalate to a point at which resolution is impossible, and the struggles become upsetting to an entire staff. This is illustrated by the case of Pat, a graduate student receiving a fellowship in a large hospital. Pat was assigned several cases on different services in the hospital. The situation was complicated by the student's husband being a radiologist on the cancer service. Other staff complained to the supervisor about Pat "taking advantage" of her husband's status in the unit and using her position as a basis for going around the rules. The supervisor attempted to discuss this with Pat by telling her to "cool it" on the ward. Pat viewed this as the supervisor "picking" on her and being "jealous" of her status. This low-grade conflict continued for several weeks and reached crisis stage when the hospital implemented a regulation that each discipline wear a designated color lab coat in the hospital. Pat refused to wear the coat, and said it "clashed with many of my clothes." Pat's husband, embarrassed by the situation, refused to get involved. The director of the social work department entered the conflict, and when Pat became verbally combative with him, he terminated her from the fellowship. The hospital administrator withdrew the fellowship and assigned it to another department. The supervisor in this case was a traditional male who had little understanding of the worker and withdrew from her. He expressed little interest in the emotional content and felt "the rules are the rules." He saw the student as a "feminist" because she had raised some feminist issues in supervision. This was not the issue, but became an excuse for the supervisor, and further isolated the student. With more openness and looking beyond slogans, the supervisor could have avoided the extreme actions that resulted.

Feminist Family Therapy

One of the most significant developments in the helping professions during the past three decades has been the increase of family therapy. This development raises a number of questions to be addressed and interpreted for the practitioner and supervisor. Some of the more salient questions are: How does the feminist therapist foster equality of the sexes in family practice? What is the effect of a feminist perspective in family treatment regarding the treatment process and outcome? How does a supervisor who is not schooled in a feminist perspective supervise a practitioner with a feminist perspective? Another related question is: Because more practitioners are entering private practice and often seek supervision from practitioners from other male dominated disciplines, how can a practitioner engage in a sustained career development process based on a feminist perspective? Because most psychiatrists are male, does the psychiatrist supervisor and psychotherapist supervisee constellation foster reinforcement of the traditional, potentially sexist model of supervision and practice? These questions need attention in the family therapy field, as well as in supervision in general.

In family therapy supervision it has been pointed out that "the supervisory process will be most successful . . . if it constantly focuses on the skills that the practitioner in training needs and must gradually begin to demonstrate" (Clarkin & Glick, 1982, p. 89). This is a good rule to follow in all forms of supervision to avoid conflict.

Administration

The feminist practitioner, as with any new and emerging approach, will have a struggle defining and building practice orientation, but this struggle will be mild compared to that of the feminist practitioner who desires to move to administration. Given the rise in the number of female practitioners and the dramatic decline of males entering the social work profession, there is increased speculation about the nature of the opportunities for and role of women in administrative positions.

Social work has lagged behind other disciplines in providing opportunities for women to move into administrative positions, and there has been a concomitant lag in documenting and investigating women's attitudes in this area (Munson, 1982). As opportunities for administration expand for women, new issues and choices are produced. New role models must be developed and supervisory opportunities and experiences provided that encourage and support women to pursue administrative positions, as well as utilizing supervision as an arena to identify women who desire administrative careers. The role of the supervisor as a model for aspiring female administrators needs more focus of attention. The importance of this area is highlighted by one study (Munson, 1982) that found female social workers in nonadministrative positions who desire to be administrators undergo more conflict and negative perceptions than other groups of women who have no desire to be administrators. This could be due to lack of encouragement, support, and adequate role models.

It is not safe to assume that because someone is a helping professional he or she will be free of sex biases. Because women in administrative positions is a relatively new development, women encounter serious biases on the part of "old-time" colleagues that can be distressing. Distortion can result, leading to lack of understanding of the basis of older colleagues' views and actions by younger women seeking role models. In the general organizational world, the woman is readily and easily made aware of the odds, resistances, and lack of role models she faces in a "man's world" (Kanter & Stein, 1979). The female professional in the clinical organizational world faces a more bewildering situation in that she is part of a profession that is moving toward a female majority, but still offers few female role models because males have gravitated to the majority of higher ranking positions. Under these circumstances, the support group concept for women becomes just as important for women in clinical settings as is the case in the business world (Faver, Fox, & Shannon, 1983:83). On the other hand, given the sex typing of occupations in our society (Pogrebin, 1980:535), the new majority status of women could enhance women's efforts to overcome the traditional sex-typing of occupations in their preparation for and movement into middle management and upper level positions of leadership. In this effort, much could be learned from patterns of women's work groups and support groups in the corporate world (Kanter, 1977:299-303).

Supervision for Career Advancement

In clinical practice it is appropriate for the supervisor of female practitioners to not only supervise job performance but to also assist the female supervisee in preparation for career advancement. Women need to be encouraged to pursue and trained to perform supervisory and management roles, and their own supervisory experience can be an excellent arena for such preparation.

The findings of one study (Munson, 1982:56) reveal that women who are practitioners with ambition to be administrators believe sexist practices exist at a high level, feel they need to be aggressive to get ahead, undergo more professional conflict, and desire more organization supports for their career goals compared to female practitioners who have no desire for administrative positions. That such perceptions exist at a significantly higher level for women with administrative ambitions raises questions for how we conceptualize and deliver supervision, since these women will be the clinical administrative leaders in the coming decades. The profession needs to establish training programs to aid women in achieving their career aspirations. Supervisors of women with clinical management career aspirations should take these aspirations into account in their supervisory practices. For example, assertiveness by women in clinical managerial positions has been described as difficult for many women to engage in, and for many other participants to accept (Drury, 1984:133-135). This is an example of one area in which supervisors can be helpful to supervisees with managerial ambitions. In order to do this, the supervisor must have experience and skill at being assertive.

Gender and Stress

The supervisor has to deal with a number of matters, but practitioner stress reactions are a significant factor. With increased practice demands brought about by more varied client problems, the practitioner today is vulnerable to work-related stress. Along with this, practitioners are expected to master more theories, develop more techniques, and possess an array of coping strategies, as illustrated by the discussion of operationalizing feminist practice. While client problems are more extensive and intensive, institutional resources are decreasing, causing many practitioners to internalize these inadequacies.

Given the practice demands and the conflicts associated with administrative opportunities feminists experience, the supervisor must be concerned with potential for stress among feminist-oriented practitioners. The empirical research on stress among clinical social workers is in the early stages. The few data-based studies have produced interesting, but sometimes confusing, results. Reiter (1980) in a study of clinical social workers found that 46 percent would not choose social work as a career if they had it to do over. This is interesting in light of the view that jobs and professions in our society have always been sex-typed, and social work has traditionally been considered a woman's profession (82 percent of the respondents in Reiter's study were women). Because socialization processes prepare people for these roles in conscious and unconscious ways (Pogrebin, 1980:535), the consciousness-raising of the feminist movement could increase the sensitivity to this regretted career choice when the reality of the practice world turns out to be radically different from the theoretical expectations and supervisors provide little assistance in making genuine feminist practice a reality.

The question of importance to the supervisor, based on Reiter's findings, is: Do women practitioners suffer higher stress reactions? Two recent studies suggest the answer to this question is no. A study by Streepy (1981) suggests that stress is associated with variables such as income level, educational level, attitude toward the profession, and amount of work experience, rather than sex of the worker. Studies of hospital social workers (Munson, 1983b) and graduate social work students (Munson, 1984) produced no significant differences in which females suffered higher levels of stress reactions than males. These findings are the opposite of those revealed in a study of the medical field in which females reported **significantly higher stress than males** (Huebner et al., 1981). Reasons for psychotherapy practitioners' and students' lower levels of stress remain in the realm of speculation. However, none of these studies controlled for feminist practice perspective. It is quite possible that the feminist suffers more or less stress when compared to others. We simply do not have enough data to currently answer this question. In such unknown areas, the role of the supervisor to promote prevention of stress is important.

The number of female students and practitioners is increasing dramatically, and the women's movement has presented new philosophical, theoretical and practical demands, conflicts and rewards in day-to-day practice activity. Increased expectations and opportunities for administrative and practice advancement are creating new career choices for women in practice organizations. The supervisor can and should be a source of support and role modeling for women.

ERGONOMICS

A section on ergonomics is included in this portion of the chapter on unique settings. Although ergonomics is unique in many agencies, it is possible that, in this period of rapid change, it could soon become a commonplace consideration in most agencies.

"Ergonomics" is a term that is being used increasingly generically to mean the relationship humans have with machines. At the macro level of technology, Toffler (1980) talks of "electronic cottages" that use machines to eliminate the need for human contact in certain areas. Naisbitt (1982) takes a somewhat different view in exploring "megatrends." He argues that high technology produces a human counter-demand for "high touch." Naisbitt calls this the "high tech/high touch formula." It is his view that much modern theory of therapy is associated with this formula. He believes that when new technology is applied to humans in institutions, there should be a built-in corresponding high touch component. From this perspective, it might be beneficial to view clinical social work as the high touch component that must accompany high technology. This is a revolutionary way of thinking of social work practice in relation to technology and will require supervisors to develop a different orientation toward technology, clients, and practitioners. Social workers are more and more involved with technology through applications to our clients as well as to ourselves personally and professionally.

Ergonomics has two implications for clinical supervision that need elaboration. First, many of our clients have relationships with machines. This is especially the case in medical settings where, for example, renal dialysis has become commonplace and, with current technology, artificial heart transplant patients live permanently attached to a machine. With the miniaturization of technology, more patients are surviving with machines implanted or strapped to their bodies.

The term "ergonomics" was derived from the term "biotechnology." Supervisors and practitioners need to be increasingly aware of the significance of ergonomics for clients. Social workers have been slow to accept and resistant to admitting that people have relationships with machines. We have seen machines as dehumanizing, and chief among these has been the computer. This has blinded us to the positive aspects of machines and retarded our advocacy for their use to benefit clients. For example, telephone electronics, hearing and sight devices, and computer hookups can have many advantages for the elderly. In this electronic age, social workers will be required to change significantly their attitudes about technology and machines if they are to provide maximum assistance to clients.

Second, machines are becoming more a part of the clinical practice and supervisory situations. The use of audio and video machines to record therapy sessions for subsequent use in therapy and supervision are becoming more common. In clinical interviews, videotape and audiotape machines are a third party to the treatment. In some settings, videotaping is considered a valuable therapeutic agent. The guidelines for the use of such machines are very limited. Used properly, such machines can enhance treatment, but improper applications can produce desultory intrusions. The supervisor has a responsibility to be skilled in the use of electronic audio and visual equipment (see Chapter 10).

Another form of technology that social workers increasingly use is communications devices, such as paging instruments. These devices have become common in hospital settings, in public welfare, and among private practitioners. There has been no study of the effects of these devices on the functioning of workers. In some cases they are used by workers voluntarily, and in others, involuntarily. Also, there have been no studies whether these instruments in fact increase response time or effectiveness of workers. Supervisors need to be more cognizant of the use of such devices and how they can be most effectively used by practitioners.

SUGGESTED READINGS

John Brendler et al. *Madness, Chaos, and Violence: Therapy with Families at the Brink*. New York: Basic Books, 1991.

>   **System of work** with families with seriously emotionally disturbed members. The system used by the authors is highly compatible with the SEES system described in this chapter.

Sophie Freud. *My Three Mothers and Other Passions*. New York: New York University Press, 1988.
Description of one person's exploration of family of origin experience that could serve as a guide for others.

Thelma Jean Goodrich et al. *Feminist Family Therapy*. New York: W.W. Norton, 1988.
Feminist conceptualization of family therapy.

Herman Holtz. *Expanding Your Consulting Practice with Seminars*. New York: John Wiley and Sons, 1987.
Ideas on how to expand consultation practice through use of seminars.

Judith Jordan et al. *Women's Growth in Connection*. New York: Guilford, 1991.
Good survey of women and treatment theory.

Kevin Leman and Randy Carlson. *Unlocking the Secrets of Your Childhood Memories*. Nashville, TN: Thomas Nelson, 1989.
Practical guide to doing family of origin work.

Monica McGoldrick et al. *Women in Families: A Framework for Family Therapy*. New York: W. W. Norton, 1991.
Broad survey of family therapy from feminist perspective.

Milton Seligman (ed.). *Group Psychotherapy and Counseling with Special Populations*. Baltimore: University Park Press, 1982.
A collection of original articles on group psychotherapy in a variety of settings.

Robin Skynner. *Institutes and How to Survive Them: Mental Health Training and Consultation*. New York: Routledge, 1989.
Perspective of consultation from a British perspective. Can provide original ideas for U.S. consultants.

> We should argue with terms, not fight
> over them.
>
> C. Wright Mills
> *The Sociological Imagination*

Chapter 15

Art and Science in Social Work Practice

In this chapter a perspective on the use of the terms *art* and *science* to describe social work is presented to aid the supervisor. The supervisor needs to be able to approach the concepts of art and science as a way to expose and explore practice issues rather than as a means of disguising them. To accomplish this, a modified conceptualization of artistic elements and scientifically based practice is substituted for art and science. The conventions of traditional art are discussed in a way that allows them to be applied in social work supervision and practice.

INTRODUCTION

In a sense, this book ends on the same note on which it began. In Chapter 2, which deals with the history of supervision, it was argued that the ideas of art and science played a key role in the evolution of practice theory and supervision's natural connection to this evolution. In this chapter an attempt is made to be more precise in the use of these two concepts in the context of modern practice theory and supervision.

The concept of art has been used loosely in many areas. Social work along with other professions uses the term without much precision. *Webster's New Collegiate Dictionary* even includes a generic definition of the term as, "skill acquired by experience, study, or observation," and then gives the example of "the art of making friends." I prefer the more specific definition of art when applying it to conveying information about our practice. The definition I use is "the conscious use of skill and creative imagination . . . in the production of aesthetic objects" (*Webster's New Collegiate Dictionary*, 1979).

The key words here are conscious, skill, creative imagination, and objects. If we are to compare our practice to art, we must be able to show how conscious use of skill was employed to produce an aesthetic object. With some reservations, the concept of "object" has been broadened in this chapter to include experiences, utterances, and actions that occur in treatment.

The most difficult task in comparing social work practice to art is the explication of our conscious use of skill in given aspects of our practice we refer to as art. A major thesis of this chapter is that in the past we have had the opposite approach to art. Rather than using the idea of art to make known our consciously used skill that resulted in an elegant piece of treatment, we have used the term art to justify the unknown, the unexplained, the unconscious, and the unverified aspects of our work.

There is a difference between the act of creating, or the process of creation, and the resulting art object, but we must remember the fact that the two are connected, and process and object in art do not exist unilaterally. One way to explore the process and object of art separately, as well as interrelating them, is to identify the conventions that surround art. Becker (1974) has pointed out that for a work of art to be created requires elaborate cooperation among many people with specialized knowledge and skill. In order for these specialized people to cooperate, certain conventions have evolved that guide their interaction and cooperative efforts, and to a large extent these conventions place strong constraints on the artist and frequently dictate what the artist does. A naive view of the artist and art produces the stereotype that the artist is an unrestrained, creative, aloof, single agent who, in a recondite way, produces objects of art. This innocent view stems from the typical childhood conception of art, in which a five-year-old confronted with a classic painting is likely to say it was produced in a factory (Gardner, 1982:103-104).

In comparing social work practice to art, it has been kept in mind there is a relationship between the creative process, works of art (objects), and conventions that surround artists and art. This constellation led to the conception of the elements of art explained in this chapter.

There is no attempt to detract from what we do as practitioners in calling attention to our vague use of the terms art and artist. What is being argued is that we develop a perspective that enhances what we do. All of the strategies suggested in this book — from audiovisual techniques to questioning techniques, for example — are designed to bring us closer to an artistic orientation rather than detracting from it.

TRADITIONS

Much has been written about the art and science of social work practice. Rarely does a book on practice fail to mention the role of art and science. The notion of social work practice as an art was fostered early in the profession:

> . . . social case work, like most professional activities, is an art, an art in which the practitioner makes use of all the knowledge, wisdom, and philosophy in his possession, but an art nevertheless whose practice cannot be patternized. Each separate bit of professional practice is a creation in itself. (Lee & Kenworthy, 1929:188)

This is the description of random activity mentioned at the beginning of this book. Mary Richmond first called attention to the difference between random activity and practice by observing that as far as social work was concerned, the public had not drawn the distinction "between going through the motions of doing things and actually getting them done" (Richmond, 1917;1965:25).

Social work has a long tradition of using the terms art and science as generalizations that are difficult to apply. In explaining social case work, Richmond said, "In any art the description of its processes is necessarily **far more clumsy than are the processes themselves**" (1917; 1965:103). In the Report of the Milford Conference, a very elegant statement about art and science is made:

Nowhere does the fact that social casework is an art appear more clearly than in treatment. Here is the blending of scientific knowledge, training and experience as in the finished picture. Here, to the vision of the artist is made an actuality through his ability to combine in effective use — not only with skill but with genius — the separate units of his knowledge. But the social case worker has no passive canvas on which to paint his picture. The client himself must be a participant in the art of social case work. (NASW, 1974:30)

Florence Hollis wrote that "casework is both an art and a science: an art in that it requires individual creativeness and skill; a science in that it is a body of systematized knowledge based upon observation, study and experimentation" (1966:265). This was the basis for her view that "casework is a scientific art" (Parad & Miller, 1963:13). Perlman contributed to the mystique of social casework as art by stating, "the art of doing cannot be taught in any complete sense" (1957:vii). Turner has raised the question: "Might it be that the complete therapist is not the theoretician but the artist whose theory is his intuition and skills his natural endowment?" He goes on to suggest that "perhaps the state of our practice is such that the artistic component is stronger than the knowledge base and for the present we should leave the two separate" (1979:9). On the other hand, Pincus and Minahan "view art and science as allies, rather than adversaries. Unfortunately they are often not seen this way" (1973:34). The Council on Social Work Education's *Standards for Accreditation of Baccalaureate Degree Programs in Social Work* summarizes all of this: "In the dissemination of and development of skill there should be, throughout the curriculum, an emphasis on . . . the profession as both a science and art."

In the 1930s "art" based on "the utilization of human skill as opposed to nature" was considered one of the "attributes" of a profession. In this sense it was observed at the time that social work was not "much understood or widely appreciated by the public" as an art, in spite of enormous success of the profession in meeting human needs. Another attribute of a profession was service based on science and learning. In this realm, social work was considered as having hopeful signs, given the technical content in the educational curricula and the emphasis on supervised field training (Chapin & Queen, 1937; 1972:99-100).

These are not descriptions of practice, and they are not even descriptions of art. This view was held up to the supervisor as essential to learning. Each student was "at the mercy of her own creative capacity," and this creative capacity could not be "produced by professional training";

its essence had to be found in the practitioner's personality (Lee & Kenworthy, 1929:188).

ART TERMINOLOGY CONFUSION

This view set up a conflict for the supervisor and the practitioner that persists to this day. If practice is art, and if creativity is innate and not learned, there is very little logic for applying prolonged, intense supervision to the practitioner's work for the purpose of "developing the capacity . . . to deal . . . with face-to-face situations" (Lee & Kenworthy, 1929:188). Only if social work practice existed solely for the entertainment of the worker and client would this view of social work as art suffice.

Since past commentators have repeatedly compared the term art in social work to the fine arts, I have taken the liberty to do the same in the following paragraphs, and to take the comparison even further in order to promote more understanding of this term and how it relates to social work. We need more clarity about this comparison; even in the fine arts there is much disagreement about what constitutes art and its conventions (Schoenwald, 1976:32). The premise of this chapter is that if social work practice is to be viewed as artistic, then we can enhance the quality of our practice by adhering more closely to the conventions of art.

There has been a tendency, as has been shown, to use the terms art and science in conjunction with one another. For example, Siporin (1975: 52-55), who has provided the most detailed analysis of these terms, exemplifies this tendency to combine the terms in his statement that "social work is . . . a . . . scientific art of practice" (Siporin, 1975:3). This is a good beginning, but we must strive to be more specific. Before we can connect these two terms, we need to be clearer about what each one means. The same approach is taken in this chapter regarding social work practice that Jarl Dyrud (1980) has taken in relation to psychoanalysis: "I shall not . . . review all the arguments centering around 'Is Psychoanalysis an Art or a Science?' We have raised it, struggled with it, and become confused by it often enough."

ARTISTIC ELEMENTS
AND SCIENTIFICALLY BASED PRACTICE

Rather than using the term art, I prefer to discuss the idea of the artistic elements of what we do in practice, and rather than science, I prefer to speak of scientifically based practice. The reasons for these distinctions are explained in the following paragraphs.

The relationship between artistic elements and scientifically based practice can be illustrated by an example from the family therapy field. If one surveys the work of the major family therapy theorists, almost all of them believe that an essential part of helping a troubled family is for the practitioner "to join" the family interactionally, and in the process of doing this, disrupt the dysfunctional interactional patterns. This is a basic, knowledge-based, routine activity that applies to almost all family intervention. How the practitioner "joins" the family and goes about breaking up the dysfunctional patterns is a matter of artistic elements. The ways of doing this are limited only by the practitioner's and supervisor's creative capabilities.

The connection between the two conceptions is also illustrated by Hamilton's view that "the art of taking histories is dependent upon the ability to relate questions to the main themes in the client's story" (Hamilton, 1951:59). The practitioner's scientifically based knowledge of human behavior determines what questions are asked. How they are asked and how they elicit understanding and change are the artistic elements of practice.

We, as social workers, have tended to look at art as a totally creative process, and since we have few conventions to guide us, our view of its artistic elements is incomplete. Perceiving art only as a creative process surrounded by mysticism is erroneous. Art in fact is surrounded by rigid conventions that often dictate creative acts (see Becker, 1974:767-776). The conventions that surround art involve collective action by support personnel. In comparing art and its conventions to social work practice, we do not normally take into account receptionists, typists, administrators, and other staff members as part of our artistic work. By considering the conventions and social organization of artistic activities and making appropriate comparisons to social work, we can foster more understanding about why some of our interventions work and others do not. For example, an untrained receptionist who offends and upsets a client in the waiting room can seriously detract from our own efforts during an interview. Supervision is one of the conventions that accompanies the practitioner's artistic efforts. Supportive supervision can enhance practitioners' artistic work; overly critical supervision can hamper it, just as poor lighting can ruin an otherwise good stage performance.

Art is a means and an end. Art exists for itself. Social work practice does not exist for itself. Its purpose is to help people change or obtain resources. These efforts are constrained by time, money, physical facilities, and many other factors. Art flourishes where there are few constraints. Even the process of treatment places constraints on the practitioner. During the diagnostic phase the practitioner is constricted in ability to do many creative acts; the diagnostic assessment must be completed. Art cannot be forced or delayed, but practice acts can.

The mention of art seems to promote profound, comprehensive statements without much detailed or practical application. I hope to add some detail where others have relied on global vagueness and abstraction. The idea of the art of practice is important to supervision because supervisors, when they have their backs to the practice wall, will frequently rely on the "art of practice" abstractions about which they have read so much in the literature.

ELEMENTS OF ART

Social work practice fails to meet the test of an art in the traditional sense. Art in the traditional sense as used here is defined as dance, writing, painting, music, and sports competition. All of these art forms, as well as others, share certain basic elements:

1. creation
2. discipline
3. rehearsal
4. audience and critics

Each of these elements is discussed separately below, after a discussion of some general principles related to art and practice.

There is no attempt to compare social work practice directly to conventional art forms; instead the comparison is of practice to the conventions that surround traditional art forms. The conventions are the four elements mentioned in the previous paragraph. In performing an art, the artist is always surrounded by this set of conventions. It is held that if practice were a true art and the practitioner were an artist, social work practice would be surrounded by these same conventions.

Although many modern day practitioners claim to be artists, Freud did not hold this view of treatment; he said, "I am not an artist; I could never have depicted the effects of light and color, only hard outlines." Picasso presented this same observation from the artist's point of view when he stated, "Anyone can take a sun and make a yellow ball out of it, but to take a yellow ball and make a sun out of it—that is art!"

Creation

Artists create. All artists produce something—a painting, a novel, a film, an on-stage performance. All genuine art forms involve an act or object of creation. Social work practice is a process that cannot be viewed as a performance. Even a recorded session of treatment does not qualify as a performance because it is one segment of a much larger and more complicated whole. No play is ever judged or considered a play on the basis of a single act.

Practitioners do engage in this convention. Practitioners create in a modified form that qualifies practice as having an artistic—a creative— element, but it is not art. There are creative ways in which practitioners engage clients, help them gain insight, and apply techniques and theory in practice. From this perspective, the practitioner uses the same processes of perceptiveness, imagination, original thinking, and recording of experience that the traditional artist uses. Once the supervisor adopts this view of artistic components of treatment, he or she is in a position to help the practitioner use theoretical orientations and philosophies to perceive and understand therapeutic action in a manner that allows him or her to be creative. The practitioner must have a theory or philosophy to guide practice, but at the same time must possess an openness to what he or she experiences in order to relate imaginatively to the uniqueness of the client. The practitioner must have a perspective that permits integration of an array of facts and actions that fit into a logical whole that makes therapeutic change possible. This highlights another difference between the practitioner and the artist. The artist produces, or more accurately, promotes change. We cannot say the practitioner creates change. Only the client can do that. In fact, from this view, the client is more the artist in treatment and the practitioner is the director, producer, or teacher of the artist. The true artist reflects and documents change, and at times produces change through his or her art. Artists mirror change and are directly involved in change that advances society.

It is interesting that comments about the creative process by creative people in the arts or sciences assign very little value to the epistemology of creativity as a concept. They espouse a certain mysticism and indescribable quality to the what-and-how of their creative work. They do not think that trying to understand it is a fruitful endeavor. Instead, they frequently mention the notion of curiosity—the desire to know more—as the more **important concept.** Curiosity is viewed as the necessary and knowable ingredient of creativity.

In supervision we could advance our knowledge by focusing more on the idea of curiosity. What is the role of curiosity in doing good diagnosis and treatment? How can curiosity be utilized to let our clients know we really care? How can curiosity enrich and advance our practice? Curiosity can be the factor that helps us enter the realm of more information and better information in a case that gives all the appearances of being just like the dozens of other cases we have treated in the past. Curiosity on the part of the supervisor can inspire the practitioner, and curiosity on the part of the practitioner can be the tool to more in-depth intervention that motivates the client to change.

One of the best discussions of the object in art is John Dewey's *Art as Experience* (1958). The reader who has special interest in interaction in the form of practice as art should read Dewey's extensive treatment of the topic. Dewey discusses experience (interaction) and object in art separately, but he does so only to illustrate that they are basic components of a unified whole. He rejects the view that experience alone or an object alone constitutes art. This leads him to reject the idea that art is some experience "in us"; but even the discussion of the concept of "in us" is based on a set of emotions that emerge from an object of art. Even though he uses examples from psychiatry, he does not equate treatment with art. In the context presented by Dewey, treatment falls short of being art. Dewey summarizes his stand quite clearly and illustrates the point that is the substance of the view presented in this chapter:

> Art denotes a process of doing or making. This is as true of fine as of technological art. Art involves molding of clay, chipping of marble, casting of bronze, laying on of pigments, construction of buildings, singing of songs, playing of instruments, enacting roles on the stage, going through rhythmic movements in dance. Every art does something with some physical material, the body or something outside the body, with or without the use of intervening tools, and with a view to production of something visible, audible or tangible. (1958:47)

Dewey also makes a distinction between art and science that can be helpful with the often-heard, vague phrase, "the art and science of practice." This statement is rarely followed by an empirical explanation and remains to be applied in any abstract sense we choose. Dewey's view is based on "drawing a distinction between expression and statement" in which "science states meanings; art expresses them." When this explanation is used as a guide, art and science can be empirically defined in clinical discussion. Science can be applied when we attempt to assign meaning to events that relate to treatment. To the extent that we can talk about art in therapy — that is, artistic activity — it occurs in relation to how one expresses feelings, thoughts, and events in treatment. This distinction can be a powerful way of organizing discussion of clinical material in supervision. Imagination combined with observation is the key to creativity in practice.

Sartre has given a micro-analysis of the importance of object in the novel, theater, and film. The object, whatever itmight be, is a sterile thing that becomes the focus of the expression of the artist. Depending on the art form, the artist's treatment of the object determines the observer's response to and interpretation of the object in the particular sense. The only perception of the object the observer brings to the artistic situation is general recognition of the object. The particular response to the generalized object is controlled by the artist, and the amount of the artist's control of the response varies with the art form (Sartre, 1976:6-20).

Discipline

Artistic creativity requires discipline. A great deal of discipline must precede a creative act. Raw talent does not assure a creative success. Art involves the unique blending of creativity and discipline. Herb Alpert has called attention to the fact that there is more to art than being technically trained by observing that, when you are a musician, "you don't get credit for just knowing the notes." If treatment has an artistic component, the practitioner must develop skill at balancing discipline and technical skill with creative reactions.

Artists, in a pure sense, have a faith in what they do, a commitment to advancing their art and their skill, and a devotion to their craft. Florence Nightingale understood the importance of devotion to art, and illustrated the point being made here when she observed:

> Nursing is an art; and if it is to be made an art, it requires as exclusive a devotion, as hard a preparation, as any painter's or sculptor's work; for what is the having to do with dead canvas or cold marble, compared with having to do with the living body . . .

In comparing this loyalty to the social work profession, we fall short. A study of clinical practitioners has revealed that almost half are disillusioned about their choice of social work as a profession (Reiter, 1980). The question that remains is how such reactions among such a large number of social workers influence their performance from an artistic perspective. Artists become disillusioned, but study of disillusioned artists demonstrates that they deal with such feelings by turning inward and using their art as an outlet for these feelings. There is evidence that many creative people are the most productive when working their way out of an episode of depression and despair (Pickering, 1974).

What remains unclear is how, and if, social workers use their work as a source of overcoming psychological reactions. Some who have studied stress among practitioners have suggested that using our work to resolve personal and professional despair leads to more stress, making such efforts self-defeating. More insight into this process could add much to our understanding of the connection between creativity and stress, as well as provide evidence that there is an artistic element to our practice.

Rehearsal

In all true art forms, the artist engages in rehearsal for the performance. This is not an element of our practice. If practitioners are to recognize the artistic elements of social work, they need to identify the equivalent of rehearsal and practice. Supervision is the place where this can occur. The use of videotape and audiotape recordings, process recordings, and case discussion can be regarded as forms of practice or rehearsal for future sessions.

Audience and Critics

All art forms have an audience. People visit galleries to view paintings; people attend plays and musical performances. The practice situation normally has no audience other than the client. Also in traditional art forms, there are critics of the art: the audience as well as professional critics.

The term "audience," with respect to social work, is being used in the conceptual sense and not the descriptive sense. Audience does not necessarily mean a group of people that sits in a music hall and observes a performance or a play. Audience in this context means the observers, the spectators, and the evaluators of the object of art. While it is a point open to debate, art cannot exist without an audience in the generic sense of the term.

In social work treatment there are rarely any critics. As has been pointed out in this book, the supervisor to some extent should and does serve as a critic. Rarely does criticism or judgment go beyond the supervisor. There is very little evaluation of outcome by individual practitioners or by agencies. Until we institute more systematic evaluation, we cannot really say we are approaching art or artistic qualities in what we do.

Art is recognized and judged through acclaim and awards. For example, painters paint to express themselves, but museums and galleries exist to reward that expression. There are numerous prizes and awards for excellence in art. The social work profession is devoid of awards and recognition of excellence in practice. Our various professional organizations have no organized programs specifically aimed at recognizing such excellence. If we are to take our artistic conceptualization of practice seriously, we will have to develop conventions for recognizing and fostering excellence in practice.

ART AS DEFENSE

Although the term art has been used to conceal our scientific shortcomings at the more general level, many practitioners will retreat into the defense of "art" at the personal level when asked to account for their performance. Haley (1980) has pointed out that it is easier to use this strategy with colleagues than with clients, but practitioners develop strategies to deal with both groups. When dealing with colleagues, practitioners insist on the importance of confidentiality, shy away from use of recordings or observation in supervision, emphasize the importance of long-term therapy, champion the idea of science in practice, and note the importance of credentials and licensing for practice (Haley, 1980:386). To guard against this the supervisor should avoid allowing supervisees to use the art defense. Supervisees should be required to justify and explain their interventions. This is a primary function of supervisors, and the supervisor should avoid shrinking from this responsibility. Some people abandon supervision rather than face this issue (see Simon, R., 1982:32).

At a difficult moment in treatment, there is a tendency to withdraw or become creative rather than to muster the discipline to exercise the tremendous technical skill that is required. Liv Ullmann has beautifully and succinctly described this phenomenon in relation to acting: "I love technical challenge. Stop on a chalk mark in the middle of a difficult emotional scene" (Ullmann, 1978:298). We must be aware of the chalk marks in treatment during powerful and significant exchanges. This takes discipline, and skill is a more constant ingredient of creative activity than cognitive insight (Abell, 1966:329). Too often supervisors emphasize cognitive insight at the expense of technical skill. The act of creation becomes a means of rationalizing failures.

Treating therapy as art assumes some highly developed approach that can be studied, mastered, applied, and judged. The way social workers have used the concept of art is the exact opposite. We use it to obscure and elevate what we do to the intangible, the unknowable. We describe what we do up to a point, but then indicate that a level of abstraction is reached that leaves us only with the alternative to call it art. Fortunately, there is a trend away from this view in psychotherapy. For example:

> . . . we believe that avoiding investigation and explicit discussion of how therapists actually deal with their patients has helped maintain an unfortunate aura of obscure complexity and magic, in which the resolution of patients' problems necessarily is seen as an art. Instead we feel that treatment is, or at least should be, much more a craft, albeit one to which the individual therapist can lend any artistry she possesses. With artistry alone, one can only stand in awe of the "gifted" therapist; with therapy viewed as a craft, one can learn to replicate effective problem-solving techniques. (Fisch et al., 1982:xiii)

Only through discipline developed over time can the practitioner be prepared to perform the task of treatment. To the extent that *creativity in use* (efforts to provide further insight, organization, and understanding of the dynamics) occurs in treatment, it should take place more at low points in the process than at high points.

PATTERNS AND ART

Patterns, although not always apparent, are the essence of art. As Ariete has pointed out, "What seems to be due to chance is totally or to a large extent the result of special combinations of biological circumstances and antecedent life experiences" (Ariete, 1976:7). At the same time, "the characteristic of uniqueness or originality in a sequence of mental events or in certain forms of behavior is not enough to qualify them as creative products" (Ariete, 1976:7). Ariete also makes a point about patterns in treatment that highlights the misguided view that creativity lacks patterns and is a single act. In discussing the technique of free association in psychoanalysis, Ariete observes:

> The aim of the technique is to remove conscious control and to allow images, feelings, and ideas to come freely into consciousness. From this free flow emerge patterns that will disclose the conflicts and then the personality of the patient . . . . These circumstances represent millions of separate events; and since they are never duplicated in their number, sequence, strength, and other characteristics, their combination is enough to explain the uniqueness or originality of the individual. When spontaneous ideas occur repeatedly or in cycles or special sequences, the analyst helps the patient recognize patterns in

them. The patterns existed before; but without the intervention of the analyst, the patient would not have discovered them or at least would have discovered them only with great difficulty. (1976:7)

Early social workers were not wrong in their description of practice; they just did not go far enough in their explanations. Such shortcomings illustrated that, at the early stages of the development of social work practice, we did not understand its essence, and perhaps because of these limitations, the idea of art was used to plug the gaps in our knowledge. Also, Ariete's description of the discovery of patterns in practice further limits the idea of art in our practice. Art must be free to take any course that presents itself, but the process of discovering preexisting patterns in treatment places restrictions on the form and direction of the treatment if it is to be of value to the client.

A question that remains to be answered through research is: Does theorizing in supervision hamper practitioner creativity? It appears that the answer depends on how the theorizing is handled by the supervisor.

There are basic, routine actions that must be done in practice; other actions are left to the discretion and creativity of the practitioner. This was illustrated in a poignant and down-to-earth comment by a social work student to a supervisor: "In my cases I think I do pretty good at the initial phase, and I can handle the termination phase okay. It is the stuff in the middle I have trouble with." The worker was expressing that the more basic, routine actions had been mastered, but the essence of the creative aspects of treatment were causing her difficulty. The supervisor must be alert to this distinction and how the creative elements of practice can be the most troublesome. The supervisor must be ready to assist the worker in balancing learning about the routine and the creative components of practice. Mary Richmond called attention to this point in *Social Diagnosis*: "The method that ignores or hampers the individuality of the worker stands condemned not only in social work but in teaching, in the ministry, in art and in every form of creative endeavor" (1917; 1965:10).

SCIENCE

Richard Cabot was one of the earliest commentators on the role of art and science in social work. In discussing "the craftsmanship of social work," he observed: "In social work the art has preceded the science, as it did in medicine and music; but neither science nor art can live well without the other. The science must back and direct the art" (1973:56). He went on to add that "the art exists, but the science has not yet gotten very far" in social work (1973:70). In Cabot's view the art must be founded on the science. This parallels the view expressed earlier that the basic and routine aspects of practice must be connected with the creative elements of practice. Science is not always the routine and art is not always the creative. Pincus and Minahan have stated succinctly the connection between artistic elements and scientifically based practice: "Although science and art will merge in the style of a particular social worker, he needs to know when he is operating from the basis of knowledge and when from creativity and intuition" (Pincus & Minahan, 1973:36). Hollis used an analogy to describe this process in a somewhat different manner:

> No blueprint of treatment can ever be given, any more than a skier can know the twists and turns he will have to take on a steep, unknown course toward a distant objective. Like the skier, the worker knows his general direction, but he can see only a little way ahead and must quickly adapt his technique to the terrain. To do this he must be a master of technique, know what to do to accomplish what, and when a given procedure is necessary. (1966:275)

Supervision is where the science of practice should be orchestrated. All that we know from research should be brought to bear on what we see in practice and used to make sense of what is in front of our noses. Supervision should be the arena in which we sort the known and familiar from the unknown and the unfamiliar. Through such a dichotomy we can begin to see supervision as the place where we forge new knowledge. Instead of hiding the unfamiliar under the cloak of "our art," we must abandon this defense and bring our failures at knowing into the open for exploration and advancement of knowledge. The blessing of science is that it reassures us that our failures can be transformed into successes if only we are willing to trust in science and use it, rather than attributing so much to art that goes unexplained and is attributed to the private knowing of the artist at work. Once we adopt this view, the science of what we do in supervision can become the source of fun and joy that the traditional scientist derives from the search for knowledge.

Science as Struggle

Judson has pointed out that "the other side of the fun of science, as of art, is pain. A problem worth solving will surely require weeks and months of lack of progress, whipsawn between hope and the blackest sense of despair" (1980:5). Unfortunately, the guise of art in our work has too often been used to avoid this pain, causing us to endure a more insidious frustration and gradual cynicism that is projected on our clients.

Lewis Thomas has provided an excellent summary of the role of science that can be applied in supervision:

> Science, then, is a model system for collective human behavior and has value because of this for all of us, for it is an activity that can be scrutinized and studied . . . . For this reason, among others, we have need of critics in science, in the sense that classical art and architecture needed the Ruskins, music the Toveys, and contemporary literature the Leavises, Eliots, and Wilsons. We need people who can tell us how science is done, down to the finest detail, and also why it is done, how the new maps of knowledge are being drawn, and how to distinguish among good science, bad science, and nonsense. (Judson, 1980:x)

In some respects "our science" of social work has been confused with "the sciences." Sullivan points out that "the sciences" are most convincing when dealing with inanimate matter, but are much less convincing when dealing with life and living (1963:125). It is interesting that we have been labeled inadequate as a science simply because we are dealing with what is admitted by scientists to be a more complex problem. In the profession we make this same error by confusing the problem with the process of dealing with the problem. When the early social workers talked about science, they did not mean that we could or should adopt the methods of the pure sciences intact. At present we spend too much time attempting to reform our efforts into a pure science. Our predecessors recognized and accepted the differences between social sciences and basic sciences in a way we would do well to come to understand today. Brackett summed this up quite adequately in 1903 when discussing supervision:

> Good administration of public aid is a part of good government . . . Whether there be a science in all this or not, theproblems are to be studied and solved in scientific ways — by openmindness, by use of the teachings of experience, by efforts to see causes and results. (1903:212)

SOCIAL WORK AND ARTISTIC QUALITIES

The idea of art should not be used to shroud what we do in mysticism and esoteric abstractions. Social work practice is not art, but it does have artistic qualities that can be specified on the basis of the criteria discussed in this chapter. Through this less general approach to our practice, we can more clearly define our technique, our theory, and our function. We can borrow conventions from art to advance what we do, but we are just obscuring what we do by simply calling it art.

Terms used in the world of art can be used to refine and define what we do, and it is in this sense that we should use art to advance our knowledge and practice. For example, Burke (1975) argues that there are five terms that can be identified as valuable in generating principles in art and science. These terms are act, scene, agent, agency, and purpose.

Another way to use ideas about art to further our practice is the common theme of seeing the particular in the universal. Schopenhauer wrote that this is a fundamental characteristic of a genius, a characteristic that is associated with art and artists (Ariete, 1976:341). Sartre stated this relationship another way:

> . . . the only way I can be connected with the tree is to see a character sit down in its shade. It is not the sight of the character, therefore, that makes the settings, but gestures; and gestures create the general rather than the particular. (1976:11)

By exploring the idea of the particular and the general or universal in our relationship with clients, we can gain much insight into what we do in practice.

Many terms used in the arts can be used to better our understanding of social work practice. This view has been expressed in relation to psychoanalysis:

> The chief hope of realizing these possibilities lies, not in psychoanalytical studies pursued in isolation, but in the combined operation of psychoanalytical insights with those derived from other and entirely different fields of knowledge. (Abell, 1966:25)

We need more precision in our use of the term art because there is a thin line between creativity and chaos. It has been observed that "art is demonic, but it is also disciplined" (Schoenwald, 1976:32). For every act committed by a practitioner, you can find support for that act as well as opposition to it. Until we have some common agreement about the basis of our interventions, we have neither art nor science.

Our propensity to confuse artistry with treatment grew out of Freud's interest in art and artists and their role in society and culture. The parallel between artists and practitioners emerged later. Freud's work gives no indication this parallel was ever a part of his view of practice. Although there are many parallels between the life and work of Freud and DaVinci, he made no effort to draw such connections in his study of DaVinci. In reading Freud's work on DaVinci, one is struck with his avoidance of such comparisons and his emphasis on the limitations of psychoanalysis in understanding the artist.

The traditional ideas of art and science have limited utility for social work, and the use of these terms in treatment and supervision ultimately presents us with a dilemma, an enigma that places us somewhere between art and science. Jung summarized all of this:

> Since self-knowledge is a matter of getting to know the individual facts, theories help very little in this respect. For the more a theory lays claim to universal validity, the less capable it is of doing justice to the individual facts. Any theory based on experience is necessarily *statistical*; that is to say, it formulates an *ideal* average which abolishes all exceptions at either end of the scale and replaces them by an abstract mean . . . . The distinctive thing about real facts, however, is their individuality . . . . At the same time man, as member of a species, can and must be described as a statistical unit; otherwise nothing general could be said about him. For this purpose he has to be regarded as a comparative unit . . . . If I want to understand an individual human being, I must lay aside all scientific knowledge of the average man and discard all theories in order to adopt a completely new and unprejudiced attitude. Now whether it is a question of understanding a fellow human being or of self-knowledge, I must in both cases leave theoretical assumptions behind me. Since scientific knowledge not only enjoys universal esteem but, in the eyes of modern man, counts as the only intellectual and spiritual authority, understanding the individual obliges me to commit *lese majeste*, so to speak, to turn a blind eye to scientific knowledge. This is a sacrifice not lightly made, for the scientific attitude cannot rid itself so easily of its sense of responsibility . . . . This conflict cannot be solved by an either-or but only by a kind of two-way

thinking: doing one thing while not losing sight of the other. (1957:16-19)

BOOK CONCLUSION

As a conclusion to this chapter and to the book, Visual 15.1 has been prepared to capture all the elements of practice style that practitioners and supervisors must take into account when analyzing supervision practices. The artistic qualities and scientific components of practice are part of each of the elements of style. Practice is not all art or all science. Some elements of practice style are more amenable to empirical measurement and scientific orientations while others are more in the realm of artistic endeavor.

As a way to unify much of the content of this book, the elements of practice style presented in Visual 15.1 are summarized below. This conceptualization of practice style can be used to explore many aspects of supervision. Whether one is trying simply to enhance and improve practice or is working to solve a specific treatment difficulty, this conceptualization can be an effective guide for conducting such analyses. It can be a valuable tool in dealing with what Greben (1985) has identified as the task of supervision that ". . . what requires examination in psychotherapy is not so much what is wrong with patients, but what is amiss with therapists." All of us go "amiss" from time to time in such a complex endeavor as clinical treatment, and guidelines are needed to organize our thoughts regarding where the difficulties reside. Analyzing the elements of our practice style can help identify the sources of the difficulty. The elements of practice style are:

1. *Philosophy of Life.* All practitioners have some philosophy of life that they can articulate in general or specific form. The person's philosophy of life can reveal much about orientation to practice. It can be helpful to practitioners to state a philosophy of life as they struggle with defining practice style. This element is predominantly in the realm of artistic qualities of practice.

2. *Philosophy of Practice.* While practitioners have a philosophy of life they can articulate if asked, all practitioners have a philosophy of practice, but they have much difficulty articulating it. It is important that the practitioner be assisted in identifying and articulating philosophy of practice as an essential aspect of practice style. A philosophy of practice and the philosophy of life do not have to be identical and completely compatible, but when philosophy of practice and philosophy of life are very different

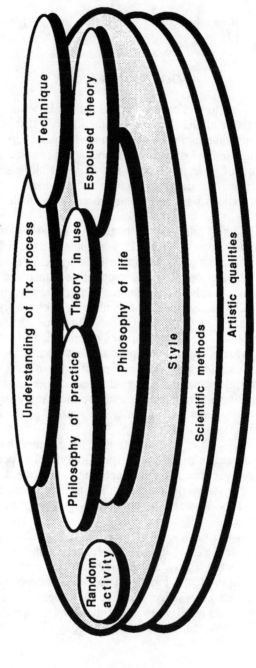

VISUAL 15.1. Elements of Practice Style

the practitioner may encounter difficulty, frustration, and callousness in practice. Philosophy of practice is primarily an artistic quality.

3. *Theory in Use.* Connected to philosophy of practice is "theory in use" which was identified by Argyris and Schon (1980). This is the theory that the practitioner uses in the actual conduct of practice. It is what the practitioner does while face to face with clients. Theory in use cannot be described. It can only be observed by others or captured on videotape (or on audiotape in a limited form). When recorded, "theory in use" can be considered artistic and subjected to scientific analysis.

4. *Espoused Theory.* "Espoused theory" was also first defined by Argyris and Schon (1980). It is connected to "theory in use" in that it is an attempt to describe or explain what the practitioner does in the actual practice situation. It can be a recognized theory from the literature or it can be the accumulation of practice wisdom developed by the individual. There should be consistency between "theory in use" and "espoused theory." If there is much disparity between the two the practitioner can become confused, can confuse clients, and can be ineffective in practice. "Espoused theory" can be a scientific aspect of practice and can be subjected to scientific scrutiny.

5. *Technique.* This element of practice style can emerge from any of the elements listed above, but should have some connection to "espoused theory" that can be described and explained by the practitioner. Technique has been covered in detail in this book and it can be considered from both artistic and scientific perspectives.

6. *Understanding of the Treatment Process.* This element is complex and can take much time and experience to develop. It is connected to all of the elements listed above. It is much more than recognizing that treatment has beginning, middle, and end phases. It is the understanding of how clients and therapists react to treatment; how trust is developed and that there are several levels of trust; how resistance occurs in the client and the therapist and the stages of this process; appreciating what dictates brief and long-term treatment; how different reactions at different stages of the treatment are connected to events inside and outside the treatment; recognizing and using the patterns of behavior the client presents; and many other factors. This understanding can have artistic qualities and can be subjected to scientific inquiry.

7. *Random Activity.* Random activity occurs when no coherent treatment activity occurs that can produce a change for the client. The therapist in this mode can have a nice conversation with the client but there is no identifiable focus or outcome. Some therapists go through entire careers

engaging in random activity, while good practitioners lapse into random activity from time to time because they are tired, upset, frustrated, frightened, or caught off guard. There are no artistic elements to random activity, but some practitioners will describe such activity in artistic terms. Random activity can be scientifically observed and measured.

SUGGESTED READINGS

Walter Abell. *The Collective Dream in Art: A Psycho Historical Theory of Culture Based on Relations Between the Arts, Psychology, and the Social Sciences*. New York: Schocken, 1966.
    An excellent intellectual discussion of the connection between art and the behavioral sciences.

Silvano Ariete. *Creativity: The Magical Synthesis*. New York: Basic Books, 1976.
    A modern parallel to Dewey's *Art as Experience*. This book can serve as background for much of the discussion in this chapter on art and practice.

Kenneth Burke. "The Five Key Terms of Dramatism." in Dennis Brissett and Charles Edgley (eds.), *Life As Theater: A Dramaturgical Sourcebook*, Chicago: Aldine, 1975.
    A series of readings on the dramatic aspects of interaction with some discussion of their relationship to intervention. Many concepts can be used to expand on the points made in this chapter.

John Dewey. *Art as Experience*. New York: Capricorn, 1958.
    An excellent, classic book that discusses art with some focus on its relation to treatment as applied in this chapter.

References

Abell, Walter. *The Collective Dream in Art: A Psycho-Historical Theory of Culture Based on Relations Between the Arts, Psychology, and the Social Sciences*. New York: Schocken, 1966.

Adler, Mortimer J.. *Six Great Ideas: Truth, Goodness, Beauty, Liberty, Equality, Justice*. New York: Macmillan, 1981.

Ajemian, Ina, and Mount, Balfour M.. *The Royal Victoria Hospital Manual on Palliative/Hospice Care*. New York: Arno, 1980.

American Board of Examiners in Clinical Social Work. *The Diplomate* 2 (June, 1989).

Anderson, S. C. and Henderson, D. C. "Working with Lesbian Alcoholics." *Social Work*, 30 (Summer 1985), pp. 518-524.

Anonymous. "Position Statement of Family Service Agencies Regarding Graduate Schools of Social Work." *Smith College Studies in Social Work* (February 1973), pp. 108-110.

Anonymous. "Supervision." *The Family* 10 (April 1929), pp. 35-45.

Argyris, Chris, and Schon, Donald A.. *Theory in Practice: Increasing Professional Effectiveness*. San Francisco: Jossey-Bass, 1980.

Ariete, Silvano. *Creativity: The Magic Synthesis*. New York: Basic Books, 1976.

Bagg, Alan R. "AV Presentations: Step by Step, Inch by Inch." *Audio-Visual Communications* 14 (January 1980), pp. 35-39.

Bailey, Joe. *Ideas and Intervention: Social Theory for Practice*. London: Routledge and Kegan Paul, 1980.

Ball, John C. et al. "The Heroin Addicts' View of Methodone Maintenance." *British Journal of Addiction* 69 (March 1974), pp. 89-95.

Barber, Bernard. "Some Problems in the Sociology of the Professions." *Daedalus* 92 (Fall 1963), pp. 669-688.

Bartlett, Harriett. *The Common Base of Social Work Practice*. Washington, DC: National Association of Social Workers, 1970.

Bartol, K. M., and Wortman, M. S., Jr. "Sex Effects in Leader Behavior Self-Description and Job Satisfaction." *Journal of Psychology* 94 (1976) pp. 177-183.

Barton, Walter E. *The History and Influence of the American Psychiatric Association*. Washington, DC: American Psychiatric Press, 1987.

Beck, Robert L. "Process and Content in the Family of Origin Group." *International Journal of Group Psychotherapy* 32 (April 1982), pp. 233-244.

Becker, Howard S. "Art as Collective Action." *American Sociological Review* 39 (December 1974), pp. 767-776.

Berger, Milton M. (ed.). *Videotape Techniques in Psychiatric Training and Treatment*. New York: Brunner/Mazel, 1978.

Bergin, Allen E., and Garfield, Sal L. (eds.). *Handbook of Psychotherapy and Behavior Change*. New York: Wiley, 1971.

Bergin, Allen E., and Strupp, Hans H.. *Changing Frontiers in the Science of Psychotherapy*. Chicago: Aldine-Atherton, 1972.

Beukenkamp, Cornelius. "Clinical Observations on the Effect of Analytically Oriented Group Therapy and Group Supervision on the Therapist." *The Psychoanalytic Review* 43 (January 1956), pp. 82-90.

Birenbaum, Arnold et al. "Training Medical Students to Appreciate the Special Problems of the Elderly." *The Gerontologist* 19 (December 1979), pp. 575-579.

Bissell, LeClair et al. "The Alcoholic Social Worker: A Survey." *Social Work in Health Care* 5 (Summer 1980), pp. 421-432.

Bloom, Fred. "Psychotherapy and Moral Culture: A Psychiatrist's Field Report," in Thomas J. Cottle and Phillip Whitten (eds.), *Psychotherapy: Current Perspectives*. New York: New Viewpoints, 1980.

Bloom, Martin. *The Paradox of Helping: Introduction to the Philosophy of Scientific Practice*. New York: Wiley, 1975.

Blum, Diane, and Euster-Fisher, Sona. "Clinical Supervisory Practice in Oncology Settings." *The Clinical Supervisor* 1 (Spring 1983), pp. 17-27.

Blumenfield, Michael. *Applied Supervision in Psychotherapy*. New York: Grune and Stratton, 1982.

Bowen, Murray. *Family Therapy in Clinical Practice*. New York: Jason Aronson, 1978.

Boyer, Ruth. *An Approach to Human Services*. San Francisco: Canfield, 1975.

Boyers, Robert (ed.). *R. D. Laing and Anti-Psychiatry*. New York: Harper and Row, 1971.

Brackett, Jeffrey Richardson. *Supervision and Education in Charity*. New York: Macmillan, 1903.

Brager, George A. "Advocacy and Political Behavior." *Social Work* 13 (April 1968), pp. 5-15.

Bramhall, Martha, and Ezell, Susan. "How Burned Out Are You?" *Public Welfare* 39 (Winter 1981a), pp. 23-55.

_____. "Working Your Way Out of Burnout." *Public Welfare* 39 (Spring 1981b), pp. 32-47.

_____. "How Agencies Can Prevent Burnout." *Public Welfare* 39 (Summer 1981c), pp. 33-47.

Brandt, Anthony. "Self-Confrontation." *Psychology Today* 14 (October 1980), pp. 78-101.

Brendler, John, et al. *Madness, Chaos, and Violence: Therapy with Families at the Brink*. New York: Basic Books, 1991.

Brennan, E. Clifford. "Expectations for Baccalaureate Social Workers." *Public Welfare* 34 (Summer 1976), pp. 19-23.

Briar, Scott. "The Current Crisis in Social Casework." in Robert W. Klenk and Robert M. Ryan (eds.), *The Practice of Social Work*, Belmont, CA: Wadsworth, 1970, pp. 85-96.

Briar, Scott, and Miller, Henry. *Problems and Issues in Social Casework*. New York: Columbia University Press, 1971.

Brodsky, A. M. "Sex Role Issues in the Supervision of Therapy," in A. K. Hess (ed.). *Psychotherapy Supervision: Theory, Research and Practice*, New York: John Wiley, 1980, pp. 509-522.

Brody, C. M. (ed.). *Women Therapists Working with Women: New Theory and Process of Feminist Therapy*. New York: Springer Publishing Co., 1984.

Brothers, Barbara Jo. *Virginia Satir: Foundational Ideas*. New York: The Haworth Press, 1991.

Brown, Esther Lucile. *Social Work as a Profession*. New York: Russell Sage Foundation, 1936.

Burgoyne, Rodney W. et al. "Who Gets Supervised? An Extension of Patient Selection Inequity." *American Journal of Psychiatry* 133 (November 1976), pp. 1313-1315.

Burke, Kenneth. "The Five Key Terms of Dramatism," in Dennis Brissett and Charles Edgely (eds.), *Life as Theater: A Dramaturgical Sourcebook*. Chicago: Aldine, 1975, pp. 370-375.

Butler, Robert N. "Age-ism: Another Form of Bigotry." *The Gerontologist* 9 (Winter 1969), pp. 243-246.

Cabot, Richard C. "Address," Proceedings of the National Conference of Charities and Corrections, Baltimore, 1915a.

_____. *Social Service and the Art of Healing*. New York: Moffat, Yard, 1915b; reprint edition, Washington, DC: National Association of Social Workers, 1973.

Caligor, Leopold et al. *Clinical Perspectives on the Supervision of Psychoanalysis and Psychotherapy*. New York: Plenum, 1984.

Caplow, Theodore. *How to Run Any Organization: A Manual of Practical Sociology*. Hinsdale, IL.: Dryden Press, 1976.

Cervantes Saavedra, Miguel de. *The Ingenious Gentleman Don Quixote de la Mancha*, 1605; reprint edition. New York: Modern Library, 1950.

Chaiklin, Harris. "Role and Utilization of the Social Worker in Clinical Practice," in George U. Balis (ed.). *Psychiatric Clinical Skills in Medical Practice*, Boston: Butterworth, 1978.

Chance, Paul. "That Drained-Out, Used-Up Feeling." *Psychology Today* 15 (January 1981), pp. 88-95.

Chapin, F. Stuart, and Queen, Stuart A. *Research Memorandum on Social Work in the Depression*. New York: Social Science Research Council, 1937; reprint edition, New York: Arno, 1972.

Cherniss, Cary, and Egnatios, Edward. "Clinical Supervision in Community Mental Health." *Social Work* 23 (May 1978), pp. 219-223.

Chescheir, Martha W. "Social Role Discrepancies as Clues to Practice." *Social Work* 24 (March 1979), pp. 89-94.

Chessick, Richard. *Great Ideas in Psychotherapy*. New York: Jason Aronson, 1977.

Clark, Ronald W. *Freud: The Man and the Cause*. New York: Random House, 1980.

Clarkin, J. F., and Glick, I. D. "Supervision of Family Therapy," in Michael Blumenfield (ed.). *Applied Supervision in Psychotherapy*. New York: Grune and Stratton, 1982, pp. 87-106.

Comstock, George A., and Tonascia, James A. "Education and Mortality in Washington County, Maryland." *Journal of Health and Social Behavior* 18 (March 1977), pp. 54-61.

Conyngton, Mary. *How to Help: A Manual of Practical Charity*. New York: Macmillan, 1909; reprint edition, New York: Arno, 1971.

Coppedge, Robert O., and Davis, Carlton G. (eds.). *Rural Poverty and the Policy Crisis*. Ames, IA: Iowa State University Press, 1977.

Corsini, Raymond J. (ed.). *Current Psychotherapies*. Itasca, IL: Peacock, 1986.

Cottle, Thomas J., and Whitten, Phillip. *Psychotherapy: Current Perspectives*. New York: New Viewpoints, 1980.

Dalali, Isobel et al. "Training of Paraprofessionals: Some Caveats." *Journal of Drug Education* 6 (1976), pp. 105-112.

Daley, Michael R. " 'Burnout': Smoldering Problem in Protective Services." *Social Work* 24 (September 1979), pp. 375-379.

Davies, Joann F. "The Country Mouse Comes into Her Own." *Child Welfare* 53 (October 1974), pp. 509-513.

Davis, Simon. "Violence by Psychiatric Inpatients: A Review." *Hospital and Community Psychiatry* 42 (June 1991), pp. 585-589.

Day, Robert C., and Hamblin, Robert L. "Some Effects of Close and Punitive Styles of Supervision," in Gerald D. Bell (ed.). *Organizations and Human Behavior: A Book of Readings*. Englewood Cliffs, NJ: Prentice-Hall, 1967, pp. 172-181.

DeSchweinitz, Karl. *The Art of Helping People Out of Trouble*. Boston: Houghton Mifflin, 1924.

Dewey, John. *Art as Experience*. New York: Capricorn, 1958.

_____. *Democracy and Education*. New York: Macmillan, 1963.

Dressler, David M. et al. "Clinical Attitudes Toward the Suicide Attempted." *Journal of Nervous and Mental Disease* 160 (February 1975), pp. 146-155.

Drury, S. S. *Assertive Supervision: Building Involved Teamwork*. Champaign, IL: Research Press, 1984.

Durkheim, Emile. *The Division of Labor in Society*. New York: Macmillan, 1933.

Dyrud, Jarl E. "Psychotherapy and the New Psychiatry," in Thomas A. Cottle and Phillip Whitten (eds.). *Psychotherapy: Current Perspectives*, New York: New Viewpoints, 1980, pp. 41-51.

Edelwich, Jerry, and Brodsky, Archie. *Burnout: Stages of Disillusionment in the Helping Professions*. New York: Human Sciences, 1980.

_____. *Sexual Dilemmas for the Helping Professional*. New York: Brunner/Mazel, 1982.

Eldridge, William D. "Coping with Accountability: Guidelines for Supervisors." *Social Casework* 63 (October 1982), pp. 489-496.

Endress, Anna H. "Being and Becoming a Professional." *Social Casework* 62 (May 1981), pp. 305-308.

Epstein, Laura. "Is Autonomous Practice Possible?" *Social Work* 18 (March 1973), pp. 5-12.

Etcheverry, Roland et al. "The Uses and Abuses of Role Playing." Paper presented at Second Group Work Symposium, Arlington, TX (November 1980), pp. 1-19.

Ewalt, Patricia L. (ed.). *Toward a Definition of Clinical Social Work*. Papers from the NASW Invitational Forum on Clinical Social Work June 7-9, 1979, Denver, CO, Washington, DC: National Association of Social Workers, 1980.

Faver, C. A. et al. "The Educational Process and Job Equity for the Sexes in Social Work." *Journal of Education for Social Work*, 19 (3), (1983), pp. 78-87.

Feibleman, James K. *Understanding Philosophy: A Popular History of Ideas*. New York: Horizon, 1973.

Finn, Peter. "Developing Critical Television Viewing Skills." *The Educational Forum* 44 (May 1980), pp. 473-482.

Fisch, Richard et al. *The Tactics of Change: Doing Therapy Briefly*. San Francisco: Jossey-Bass, 1982.

Fisher, Jacob. *The Response of Social Work to the Depression*. Cambridge, MA: Schenkman, 1980.

Fisher, Joel. "Training for Effective Therapeutic Practice." *Psychotherapy: Theory, Research and Practice* 12 (Spring 1975), pp. 118-123.

Fosdick, Harry Emerson. *On Being a Real Person*. New York: Harper and Row, 1943.

Freeman, Edith M. "The Importance of Feedback in Clinical Supervision: Implications for Direct Practice." *The Clinical Supervisor* 3 (Spring 1985), pp. 5-26.

Freeman, Lucy. *Freud Rediscovered*. New York: Arbor House, 1980.

Freud, Sigmund. *Moses and Monotheism*, 1939; reprint edition. New York: Vintage, 1967.

Freud, Sophie. *My Three Mothers and Other Passions*. New York: New York University Press, 1988.

Freudenberger, Herbert J. "Burnout: Occupational Hazard of the Child Care Worker." *Child Care Quarterly* 6 (Summer 1977), pp. 90-99.

Freudenberger, Herbert J., and Richelsen, Geraldine. *Burn-Out: The High Cost of High Achievement*. New York: Anchor, 1980.

Fritz, Gregory K., and Poe, Richard O. "The Role of a Cinema Seminar in Psychiatric Education." *American Journal of Psychiatry* 136 (February 1979), pp. 207-210.

Gallant, J. Paul, and Thyer, Bruce A. "The 'Bug-in-the-Ear' in Clinical Supervision." *The Clinical Supervisor* 7 (Fall/Winter 1989), pp. 43-58.

Gallessich, June. *The Professional Practice of Consultation*. San Francisco: Jossey Bass, 1982.

Gardner, Howard. *Art, Mind and Brain: A Cognitive Approach to Creativity*. New York: Basic Books, 1982.

Garrett, Annette. *Learning Through Supervision*. Northampton, MA: Smith College Studies in Social Work, 1954.

Geiger, Deborah L. "Note: How Future Professionals View the Elderly: A Comparative Analysis of Social Work, Law, and Medical Students' Perceptions." *The Gerontologist* 18 (December 1978), pp. 591-594.

Geismar, Ludwig L., and Wood, Katherine M. "Evaluating Practice: Science as Faith." *Social Casework* 63 (May 1982), pp. 266-272.

Gelfand, Bernard et al. "An Andragogical Application to the Training of Social Workers." *Journal of Education for Social Work* 11 (Fall 1975), pp. 55-61.

Gibbs, M. S. "The Therapist as Imposter," in C. M. Brody (ed.), *Women Therapists Working with Women: New Theory and Process of Feminist Therapy*. New York: Springer Publishing Co, 1984, pp. 22-33.

Ginsberg, Leon (ed.). *Social Work in Rural Communities: A Book of Readings*. New York: Council on Social Work Education, 1976.

Gitterman, Alex (ed.). *Handbook of Social Work Practice with Vulnerable Populations*. New York: Columbia University Press, 1991.

Goldenberg, Irene, and Goldenberg, Herbert. *Family Therapy: An Overview*. Monterey, CA: Brooks/Cole, 1980.

Goldstein, Eda G. "Knowledge Base of Clinical Social Work." *Social Work* 25 (May 1980), pp. 173-178.

Goldstein, Howard. *Social Work Practice: A Unitary Approach*. Columbia, SC: University of South Carolina Press, 1973.

Goodrich, Thelma Jean et al. *Feminist Family Therapy: A Casebook*. New York: W.W. Norton and Company, 1988.

Goodyear, Rodney K. "Gender Configurations in Supervisory Dyads: Their Relation to Supervisee Influence Strategies and to Skill Evaluations of the Supervisee." *The Clinical Supervisor* 8 (Summer 1990, pp. 67-79.

Gordon, William E. "A Natural Classification System for Social Work Literature and Knowledge." *Social Work* 26 (March 1981), pp. 134-138.

Gould, K. H. "Original Works of Freud on Women: Social Work References." *Social Casework*, 65, 1984, pp. 94-101.

Gould, Stephen Jay. *The Panda's Thumb: More Reflections in Natural History*. New York: Norton, 1980.

Greben, S. E. "Dear Brutus: Dealing with Unresponsiveness Through Supervision." *Canadian Journal of Psychiatry* 30 (February 1985), pp. 48-53.

Greenberg, Harold. *Social Environment and Behavior*. New York: Schenkman, 1971.

Grinder, John, and Bandler, Richard. *The Structure of Magic II*. Palo Alto, CA: Science and Behavior Books, 1976.

Grinnell, Richard M., Jr. (ed.). *Social Work Research and Evaluation*. Itasca, IL: Peacock, 1981.

Grosser, Charles. "Community Development Programs Serving the Urban Poor." *Social Work* 10 (July 1965), pp. 15-21.

Grotjahn, Martin. *The Art and Technique of Analytic Group Therapy*. New York: Jason Aronson, 1977.

Groves, Ernest R. "A Decade of Marriage Counseling." *The Annals of the American Academy of Political and Social Science* 212 (November 1940), pp. 72-80.

Guerin, Philip J. *Family Therapy: Theory and Practice*. New York: Gardner, 1976.

Gurman, Alan S., and Razin, Andrew M. *Effective Psychotherapy: A Handbook of Research*. New York: Pergamon, 1977.

Gurman, Alan S. (ed.). *Questions and Answers in the Practice of Family Therapy*. New York: Brunner/Mazel, 1981a.

Gurman, Alan S. "Integrative Marital Therapy: Toward the Development of an Interpersonal Approach," in S. H. Budman (ed.), *Forms of Brief Therapy*. New York: Guilford Press, 1981b, pp. 415-457.

Haley, Jay. "Marriage Therapy," in H. Greenwald (ed.), *Active Psychotherapy*. New York: Atherton, 1967, pp. 189-223.

_____. "How to Be a Marriage Therapist Without Knowing Practically Anything," *Journal of Marital and Family Therapy* (October 1980), pp. 385-391.

_____. (ed.). *Changing Families: A Family Therapy Reader*. New York: Grune and Stratton, 1971.

_____. *Uncommon Therapy: The Psychiatric Techniques of Milton H. Erickson, MD*. New York: Norton, 1973.

_____. *Problem-Solving Therapy: New Strategies for Effective Family Therapy*. New York: Harper Colophon, 1976.

Hall, Calvin S., and Lindzey, Gardner. *Theories of Personality*. New York: Wiley, 1970.

Halmos, Paul. *The Faith of the Counsellors: A Study in the Theory and Practice of Social Case Work and Psychotherapy*. New York: Schocken, 1970.

Hamilton, Gordon. *Theory and Practice of Social Case Work*. New York: Columbia University Press, 1951.

Hamlin, Elwood R., and Timberlake, Elizabeth M. "Peer Group Supervision for Supervisors." *Social Casework* 63 (February 1982), pp. 82-87.

Handler, Ellen. "Residential Treatment Programs for Juvenile Delinquents." *Social Work* 20 (May 1975), pp. 217-222.

Handley, Patrick. "Relationship Between Supervisors' and Trainees' Cognitive Styles and the Supervision Process." *Journal of Counseling Psychology* 29 (1982), pp. 508-515.

Hansen, James C., and Warner, Richard W. "Review of Research on Practicum Supervision." *Counselor Education and Supervision* 10 (Spring 1971), pp. 261-272.

Harrison, Allen F., and Bramson, Robert M. *Styles of Thinking: Strategies for Asking Questions, Making Decisions, and Solving Problems.* Garden City, NY: Anchor Press/Doubleday, 1982.

Harrison, W. David. "Role Strain and Burnout in Child Protective Service Workers." *Social Service Review* 54 (March 1980), pp. 31-44.

Hart, Gordon M. *The Process of Clinical Supervision.* Baltimore: University Park Press, 1982.

Hart, Hornell, and Hart, Ella B. *Personality and the Family.* Boston: Heath, 1935.

Hawkins, Dorothy. "Mental Hygiene Problems of the Adolescent Period." *The Annals of the American Academy of Political and Social Service* 236 (November 1944), pp. 128-135.

Hawthorne, Lillian. "Games Supervisors Play." *Social Work* 20 (May 1975), pp. 179-183.

Heidegger, Martin. *What Is Called Thinking?* New York: Harper and Row, 1968, p. 15.

Hersen, Michel, and Barlow, David H. *Single-Case Experimental Designs: Strategies for Studying Behavior Change.* New York: Pergamon, 1976.

Hess, Allen K. (ed). *Psychotherapy Supervision: Theory, Research, and Practice.* New York: Wiley, 1980.

Heston, Alice H. "The Staff Conference as a Method of Supervision." *The Family* 10 (April 1929), pp. 46-48.

Hewitt, John P. *Self and Society: A Symbolic Interactionist Social Psychology.* Boston: Allyn and Bacon, 1976.

Hoffman, Ludmila. *Old Scapes, New Maps: A Training Program for Psychotherapy Supervisors.* Cambridge, MA: Milusik, 1990.

Hollis, Ernest V., and Taylor, Alice L. *Social Work Education in the United States: The Report of a Study Made for the National Council on Social Work Education.* New York: Columbia University Press, 1951.

Hollis, Florence. *Casework: A Psychosocial Therapy.* New York: Random House, 1966.

Holloway, Stephen, and Brager, George. *Supervising in the Human Services.* New York: The Free Press, 1989.

Holtz, Herman. *Expanding Your Consulting Practice with Seminars.* New York: John Wiley and Sons, 1987.

Holzner, Burkart, and Marx, John H. *Knowledge Application: The Knowledge System in Society.* Boston: Allyn and Bacon, 1979.

Horney, Karen. *Self-Analysis*. New York: Norton, 1942.

Howe, David. *The Consumers' View of Family Therapy*. Hants, England: Gower, 1989.

Hudson, Walter W. *The Clinical Measurement Package: A Field Manual*. Homewood, IL: Dorsey, 1982.

Huebner, L. et al. "Stress Management Training in Medical School," *Journal of Medical Education*, 56 (1981), pp. 547-558.

Hughes, Everett C., "Professions," *Daedalus* 92 (Fall 1963), pp. 655-668.

Hutchinson, Dorothy. "Supervision in Social Case Work." *The Family* 16 (April 1935), pp. 44-47.

Jayaratne, Srinika, and Levy, Rona L. *Empirical Clinical Practice*. New York: Columbia University Press, 1979.

Jones, James H. *Bad Blood: The Tuskegee Syphilis Experiment*. New York: The Free Press, 1981.

Jones, Robin W. "Social Values and Social Work Education," in Katherine A. Kendall (ed.), *Social Work Values in an Age of Discontent*. New York: Council on Social Work Education, 1970, pp. 35-45.

Jordan, Judith V. et al. *Women's Growth in Connection*. New York: The Guilford Press, 1991.

Judson, Horace Freeland. *The Search for Solutions*. New York: Holt, Rinehart and Winston, 1980.

Jung, Carl G. *The Undiscovered Self*. New York: Mentor, 1957.

Kadushin, Alfred. "Games People Play in Supervision," *Social Work* 8 (March 1968), pp. 23-32.

————. *The Social Work Interview*. New York: Columbia University Press, 1972.

————. "Supervisor-Supervisee," *Social Work* 19 (May 1974), pp. 288-297.

————. *Supervision in Social Work*. New York: Columbia University Press, first edition, 1976.

————. *Supervision in Social Work*. New York: Columbia University Press, third edition, 1991.

————. "Men in A Women's Profession," *Social Work*, 21, pp. 440-447, 1976.

————. *Consultation in Social Work*. New York: Columbia University Press, 1977.

Kahn, Alfred (ed.). *Shaping the New Social Work*. New York: Columbia University Press, 1973.

Kahn, Eva M. "The Parallel Process in Social Work Treatment and Supervision," *Social Casework* 60 (November 1979), pp. 520-528.

Kanter, R. M. *Men and Women of the Corporation*. New York: Basic Books, 1977.

Kanter, R. M., and Stein, B. A. "The Gender Pioneers: Women in an Industrial Sales Force," in R. M. Kanter and B. A. Stein (eds.), *Life in Organizations: Work Places as People Experience Them*, pp. 134-160. New York: Basic Books, 1979.

Kaplan, Abraham. *The Conduct of Inquiry: Methodology for Behavioral Science*. San Francisco: Chandler, 1964.

Kaplan, A. G. et al. "Women and Anger in Psychotherapy," in J. H. Robbins & R. J. Siegel (eds.), *Women Changing Therapy*. New York: The Haworth Press, 1983, pp. 29-40.

Kaslow, Florence (ed.). *Issues in the Human Services*. San Francisco: Jossey-Bass, 1972.

_____. *Supervision, Consultation, and Staff Training in the Helping Professions*. San Francisco: Jossey-Bass, 1979.

Keefe, T., and Maypole, D. E. *Relationships in Social Service Practice*. Monterey, CA: Brooks/Cole, 1983.

Kendall, Katherine A. "A Sixty Year Perspective of Social Work." *Social Casework* 63 (September 1982), pp. 424-428.

Kenemore, Thomas K. "Board Certified Diplomate: Who Cares?", *Clinical Social Work Journal* 19 (Spring 1991), pp. 83-93.

Kets de Vries, M. F. R. (ed.). *The Irrational Executive: Psychoanalytic Studies in Management*. New York: International Universities Press, 1984.

Kets de Vries, M. F. R., and Miller, D. *The Neurotic Organization: Diagnosing and Revitalizing Unhealthy Companies*. New York: Harper Business, 1984.

Kirk, Stuart A., and Fischer, Joel. "Do Social Workers Understand Research?" *Journal of Education for Social Work* 12 (Winter 1976), pp. 63-70.

Knowles, Malcolm. *The Modern Practice of Adult Education: Andragogy Versus Pedagogy*. New York: Association Press, 1970.

Kopp, Sheldon. *The Naked Therapist: A Collection of Embarrassments*. San Diego: EDITS, 1976.

Kramer, Charles H. *Becoming a Family Therapist: Developing an Integrated Approach to Working with Families*. New York: Human Sciences Press, 1980.

Kramer, Ernest. *A Beginning Manual for Psychotherapists*. New York: Grune and Stratton, 1978.

Kramer, Jonathan. *Stepping Up: How to Fight Your Boss and Win*. New York: Arbor House, 1985.

Krause, Elliott A. *Power and Illness: The Political Sociology of Health and Medical Care*. New York: Elsevier, 1977.

Krumboltz, John D., and Thoresen, Carl E. *Counseling Methods*. New York: Holt, Rinehart and Winston, 1976.

Lachman, Roy et al. *Cognitive Psychology and Information Processing: An Introduction*. Hillside, NJ: Lawrence Erlbaum, 1979.

Langs, Robert. *The Therapeutic Interaction, Volume II: A Critical Overview and Synthesis*. New York: Jason Aronson, 1976.

_____. *The Supervisory Experience*. New York: Jason Aronson, 1979.

_____. *The Psychotherapeutic Conspiracy*. New York: Jason Aronson, 1982.

Lastrucci, Carlo L. *The Scientific Approach: Basic Principles of the Scientific Method*. Cambridge, MA: Schenkman, 1967.

Lecker, S. "Family Therapies," in B. B. Wolman (ed.). *The Therapist's Handbook: Treatment Methods of Mental Disorders*. New York: Van Nostrand Reinhold, 1976, pp. 184-198.

Lee, Porter R., and Kenworthy, Marion E. *Mental Hygiene and Social Work*. New York: Commonwealth Fund, 1929.

Leman, Kevin and Carlson, Randy. *Unlocking the Secrets of Your Childhood Memories*. Nashville, TN: Thomas Nelson Publishers, 1989.

Levi-Strauss, Claude. "Science: Forever Incomplete." *Johns Hopkins Magazine* 39 (July 1978), p. 30.

Levy, Charles. "The Ethics of Supervision." *Social Work* 18 (March 1973), pp. 14-21.

Lewin, Karl Kay. *Brief Psychotherapy: Brief Encounters*. St. Louis, MO: Warren H. Green, 1970.

Lewis, Jerry M. *To Be a Therapist: The Teaching and Learning*. New York: Brunner/Mazel, 1978.

Lief, Alfred. *The Commonsense Psychiatry of Dr. Adolf Meyer*. New York: McGraw-Hill, 1948.

Lowenburg, Frank, and Dolgoff, Ralph. *Ethical Decisions for Social Work Practice*. Itasca, IL.: Peacock, 1988.

Lowy, Louis. *Social Work with the Aging: The Challenge and Promise of the Later Years*. New York: Harper and Row, 1979.

Luthman, Shirley Gehrke, and Kirschenbaum, Martin. *The Dynamic Family*. Palo Alto, CA: Science and Behavior Books, 1974.

Magee, James J. "Integrating Research Skills with Human Behavior and Social Environment: Assessing Historical and Cultural Influences on Students' Family Structure." *Journal of Education for Social Work* 18 (Winter 1982), pp. 14-19.

Mandell, Betty. "The 'Equality' Revolution and Supervision." *Journal of Education for Social Work* 9 (Winter 1973), pp. 43-54.

Marcus, Philip M., and Marcus, Dora. "Control in Modern Organizations," in Merlin B. Brinkenhoff and Phillip R. Kung (eds.), *Complex Organizations and Their Environments*. Dubuque, IA: W. C. Brown, 1972, pp. 234-243.

Marecek, J., and Kravetz, D. "Women and Mental Health: A Review of Feminist Change Efforts," in H. Rubenstein and M. H. Bloch (eds.). *Things That Matter*. New York: Macmillan, 1982, pp. 296-303.

Marsh, Robert C. (ed.). *Bertrand Russell: Logic and Knowledge*. New York: Capricorn, 1971.

Martin, Shan. *Managing Without Managers: Alternative Work Arrangements in Public Organizations*. Beverly Hills, CA.: Sage Publications, 1983.

McGoldrick, Monica et al. *Women in Families, A Framework for Family Therapy*. New York: W.W. Norton and Company, 1991.

McQuade, Walter, and Aikman, Ann. *Stress*. New York: Bantam, 1974.

Merdinger, Joan. "Socialization into the Profession: The Case of Undergraduate Social Work Students." *Journal of Education for Social Work* 18 (Spring 1982), pp. 12-19.

Meyer, Robert G. et al. *Law for the Psychotherapist*. New York: W.W. Norton, 1988.

Mills, C. Wright. *The Sociological Imagination*. New York: Oxford University Press, 1959.

Milwid, B. "Breaking In: Experience in Male-Dominated Professions," in J. H. Robbins and R. J. Siegel (eds.). *Women Changing Therapy: New Assessments, Values and Strategies in Feminist Therapy*. New York: The Haworth Press, 1983, pp. 67-79.

Minahan, Anne. "What Is Clinical Social Work?" *Social Work* 25 (May 1980), p. 171.

Minuchin, Salvador. *Families and Family Therapy*. Cambridge, MA.: Harvard University Press, 1974.

Mishne, Judith. *Psychotherapy and Training in Clinical Social Work*. New York: Gardner, 1980.

Munson, Carlton E. "Definition of the Situation and Viewing Television Newscasts." *Sociological Research Symposium Proceedings IV*, Richmond, VA: Virginia Commonwealth University, 1974, pp. 452-459.

_____. "The Uses of Structural, Authority and Teaching Models in Social Work Supervision," DSW dissertation, University of Maryland, 1975; Ann Arbor, MI: University Microfilms International, 1975.

_____. "Professional Autonomy and Social Work Supervision," *Journal of Education for Social Work* 12 (Fall 1976), pp. 95-02.

_____. "Consultation in an Adolescent Group Home Using a Role Theory Perspective," *Offender Rehabilitation* 2 (Fall 1977), pp. 65-78.

_____. "The Concepts of Effectiveness and Efficiency Applied to the Social Work Profession: An Historical Perspective," *Journal of Education for Social Work* 14 (Spring 1978), pp. 90-97.

_____. (ed.). *Social Work Supervision: Classic Statements and Critical Issues*. New York: The Free Press, 1979a.

_____. "Evaluation of Male and Female Supervisors," *Social Work* 24 (March 1979b), pp. 104-110.

_____. "Symbolic Interaction and Social Work Supervision," *Journal of Sociology and Social Welfare* 6 (January 1979c), pp. 8-18.

_____. "Supervision and Consultation in Rural Mental Health Practice," in *Proceedings, Fourth National Institute on Social Work in Rural Areas*, University of Wyoming (1979d), pp. 87-93.

_____. "Applied Sociology and Social Work: Manpower and Theoretical Issues," *Journal of Sociology and Social Welfare* 6 (September 1979e), pp. 611-621.

_____. "Supervising the Family Therapist," *Social Casework* 61 (March 1980a), pp. 131-137.

_____. "Differential Impact of Structure and Authority in Supervision," *Arete* 6 (Spring 1980b), pp. 3-15.

_____. "Social Work in Aging," *Gerontology and Geriatric Education* 1 (September 1980c), pp. 17-29.

_____. "Urban Rural Differences: Implications for Social Work Education and Training," *Journal of Education for Social Work* 16 (Winter 1980d), pp. 95-103.

_____. "Supervision for Clinical Practice," paper presented at Fifth Annual State Convention, National Association of Social Workers, El Paso, TX, October 21-23, 1981a.

_____. "Social Work Educational Consultation in Church-Related Nursing Homes," *Gerontology and Geriatric Education* 1 (Spring 1981b), pp. 175-180.

_____. "A Study of Distress Reactions in Public Welfare Practitioners," Unpublished manuscript, 1982.

_____. *An Introduction to Clinical Social Work Supervision*. New York: The Haworth Press, 1983a.

_____. *Stress Among Hospital Social Workers: An Empirical Study*, Unpublished manuscript, 1983b.

_____. "Perceptions of Female Social Workers Toward Administrative Positions," *Social Casework*, 63, (1982), pp. 54-59.

_____. "Stress Among Graduate Social Work Students: An Empirical Study," *Journal of Education for Social Work*, 20(3), (1984), pp. 20-29.

_____. "Editorial: A Study of Ethics," *The Clinical Supervisor* 4 (Fall 1986), pp. 1-5.

Munson, Carlton E., and Balgopal, Pallassana. "The Worker/Client Relationship: Relevant Role Theory," *Journal of Sociology and Social Welfare* 5 (May 1978), pp. 404-417.

Murphy, John W., and Pardeck, John T. "The 'Burnout Syndrome' and Management Style," *The Clinical Supervisor* 4 (Winter 1986), pp. 35-44.

Naisbitt, John. *Megatrends: Ten New Directions Transforming Our Lives*. New York: Warner Books, 1982.

National Association of Social Workers. *A Membership Sketch*. Washington, DC: NASW, 1991.

National Association of Social Workers (NASW). *Social Casework: Generic and Specific: A Report of the Milford Conference*. Washington, DC: NASW, Classic Series, 1974.

_____. "Ethics Violator Gets a Suspension," *NASW News* (October 1982), p. 12.

_____. *NASW Register of Clinical Social Workers, 1987*. Washington, DC: NASW, 1987.

National Institute for Clinical Social Work Advancement. *National Registry of Health Care Providers in Clinical Social Work and National Registry of Board Certified Clinical Social Workers, 1987-1989*, San Antonio: NICSWA, 1987.

Nelson, Gary L. "Psychotherapy Supervision from the Trainee's Point of View: A Survey of Preferences," *Professional Psychology* (November 1978), pp. 539-549.

O'Neill, Patrick, and Trickett, Edison J. *Community Consultation: Strategies for Facilitating Change in Schools, Hospitals, Prisons, Social Service Programs, and Other Community Settings*, San Francisco: Jossey-Bass, 1982.

Palmer, James O. *A Primer of Eclectic Psychotherapy*. Monterey, CA: Brooks/Cole, 1980.

Parad, Howard J., and Miller, Roger R. *Ego-Oriented Casework: Problems and Perspectives*. New York: Family Service Association of America, 1963.

Parkinson, C. Northcote. *Parkinson's Law and Other Studies in Administration*. Boston: Houghton Mifflin, 1957.

Patterson, James, and Kim, Peter. *The Day America Told the Truth*. New York: Prentice Hall, 1991.

Peake, Thomas H., and Ball, John D. *Psychotherapy Training: Contextual and Developmental Influences in Settings, Stages and Mind Sets*. New York: The Haworth Press, 1991.

Pearlin, Leonard I., and Schooler, Carmi. "The Structure of Coping," *Journal of Health and Social Behavior* 19 (March 1978), pp. 2-21.

Perkins, John F. "Common Sense and Bad Boys," *Atlantic Monthly* 173 (May 1944), pp. 43-47.

Perlman, Helen H., *Social Casework: A Problem-solving Process*. Chicago: The University of Chicago Press, 1957.

Perlman, Helen Harris. *Social Casework: A Problem-Solving Process*. Chicago: University of Chicago Press, 1969.

———. *Helping: Charlotte Towle on Social Work and Social Casework*. Chicago: University of Chicago Press, 1969.

Pettes, Dorothy. *Supervision in Social Work: A Method of Student Training and Staff Development*. London: Allen and Unwin, 1967.

Pettes, D. E. *Student and Staff Supervision: A Task-Centered Approach*, London: Allen and Unwin, 1979.

Pickering, George. *Creative Malady: Illness in the Lives and Minds of Charles Darwin, Florence Nightingale, Mary Baker Eddy, Sigmund Freud, Marcel Proust, Elizabeth Barrett Browning*. New York: Dell, 1974.

Pincus, Allen, and Minahan, Anne. *Social Work Practice: Model and Method*. Itasca, IL: Peacock, 1973.

Pine, Fred. *Drive, Ego, Object, and Self: A Synthesis for Clinical Work*. New York: Basic Books, 1990.

Plant, James. "Social Significance of War Impact on Adolescents." *The Annals of the American Academy of Political and Social Science* 236 (November 1944), pp. 1-7.

Pogrebin, L. C. *Growing Up Free*. New York: Bantam, 1980.

Porter, N. "New Perspectives on Therapy Supervision," in L. B. Rosewater and L. E. A. Walker (eds.). *Handbook of Feminist Therapy: Women's Issues in Psychotherapy*, pp. 332-343. New York: Springer Publishing Co., 1985.

Powell, David J. *Clinical Supervision: Skills for Substance Abuse Counselors*. New York: Human Sciences Press, 1980.

Powicke, Frederick. *Modern Historians and the Study of History*. London: Odhams, 1955.

Pratt, Lois. "Levels of Sociological Knowledge Among Health and Social Workers." *Journal of Health and Social Behavior* 10 (March 1969), pp. 59-65.

Pruger, Robert. "The Good Bureaucrat." *Social Work* 18 (July 1973), pp. 26-32.

Rabin, Herbert M. "How Does Co-Therapy Compare with Regular Group Therapy?" *American Journal of Psychotherapy* 21 (April 1967), pp. 244-255.

Reamer, Fred. "AIDS and Ethics: The Agenda for Social Workers." *Social Work* 33 (May 1988), pp. 460-464.

Redl, Fritz, and Wineman, David. *Children Who Hate*. New York: The Free Press, 1951.

_____. *Controls from Within: Techniques for the Treatment of the Aggressive Child*. New York: The Free Press, 1952.

Reeves, Elton T. *So You Want to Be a Supervisor!* New York: AMACOM, American Management Associations, 1980.

Reid, William. "Mapping the Knowledge Base of Social Work." *Social Work* 26 (March 1981), pp. 124-132.

Reiter, Laura. "Professional Morale and Social Work Training: A Study." *Clinical Social Work Journal* 8 (Fall 1980), pp. 198-209.

Reynolds, Bertha Capen. *Learning and Teaching in the Practice of Social Work*, 1942; reprint edition. New York: Russell and Russell, 1965.

_____. *Between Client and Community: A Study in Responsibility in Social Casework*. The Smith College Studies in Social Work 5 (1934); reprint edition. New York: Oriole, 1973.

Rice, David G. et al. "Therapist Experience and Style as Factors in Cotherapy." *Family Process* 11 (March 1972), pp. 1-12.

Richmond, Mary. *Social Diagnosis*. New York: Russell Sage Foundation, 1917; reprint edition. New York: The Free Press, 1965.

Rippere, Vicky, and Williams, Ruth. *Wounded Healers: Mental Health Workers' Experiences of Depression*. New York: John Wiley and Sons, 1985.

Roazen, Paul. *Freud and His Followers*. New York: Knopf, 1974.

Robbins, J. H., and Siegel, R. J. (eds.). *Women Changing Therapy: New Assessments, Values and Strategies in Feminist Therapy*. New York: The Haworth Press, 1983.

Roberts, Albert R. *Crisis Intervention Handbook: Assessment, Treatment and Research*. Belmont, CA: Wadsworth Publishing Company, 1990.

Robinson, Virginia P. *A Changing Psychology in Social Case Work*. Chapel Hill, NC: University of North Carolina Press, 1930.

Rock, Barry. "Social Worker Autonomy in an Age of Accountability." *The Clinical Supervisor* 8 (Summer 1990), pp. 19-31.

Rosenblatt, Aaron. "The Practitioner's Use and Evaluation of Research." *Social Work* 13 (January 1968), pp. 53-59.

Rossman, Parker. *Hospice*. New York: Fawcett, 1977.

Ruckdeschel, Roy A., and Farris, Buford E. "Science: Critical Faith or Dogmatic Ritual." *Social Casework* 63 (May 1982), pp. 272-275.

Sales, Esther, and Navarre, Elizabeth. *Individual and Group Supervision in Field Instruction: A Research Report*. Ann Arbor, MI: University of Michigan, School of Social Work, 1970.

Samantrai, Krishna. "Clinical Social Work in Public Child Welfare Practice." *Social Work*, 36 (July 1991), pp. 359-361.

Sands, Roberta G. *Clinical Social Work Practice in Community Mental Health*. New York: Macmillan, 1991.

Sartre, Jean-Paul. *Sartre on Theater*. New York: Pantheon, 1976.

Schafer, Roy. *A New Language for Psychoanalysis*. New Haven, CT: Yale University Press, 1976.

Scheflen, Albert E. *Body Language and the Social Order: Communication as Behavior Control*. Englewood Cliffs, NJ: Prentice-Hall, 1972.

Scheibe, Karl E. *Beliefs and Values*. New York: Holt, Rinehart and Winston, 1970.

Schoenwald, Richard L. "Belly Dancing or Baudelaire?", *The Chronicle of Higher Education* 13 (December 6, 1976), p. 32.

Schuler, Edgar A. et al. (eds.). *Readings in Sociology*. New York: Crowell, 1971.

Schumacher, E. F. *A Guide for the Perplexed*. New York: Perennial Library, 1977.

Schutz, Benjamin M. *Legal Liability in Psychotherapy: A Practitioner's Guide to Risk Management*. San Francisco: Jossey-Bass, 1982.

Scotch, B. C. "Sex Status in Social Work: Grist for Women's Liberation." *Social Work*, 16, pp. 5-11, 1971.

Seefeldt, Carol et al. "Using Pictures to Explore Children's Attitudes Toward the Elderly." *The Gerontologist* 17 (December 1977), pp. 506-512.

Seiden, A. M. "Overview: Research on the Psychology of Women." In H. Rubenstein and M. H. Bloch (Eds.). *Things That Matter: Influences on Helping Relationships*, pp. 285-295. New York: Macmillan, 1982.

Seligman, Milton. (ed.). *Group Psychotherapy and Counseling with Special Populations*. Baltimore: University Park Press, 1982.

Selye, Hans. *Stress Without Distress*. New York: New American Library, 1974.

Sennett, Richard. *Authority*. New York: Knopf, 1980.

Shea, Shawn. *Psychiatric Interviewing: The Art of Understanding*. Philadelphia: W. B. Saunders Company, 1988.

Shulman, Lawrence. *Skills of Supervision and Staff Management*. Itasca, IL: Peacock, 1982.

Simon, Bernece K. "Diversity and Unity in the Social Work Profession." *Social Work* 22 (September 1977), pp. 395-400.

Simon, Richard. "'Always with Guts': An Interview with Mara Selvini Palazzoli." *The Family Therapy Networker* 6 (May-June 1982), pp. 29-32.

Siporin, Max. "Dual Supervision of Psychiatric Social Workers." *Social Work* 1 (April 1956), pp. 32-42.

_____. *Introduction to Social Work Practice*. New York: Macmillan, 1975.

_____. "Marriage and Family Therapy in Social Work," *Social Casework* 61 (January 1980), pp. 11-21.

Skynner, Robin. *Institutes and How to Survive Them: Mental Health Training and Consultation*. New York: Routledge, 1989.

Sobel, Dava. "Psychotherapy from A to Z." *Houston Post* (November 16, 1980), p. 3.

Spencer, Herbert. *The Data of Ethics*. New York: P. F. Collier, 1902.

Stein, Morris I. (ed.). *Contemporary Psychotherapies*. New York: The Free Press, 1961.

Stein, Ronald H. *Ethical Issues in Counseling*. New York: Prometheus, 1990.

Steininger, M. et al. *Ethical Issues in Psychology*. Homewood, IL: The Dorsey Press, 1984.

Sternberg, Robert J., and Davidson, Janet E. "The Mind of the Puzzler," *Psychology Today* 16 (June 1982), pp. 37-44.

Stevenson, George S. "Mental Hygiene of Children," *The Annals of the American Academy of Political and Social Science*, 212 (November 1940), pp. 130-137.

Stevenson, Leslie. *Seven Theories of Human Nature*. New York: Oxford University Press, 1974.

Strean, Herbert S. *Clinical Social Work: Theory and Practice*. New York: The Free Press, 1978.

Strean, Herbert S. *Psychoanalytic Theory and Social Work Practice*. New York: The Free Press, 1979.

Streepy, Joan. "Direct-Service Providers and Burnout," *Social Casework* 62 (June 1981), pp. 352-361.

Strupp, Hans H. et al. *Psychotherapy for Better or Worse: The Problem of Negative Effects*. New York: Jason Aronson, 1977.

Sturdivant, S. *Therapy with Women: A Feminist Philosophy of Treatment*. New York: Springer, 1980.

Sullivan, Harry Stack. *The Psychiatric Interview*. New York: Norton, 1954.

Sullivan, J. W. N. *The Limits of Science*. New York: New American Library, 1963.

Svechs, Ilga, and Donald Zall. *A Curriculum Guide for the Advanced Level Review and Update Course*. The National Institute for Clinical Social Work Advancement, 1989.

Taft, Jessie. "Foster Care for Children," *The Annals of the American Academy of Political and Social Science* 212 (November 1940), 179-185.

Tessler, Richard C., and Polansky, Norman A. "Perceived Similarity: A Paradox in Interviewing," *Social Work* 20 (September 1975), pp. 359-363.

Thigpen, Joe D. "Perceptional Differences in the Supervision of Paraprofessional Mental Health Workers," *Community Mental Health Journal* 15 (Summer 1979), pp. 139-148.

Thistle, Pamela. "The Therapist's Own Family: Focus of Training for Family Therapists," *Social Work* 26 (May 1981), pp. 248-250.

Toffler, Alvin. *The Third Wave*. New York: Bantam Books, 1980.

Towle, Charlotte. *Common Human Needs*. Washington, DC: National Association of Social Workers, 1965.

Trader, Harriet. "A Professional School's Role in Training Ex Addict Counselors," *Journal of Education for Social Work* 10 (Fall 1974), pp. 99-106.

Turner, Francis J. (ed.). *Differential Diagnosis and Treatment in Social Work*. New York: The Free Press, 1976.

———. *Psychosocial Therapy: A Social Work Perspective*. New York: The Free Press, 1978.

——— (ed.). *Social Work Treatment: Interlocking Theoretical Approaches*. New York: The Free Press, 1979.

——— (ed.). *Social Work Treatment: Interlocking Theoretical Approaches*. New York: The Free Press, second edition 1985.

Ullmann, Liv. *Changing*. New York: Bantam, 1978.

Utz, Peter. *Video User's Handbook*. Englewood Cliffs, NJ: Prentice-Hall, 1980.

Veeder, Nancy. "Autonomy, Accountability, and Professionalism: The Case Against Close Supervision in Social Work." *The Clinical Supervisor* 8 (Summer 1990), pp. 33-65.

Veroff, Joseph et al. *Mental Health in America: Patterns of Help Seeking From 1957 to 1976*. New York: Basic Books, 1981.

Wallace, Jean E., and Brinkerhoff, Merlin E. "The Measurement of Burnout Revisited," *Journal of Social Service Research* 14 (Spring/Summer 1991), pp. 85-111.

Wallace, Marquis Earl. "A Framework for Self-Supervision in Social Work Practice," *Social Casework* 62 (May 1981), pp. 293-304.

_____. "Private Practice: A Nationwide Study," *Social Work* 27 (May 1982), pp. 262-267.

Webster's New Collegiate Dictionary. Springfield, MA: G. C. Merriam, 1979.

Webster, Elizabeth, and Haler, Paul. "Effects of Two Types of Direct Supervisory Feedback on Student Clinicians' Use of Consequation." *The Clinical Supervisor* 7 (Spring 1989), pp. 7-26.

Weinberg, George. *Self-Creation*. New York: St. Martin's, 1978.

Weinberger, Paul E. *Perspectives on Social Welfare: An Introductory Anthology*. New York: Macmillan, 1974.

Weisinger, Hendrie, and Lobsenz, Norman M. *Nobody's Perfect: How to Give Criticism and Get Results*. Los Angeles: Stratford, 1981.

Weisman, Avery. *On Dying and Denying*. New York: Behavioral Publications, 1972.

Weissman, Harold, and Epstein, Irwin. *Agency-Based Social Work: Neglected Aspects of Clinical Practice*. Philadelphia: Temple University Press, 1983.

Weppner, Robert S. et al. "Effects of Criminal Justice and Medical Definitions of a Social Problem upon the Delivery of Treatment: The Case of Drug Abuse," *Journal of Health and Social Behavior* 17 (June 1976), pp. 170-177.

Whiffen, Rosemary, and Byng-Hall, John. *Family Therapy Supervision: Recent Developments in Practice*. New York: Grune and Stratton, 1982.

Whyte, William H. *The Organization Man*. New York: Simon and Schuster, 1956.

Widen, Paul. "Organizational Structure for Casework Supervision," *Social Work* 7 (October 1962), pp. 78-85.

Wijnberg, Marion H., and Schwartz, Mary C. "Models of Student Supervision: The Apprentice, Growth, and Role Systems Models," *Journal of Education for Social Work* 13 (Fall 1977), pp. 110-112.

Wilensky, H. L., and Lebeaux, C. N. *Industrial Society and Social Welfare*. New York: The Free Press, 1975.

Williams, M., Ho, L., and Fielder, L. "Career Patterns: More Grist for Women's Liberation," *Social Work* 19 (1974), pp. 463-466.

Williams, Robert H. "Is Plato Only Worth Five Points?", *The Educational Forum* 46 (Winter 1982), pp. 167-179.

Wilson, Suanna J. *Confidentiality in Social Work: Issues and Principles*. New York: The Free Press, 1978.

————. *Field Instruction: Techniques for Supervisors*. New York: The Free Press, 1981.

Wiseman, Personal Communication, 1979.

Wodarski, John S. *The Role of Research in Clinical Practice: A Practical Approach for the Human Services*. Baltimore: University Park Press, 1981.

Wolman, Benjamin B. *The Therapist's Handbook: Treatment Methods of Mental Disorders*. New York: Van Nostrand Reinhold, 1976.

Woolf, Virginia. *The Second Common Reader*. New York: Harcourt, Brace and Co., 1932; reprint edition, New York: Harcourt Brace Jovanovich, 1960.

Yankelovich, Daniel. *New Rules: Searching for Self-Fulfillment in a World Turned Upside Down*. New York: Random House, 1981.

Zischka, Pauline C. "The Effects of Burnout on Permanency Planning and the Middle Management Supervisor in Child Welfare Agencies," *Child Welfare* 60 (November 1981), pp. 611-616.

Appendix 1

Assessment Scale for Becoming a Clinical Supervisor

ASSESSMENT SCALE FOR BECOMING
A CLINICAL SUPERVISOR

Deciding to become a clinical supervisor can be a difficult decision. To offer some guides to consider this instrument is provided. Circle the response to the right of each factor.

FACTOR	RATING (Circle one for each factor)	
The following is descriptive of me:	PLUS	MINUS
1. Enjoy teaching others	Yes	No
2. Patient when others don't understand	Yes	No
3. Skilled at indirect suggestion	Yes	No
4. Commitment to helping others do better	Yes	No
5. Patient when listening to others' complaints	Yes	No
6. Enjoy planning ahead	Yes	No
7. Willing to decrease my own practice activity	Yes	No
8. Enjoy answering questions	Yes	No
9. Comfortable asking questions	Yes	No
10. Can discuss organizational problems without anger	Yes	No
11. Can tolerate others making mistakes	Yes	No
12. Can accept criticism	Yes	No
13. Can accept it when others do not take my advice	Yes	No
14. Enjoy making decisions	Yes	No
15. Like discussing theory	Yes	No
16. Need a lot of support for decisions I make	No	Yes
17. Dislike evaluating others' practice	No	Yes
18. Prefer to work alone	No	Yes
19. Find paperwork a source of frustration	No	Yes
20. Prefer action to speculation	No	Yes

TOTAL circles in each column   =   _____ _____

If the total of the PLUS column is larger than the total of the MINUS column you will most likely find supervision rewarding. If the MINUS column exceeds the PLUS column you should review the factors in this column and find ways to alter your attitudes and behavior in these areas as you enter supervision practice.

Appendix 2

Educational Assessment Scale

EDUCATIONAL ASSESSMENT SCALE
by Dr. Carlton E. Munson

The following questions are to help your supervisor plan your educational program. There are no correct or incorrect answers. Answer the questions factually. The objective is to be able to assess what you presently know and what areas that need development. It is expected there will be a number of areas in which you will have no knowledge or limited knowledge. Do not feel bad that you have limited knowledge in a given area. This instrument will be helpful only if you identify accurately what you know and do not know.

1. Previous Experience
Total years social work paid experience: List job responsibilities:

Total years volunteer social work experience: List job responsibilities:

Total years non social work experience: List job responsibilities:

2. Ethical Awareness
Have you read the Social work code of ethics:
If yes how many years has it been since you read the code of ethics:
Have you taken the Munson Code of Ethics Scale:
If yes how many years ago: If yes what was your score:

Circle the number to the right in each area to indicate your level of knowledge or ability:
3. Theoretical Knowledge

	None	Little	Some		Moderate		Strong			Thorough
Psychoanalytic	1	2	3	4	5	6	7	8	9	10
Adlerian	1	2	3	4	5	6	7	8	9	10
Jungian	1	2	3	4	5	6	7	8	9	10
Person-Centered	1	2	3	4	5	6	7	8	9	10
Rational-Emotive	1	2	3	4	5	6	7	8	9	10
Behavioral	1	2	3	4	5	6	7	8	9	10
Gestalt	1	2	3	4	5	6	7	8	9	10
Reality Therapy	1	2	3	4	5	6	7	8	9	10
Existential	1	2	3	4	5	6	7	8	9	10
Transactional Analysis	1	2	3	4	5	6	7	8	9	10
Psychodrama	1	2	3	4	5	6	7	8	9	10
Family Therapy	1	2	3	4	5	6	7	8	9	10
Human Potential	1	2	3	4	5	6	7	8	9	10
Communication	1	2	3	4	5	6	7	8	9	10

Indicate theories not listed above that you have utilized or know. Use the number scale to indicate your knowledge level of each theory you list:

4. Assessment and Diagnosis

	None	Some	Average	Extensive	Thorough
Social assessment	1	2	3	4	5
Use of DSM III-R	1	2	3	4	5
Initial data base	1	2	3	4	5
Initial treatment plans	1	2	3	4	5
Review treatment plans	1	2	3	4	5
Evaluating mental status	1	2	3	4	5
Interview evaluation	1	2	3	4	5
Social assessment	1	2	3	4	5
Social assessment	1	2	3	4	5

5. Intervention

	None	Some	Average	Extensive	Thorough
Forming alliances	1	2	3	4	5
Client engagement	1	2	3	4	5
Client confusion	1	2	3	4	5
Client hostility	1	2	3	4	5
Client resistance	1	2	3	4	5
interpretations	1	2	3	4	5
Seeking clarification	1	2	3	4	5
Being supportive	1	2	3	4	5
Asking sensitive questions	1	2	3	4	5
Transference	1	2	3	4	5
Counter-transference	1	2	3	4	5
Termination	1	2	3	4	5

6. Record Keeping

	None	Some	Average	Extensive	Thorough
Initial data Bases (IDBs)	1	2	3	4	5
Initial Tx plans (ITPs)	1	2	3	4	5
Review Tx plans (RTPs)	1	2	3	4	5
Progress notes	1	2	3	4	5
Invoicing	1	2	3	4	5
Service tickets	1	2	3	4	5
Case management	1	2	3	4	5

7. General

List any other areas of learning you can identify that you desire as part of your educational field instruction experience/supervisory experience:

Appendix 3

Credentialing, Accrediting, and Service Organizations in Social Work

CREDENTIALING, ACCREDITING, AND SERVICE ORGANIZATIONS IN SOCIAL WORK

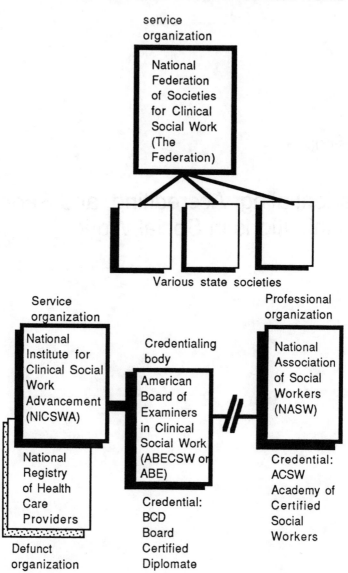

service organization

National Federation of Societies for Clinical Social Work (The Federation)

Various state societies

Service organization

National Institute for Clinical Social Work Advancement (NICSWA)

National Registry of Health Care Providers

Defunct organization

Credentialing body

American Board of Examiners in Clinical Social Work (ABECSW or ABE)

Credential: BCD Board Certified Diplomate

Professional organization

National Association of Social Workers (NASW)

Credential: ACSW Academy of Certified Social Workers

Accrediting
body

Council
on Social
Work
Education
(CSWE)

Accredits BSW & MSW
education programs

Service
organization

American
Association
of State
Social Work
Boards
(AASWB)

AASWB prepares and administers
examinations for state boards

Voluntary association
State board members are
appointed to AASWB Board

Various state licensing boards
Numerous names with numerous credentials
such as CSW, LCSW, ACP, LPC, ETC.

Appendix 4

Code of Ethics of the National Association of Social Workers

CODE OF ETHICS OF THE NATIONAL ASSOCIATION OF SOCIAL WORKERS

As adopted by the 1979 NASW Delegate Assembly and revised by the 1990 NASW Delegate Assembly.

National Association of Social Workers, Inc.
7981 Eastern Avenue
Silver Spring, MD 20910

Contents

Preamble

Summary of Major Principles

Code of Ethics

I. The Social Worker's Conduct and Comportment as a Social Worker
II. The Social Worker's Ethical Responsibility to Clients
III. The Social Worker's Ethical Responsibility to Colleagues
IV. The Social Worker's Ethical Responsibility to Employers and Employing Organizations
V. The Social Worker's Ethical Responsibility to the Social Work Profession
VI. The Social Worker's Ethical Responsibility to Society

Preamble

This code is intended to serve as a guide to the everyday conduct of members of the social work profession and as a basis for the adjudication of issues in ethics when the conduct of social workers is alleged to deviate from the standards expressed or implied in this code. It represents standards of ethical behavior for social workers in professional relationships with those served, with colleagues, with employers, with other individuals and professions, and with the community and society as a whole. It also embodies standards of ethical behavior governing individual conduct to the extent that such conduct is associated with an individual's status and identity as a social worker.

This code is based on the fundamental values of the social work profes-

---

sion that include the worth, dignity, and uniqueness of all persons as well as their rights and opportunities. It is also based on the nature of social work, which fosters conditions that promote these values.

In subscribing to and abiding by this code, the social worker is expected to view ethical responsibility in as inclusive a context as each situation demands and within which ethical judgement is required. The social worker is expected to take into consideration all the principles in this code that have a bearing upon any situation in which ethical judgement is to be exercised and professional intervention or conduct is planned. The course of action that the social worker chooses is expected to be consistent with the spirit as well as the letter of this code.

In itself, this code does not represent a set of rules that will prescribe all the behaviors of social workers in all the complexities of professional life. Rather, it offers general principles to guide conduct, and the judicious appraisal of conduct, in situations that have ethical implications. It provides the basis for making judgements about ethical actions before and after they occur. Frequently, the particular situation determines the ethical principles that apply and the manner of their application. In such cases, not only the particular ethical principles are taken into immediate consideration, but also the entire code and its spirit. Specific applications of ethical principles must be judged within the context in which they are being considered. Ethical behavior in a given situation must satisfy not only the judgement of the individual social worker, but also the judgement of an unbiased jury of professional peers.

This code should not be used as an instrument to deprive any social worker of the opportunity or freedom to practice with complete professional integrity; nor should any disciplinary action be taken on the basis of this code without maximum provision for safeguarding the rights of the social worker affected.

The ethical behavior of social workers results not from edict, but from a personal commitment of the individual. This code is offered to affirm the will and zeal of all social workers to be ethical and to act ethically in all that they do as social workers.

The following codified ethical principles should guide social workers in the various roles and relationships and at the various levels of responsibility in which they function professionally. These principles also serve as a basis for the adjudication by the National Association of Social Workers of issues in ethics.

In subscribing to this code, social workers are required to cooperate in its implementation and abide by any disciplinary rulings based on it. They should also take adequate measures to discourage, prevent, expose, and

correct the unethical conduct of colleagues. Finally, social workers should be equally ready to defend and assist colleagues unjustly charged with unethical conduct.

Summary of Major Principles

I. The Social Worker's Conduct and Comportment as a Social Worker

A. Propriety. The social worker should maintain high standards of personal conduct in the capacity or identity as social worker.

B. Competence and Professional Development. The social worker should strive to become and remain proficient in professional practice and the performance of professional functions.

C. Service. The social worker should regard as primary the service obligation of the social work profession.

D. Integrity. The social worker should act in accordance with the highest standards of professional integrity.

E. Scholarship and Research. The social worker engaged in study and research should be guided by the conventions of scholarly inquiry.

II. The Social Worker's Ethical Responsibility to Clients

F. Primacy of Clients' Interests. The social worker's primary responsibility is to clients.

G. Rights and Prerogatives of Clients. The social worker should make every effort to foster maximum self-determination on the part of clients.

H. Confidentiality and Privacy. The social worker should respect the privacy of clients and hold in confidence all information obtained in the course of professional service.

I. Fees. When setting fees, the social worker should ensure that they are fair, reasonable, considerate, and commensurate with the service performed and with due regard for the clients' ability to pay.

III. The Social Worker's Ethical Responsibility to Colleagues

J. Respect, Fairness, and Courtesy. The social worker should treat colleagues with respect, courtesy, fairness, and good faith.

K. Dealing with Colleagues' Clients. The social worker has the responsibility to relate to the clients of colleagues with full professional consideration.

IV. The Social Worker's Ethical Responsibility to Employers and Employing Organizations

L. Commitments to Employing Organizations. The social worker should adhere to commitments made to the employing organizations.

V. The Social Worker's Ethical Responsibility to the Social Work Profession

M. Maintaining the Integrity of the Profession. The social worker should uphold and advance the values, ethics, knowledge, and mission of the profession.

N. Community Service. The social worker should assist the profession in making social services available to the general public.

O. Development of Knowledge. The social worker should take responsibility for identifying, developing, and fully utilizing knowledge for professional practice.

VI. The Social Worker's Ethical Responsibility to Society

P. Promoting the General Welfare. The social worker should promote the general welfare of society.

The NASW Code of Ethics

I. The Social Worker's Conduct and Comportment as a Social Worker

A. Propriety. The social worker should maintain high standards of personal conduct in the capacity or identity as social worker.

1. The private conduct of the social worker is a personal matter to the same degree as is any other person's, except when such conduct compromises the fulfillment of professional responsibilities.
2. The social worker should not participate in, condone, or be associated with dishonesty, fraud, deceit, or misrepresentation.
3. The social worker should distinguish clearly between statements and actions made as a private individual and as a representative of the social work profession or an organization or group.

B. Competence and Professional Development. The social worker should strive to become and remain proficient in professional practice and the performance of professional functions.

1. The social worker should accept responsibility or employment only on the basis of existing competence or the intention to acquire the necessary competence.
2. The social worker should not misrepresent professional qualifications, education, experience, or affiliations.

C. *Service.* The social worker should regard as primary the service obligation of the social work profession.

1. The social worker should retain ultimate responsibility for the quality and extent of the service that individual assumes, assigns, or performs.
2. The social worker should act to prevent practices that are inhumane or discriminatory against any person or group of persons.

D. *Integrity.* The social worker should act in accordance with the highest standards of professional integrity and impartiality.

1. The social worker should be alert to and resist the influences and pressures that interfere with the exercise of professional discretion and impartial judgement required for the performance of professional functions.
2. The social worker should not exploit professional relationships for personal gain.

E. *Scholarship and Research.* The social worker engaged in study and research should be guided by the conventions of scholarly inquiry.

1. The social worker engaged in research should consider carefully its possible consequences for human beings.
2. The social worker engaged in research should ascertain that the consent of participants in the research is voluntary and informed without any implied deprivation or penalty for refusal to participate, and with due regard for participants' privacy and dignity.
3. The social worker engaged in research should protect participants from unwarranted physical or mental discomfort, distress, harm danger, or deprivation.
4. The social worker who engages in the evaluation of services or cases should discuss them only for the professional purposes and only with persons directly and professionally concerned with them.
5. Information obtained about participants in research should be treated as confidential.
6. The social worker should take credit only for work actually done in

connection with scholarly and research endeavors and credit contributions made by others.

II. The Social Worker's Ethical Responsibility to Clients

F. *Primacy of Clients' Interests.* The social worker's primary responsibility is to clients.

1. The social worker should serve clients with devotion, loyalty, determination, and the maximum application of professional skill and competence.
2. The social worker should not exploit relationships with clients for personal advantage.
3. The social worker should not practice, condone, facilitate or collaborate with any form of discrimination on the basis of race, color, sex, sexual orientation, age, religion, national origin, marital status, political belief, mental or physical handicap, or any other preference or personal characteristic, condition or status.
4. The social worker should avoid relationships or commitments that conflict with the interests of clients.
5. The social worker should under no circumstances engage in sexual activities with clients.
6. The social worker should provide clients with accurate and complete information regarding the extent and nature of the services available to them.
7. The social worker should apprise clients of their risks, rights, opportunities, and obligations associated with social service to them.
8. The social worker should seek advice and counsel of colleagues and supervisors whenever such consultation is in the best interest of clients.
9. The social worker should terminate service to clients, and professional relationships with them, when such service and relationships are no longer required or no longer serve the clients' needs or interests.
10. The social worker should withdraw services precipitously only under unusual circumstances, giving careful consideration to all factors in the situation and taking care to minimize possible adverse effects.
11. The social worker who anticipates the termination or interruption of service to clients should notify clients promptly and seek the transfer, referral, or continuation of service in relation to the clients' needs and preferences.

G. *Rights and Prerogatives of Clients.* The social worker should make every effort to foster maximum self-determination on the part of clients.

1. When the social worker must act on behalf of a client who has been adjudged legally incompetent, the social worker should safeguard the interests and rights of that client.
2. When another individual has been legally authorized to act in behalf of a client, the social worker should deal with that person always with the client's best interest in mind.
3. The social worker should not engage in any action that violates or diminishes the civil or legal rights of clients.

H. *Confidentiality and Privacy.* The social worker should respect the privacy of clients and hold in confidence all information obtained in the course of professional service.

1. The social worker should share with others confidences revealed by clients, without their consent, only for compelling professional reasons.
2. The social worker should inform clients fully about the limits of confidentiality in a given situation, the purposes for which information is obtained, and how it may be used.
3. The social worker should afford clients reasonable access to any official social work records concerning them.
4. When providing clients with access to records, the social worker should take due care to protect the confidences of others contained in those records.
5. The social worker should obtain informed consent of clients before taping, recording, or permitting third party observation of their activities.

I. *Fees.* When setting fees, the social worker should ensure that they are fair, reasonable, considerate, and commensurate with the service performed and with due regard for the clients' ability to pay.

1. The social worker should not accept anything of value for making a referral.

III. *The Social Worker's Ethical Responsibility to Colleagues*

J. *Respect, Fairness, and Courtesy.* The social worker should treat colleagues with respect, courtesy, fairness, and good faith.

1. The social worker should cooperate with colleagues to promote professional interests and concerns.
2. The social worker should respect confidences shared by colleagues in the course of their professional relationships and transactions.
3. The social worker should create and maintain conditions of practice that facilitate ethical and competent professional performance by colleagues.
4. The social worker should treat with respect, and represent accurately and fairly, the qualifications, views, and findings of colleagues and use appropriate channels to express judgements on these matters.
5. The social worker who replaces or is replaced by a colleague in professional practice should act with consideration for the interest, character, and reputation of that colleague.
6. The social worker should not exploit a dispute between a colleague and employers to obtain a position or otherwise advance the social worker's interest.
7. The social worker should seek arbitration or mediation when conflicts with colleagues require resolution for compelling professional reasons.
8. The social worker should extend to colleagues of other professions the same respect and cooperation that is extended to social work colleagues.
9. The social worker who serves as an employer, supervisor, or mentor to colleagues should make orderly and explicit arrangements regarding the conditions of their continuing professional relationship.
10. The social worker who has the responsibility for employing and evaluating the performance of other staff members, should fulfill such responsibility in a fair, considerate, and equitable manner, on the basis of clearly enunciated criteria.
11. The social worker who has the responsibility for evaluating the performance of employees, supervisees, or students should share evaluations with them.

K. Dealing with Colleagues' Clients. The social worker has the responsibility to relate to the clients of colleagues with full professional consideration.

1. The social worker should not assume professional responsibility for the clients of another agency or a colleague without appropriate communication with that agency or colleague.
2. The social worker who serves the clients of colleagues, during a temporary absence or emergency, should serve those clients with the same consideration as that afforded any client.

IV. The Social Worker's Ethical Responsibility to Employers and Employing Organizations

L. Commitments to Employing Organizations. The social worker should adhere to commitments made to the employing organizations.

1. The social worker should work to improve the employing agency's policies and procedures, and the efficiency and effectiveness of its services.
2. The social worker should not accept employment or arrange student field placements in an organization which is currently under public sanction by NASW for violating personnel standards, or imposing limitations on or penalties for professional actions on behalf of clients.
3. The social worker should act to prevent and eliminate discrimination in the employing organization's work assignments and in its employment policies and practices.
4. The social worker should use with scrupulous regard, and only for the purpose for which they are intended, the resources of the employing organization.

V. The Social Worker's Ethical Responsibility to the Social Work Profession

M. Maintaining the Integrity of the Profession. The social worker should uphold and advance the values, ethics, knowledge, and mission of the profession.

1. The social worker should protect and enhance the dignity and integrity of the profession and should be responsible and vigorous in discussion and criticism of the profession.
2. The social worker should take action through appropriate channels against unethical conduct by any other member of the profession.
3. The social worker should act to prevent the unauthorized and unqualified practice of social work.

4. The social worker should make no misrepresentation in advertising as to qualifications, competence, service, or results to be achieved.

N. Community Service. The social worker should assist the profession in making social services available to the general public.

1. The social worker should contribute time and professional expertise to activities that promote respect for the utility, the integrity, and the competence of the social work profession.
2. The social worker should support the formulation, development, enactment and implementation of social policies of concern to the profession.

O. Development of Knowledge. The social worker should take responsibility for identifying, developing, and fully utilizing knowledge for professional practice.

1. The social worker should base practice upon recognized knowledge relevant to social work.
2. The social worker should critically examine, and keep current with emerging knowledge relevant to social work.
3. The social worker should contribute to the knowledge base of social work and share research knowledge and practice wisdom with colleagues.

VI. The Social Worker's Ethical Responsibility to Society

P. Promoting the General Welfare. The social worker should promote the general welfare of society.

1. The social worker should act to prevent and eliminate discrimination against any person or group on the basis of race, color, sex, sexual orientation, age, religion, national origin, marital status, political belief, mental or physical handicap, or any other preference or personal characteristic, condition, or status.
2. The social worker should act to ensure that all persons have access to the resources, services, and opportunities which they require.
3. The social worker should act to expand choice and opportunity for all persons, with special regard for disadvantaged or oppressed groups and persons.
4. The social worker should promote conditions that encourage respect for the diversity of cultures which constitute American society.

5. The social worker should provide appropriate professional services in public emergencies.
6. The social worker should advocate changes in policy and legislation to improve social conditions and to promote social justice.
7. The social worker should encourage informed participation by the public in shaping social policies and institutions.

Appendix 5

Knowledge Survey for the NASW Code of Ethics

KNOWLEDGE SURVEY FOR THE
NASW CODE OF ETHICS

by Carlton E. Munson

The following true-false questions are to measure your familiarity with the NASW code of ethics. This is not a test. Please answer all questions. If you do not know the answer to a question, select what you consider the most reasonable answer. Check the box to the left of the question to indicate your answer. Before answering the questions, we would like for you to provide some background information.

Please begin . . . . .

NAME: _____

SEX: ___MALE ___FEMALE AGE: ___

HIGHEST DEGREE: ___ BA ___ MSW ___ PHD ___ OTHER

HAVE YOU READ THE NASW CODE OF ETHICS? ___ YES ___ NO

IF YOU ANSWERED YES ABOVE, HOW LONG AGO DID YOU READ IT? ___

WERE YOU REQUIRED TO READ THE NASW CODE OF ETHICS AS PART OF YOUR SOCIAL WORK EDUCATION PROGRAM?

___ YES ___ NO

CHECK YOUR ANSWER IN THE BLANK TO THE LEFT OF EACH QUESTION.

THE NASW CODE OF ETHICS. . . .

TRUE__ FALSE__ 01. does not cover research activities of social workers.

TRUE__ FALSE__ 02. requires social workers make every effort to foster self-determination of clients.

TRUE__ FALSE__ 03. makes a social worker's primary responsibility to serve clients.

TRUE__ FALSE__ 04. requires respect for clients' privacy.

TRUE__ FALSE__ 05. does not address the issue of fees.

TRUE__ FALSE__ 06. does not offer guidelines for disputes among colleagues.

TRUE__ FALSE__ 07. urges practitioners to adhere to commitments made to employing organizations.

TRUE__ FALSE__ 08. is a set of rules that prescribes all behaviors of social workers in all complexities of professional life.

TRUE__ FALSE__ 09. requires that judgment of ethical behavior be conducted by a jury of professional peers.

TRUE__ FALSE__ 10. is simply a guide for conduct in situations that have ethical implications.

TRUE__ FALSE__ 11. directs social workers to report knowledge of unethical conduct.

TRUE__ FALSE__ 12. draws a distinction between private individual statements and those made as a representative of a professional organization.

TRUE__ FALSE__ 13. urges social workers to accept only jobs they have skills to perform.

TRUE__ FALSE__ 14. declares the social worker should retain ultimate responsibility for the quality and extent of services they perform.

TRUE__ FALSE__ 15. does not address the issue of the methods by which social workers obtain income.

TRUE__ FALSE__ 16. makes exceptions of confidentiality rules when clients are participating in federally funded research projects.

TRUE__ FALSE__ 17. does not address the issue of plagiarism in research and writing.

TRUE__ FALSE__ 18. advises social workers not to solicit the clients of one's agency for private practice.

TRUE__ FALSE__ 19. warns against refusing to treat someone because they believe in a fundamental religion.

TRUE__ FALSE__ 20. holds that social workers should avoid relationships that conflict with the interests of clients.

TRUE__ FALSE__ 21. states that social workers should not engage in sexual activities with clients.

TRUE__ FALSE__ 22. states that supervisors should not have sexual relationships with supervisees.

TRUE__ FALSE__ 23. requires that social workers provide clients with full information regarding services available to them.

TRUE__ FALSE__ 24. requires practitioners to seek advice of supervisors and colleagues whenever they are in doubt about practice.

TRUE__ FALSE__ 25. does not cover when or how to terminate with clients.

TRUE__ FALSE__ 26. allows revealing confidential client information when there are compelling professional reasons.

TRUE__ FALSE__ 27. permits clients access to records concerning them.

TRUE__ FALSE__ 28. mandates informed consent before clients are taped.

TRUE__ FALSE__ 29. requires practitioners fees be fair and based on client's income.

TRUE__ FALSE__ 30. requires respecting confidences shared by colleagues.

TRUE__ FALSE__ 31. requires reporting unethical colleagues, but does not tell you who to report them to.

TRUE__ FALSE__ 32. suggests seeking arbitration or mediation in disputes with colleagues.

TRUE__ FALSE__ 33. requires social workers to treat psychiatrists and psychologists with respect.

TRUE__ FALSE__ 34. makes clear the confidentiality rule is absolute.

TRUE__ FALSE__ 35. allows practitioners to receive fees for making referrals.

TRUE__ FALSE__ 36. requires supervisors to make orderly and explicit arrangements regarding relationships with supervisees.

TRUE__ FALSE__ 37. indicates performance evaluations should be based on practice criteria only.

TRUE__ FALSE__ 38. indicates performance evaluations should be shared with those being evaluated.

TRUE__ FALSE__ 39. prohibits soliciting the clients of colleagues.

TRUE__ FALSE__ 40. does not require practitioners to become involved in establishing agency policy.

TRUE__ FALSE__ 41. does not make clear whether students can be placed in agencies that are under public sanction from NASW.

TRUE__ FALSE__ 42. does not allow social workers to accept jobs in agencies that are under public sanction from NASW.

TRUE__ FALSE__ 43. encourages social workers to criticize the social work profession.

TRUE__ FALSE__ 44. urges against advertising/marketing of services by social workers.

TRUE__ FALSE__ 45. requires social workers to keep current on practice knowledge developments.

TRUE__ FALSE__ 46. requires social workers to contribute their services during public emergencies.

TRUE__ FALSE__ 47. encourages public participation in shaping social policy through support of social workers.

TRUE__ FALSE__ 48. requires clients be informed of their rights regarding services, but does not require identification of risks because they are unknown.

TRUE__ FALSE__ 49. holds supervisors responsible for the acts of their supervisees.

TRUE__ FALSE__ 50. does not mention students anyplace in the code.

Appendix 6

Practitioner Self-Assessment Form

PRACTITIONER SELF-ASSESSMENT FORM

1. How long did the interview last?

2. Do you feel the interview was:

   A. Too short?
   B. Too long?
   C. Just about right?

   If you checked A or B, explain what factors contributed to the interview being too short or too long. Who contributed most to this?

What could have been done to overcome this?

3. Did the interview have a focus?

   If yes, what was the focus?

   If no, what prevented a focus being developed?

   What could have been done to focus the interview more?

4. Do you feel the client(s) got what he, she, or they came for?

   If yes, what did he, or she, or they get?

   If no, what prevented it?

5. Did the interview have a flow or interaction or continuity?

If yes, generally describe this flow and how it was achieved.

If no, what prevented flow and continuity?

6. Describe generally how you felt prior to the interview.

7. Describe generally how you felt during the interview.

8. Describe generally how you felt after the interview.

9. Describe your behaviors during the interview you felt good about.

10. Describe client behaviors during the interview you felt good about.

11. Describe your behaviors during the interview you felt were not effective.

12. Describe client behaviors during the interview you felt were distracting or disturbing.

13. Are there any gestures cr behaviors that you believe enhanced the communication process?

14. Are there any gestures or behaviors on the part of the client(s) that enhanced the communication process?

15. Are there any gestures or behaviors on your part that distracted from the communication process?

16. Are there any gestures or behaviors on the part of the client(s) that distracted from the communication process?

17. Are there any problems associated with this interview you would like help with?

18. What would you do differently if you could do the interview again?

19. Base on this interview, what actions do you think the client(s) needs to take to make significant changes?

20. Based on what you know now, what are the plans for the next interview?

Appendix 7

Short Form Stress Scale

SHORT FORM STRESS SCALE
by Carlton E. Munson

This questionnaire is to measure stress associated with your work. The instrument has a self-scoring component. With the aid of the seminar leader you can score the answers and get immediate feedback about your stress level. This instrument is for diagnostic purposes only and is not intended to substitute for treatment of stress reactions. Persons who score high on the following scales are encouraged to seek professional help. When stress reactions are recognized early and treated, positive outcomes are more likely.

The first part of the questionnaire deals with some basic background information:

Name (optional):_____

Address (optional):_____

_____

Sex: _____Male _____Female   Age: _____   Religion: _____

Marital status: ___Single ___Married ___Divorced ___Widowed

Number of children:_____

How often do you attend religious services: _____

Education: _____

Years employed by this agency: _____

Job title: _____

Circle the number on the scale to the right of the question that best describes your experience.

	1	2	3	4	5
1. Headaches	1 N	2 R	3 S	4 O	5 A
2. Colds	1 E	2 A	3 O	4 F	5 L
3. Stomach problems	1 V	2 R	3 M	4 T	5 W
4. Dizzy spells	1 E	2 E	3 E	4 E	5 A
5. Crying	1 R	2 L	3 T	4 N	5 Y
6. Muscle tension or cramps	1	2 Y	3 I	4	5 S
7. Trouble falling to sleep	1	2	3 M	4	5
8. Waking too early	1	2	3 E	4	5
9. Tense at end of work day	1	2	3 S	4	5
10. Lose track of what day it is	1	2	3	4	5

SYMPTOMS TOTALS (ITEMS 1 TO 10) = ___ + ___ + ___ + ___ +___ = _____

Please continue to next page.........

454

11. Drink too much...	1	2	3	4	5
12. Smoke too much...	1	2	3	4	5
13. Use drugs...	1	2	3	4	5
14. Lack of adequate daily exercise...................	1	2	3	4	5
15. Watch too much television..........................	1	2	3	4	5
16. Do not eat balanced meals..........................	1	2	3	4	5
17. Eat too fast...	1	2	3	4	5
18. Try to do too many things at once..............	1	2	3	4	5
19. Spend too much time alone..........................	1	2	3	4	5
20. Watch television to get to sleep..................	1	2	3	4	5

UNHEALTHY ACTIVITIES TOTALS (ITEMS 11 TO 20)   = ___ +   ___ +   ___ +   ___ +___ =   __

21. Feel unappreciated and used by clients.........................	1	2	3	4	5
22. Feel clients create their own problems........................	1	2	3	4	5
23. Apprehensive when meeting new clients.......................	1	2	3	4	5
24. Clients make me nervous...	1	2	3	4	5
25. Get mad when clients do not follow instructions...........	1	2	3	4	5
26. Daydream while interviewing clients............................	1	2	3	4	5
27. Fail to be helpful to clients.......................................	1	2	3	4	5
28. Do not understand clients' anger................................	1	2	3	4	5
29. Delay appointments and returning telephone messages...	1	2	3	4	5
30. Feel clients really do not want to change....................	1	2	3	4	5

PRACTICE PERFORMANCE TOTALS (ITEMS 21 TO 30) = ___ +   ___ +   ___ +   ___ +___ =   ___

31. Feel my job is boring...................................	1	2	3	4	5
32. Feel trapped in my job................................	1	2	3	4	5
33. Become easily irritated at work....................	1	2	3	4	5
34. Things at work depress me...........................	1	2	3	4	5
35. Feel overwhelmed by my job........................	1	2	3	4	5
36. Do not not have enough training to do my job.............	1	2	3	4	5
37. Job tasks are not clearly defined.................	1	2	3	4	5
38. Work overtime or take work home...............	1	2	3	4	5
39. Avoid my coworkers....................................	1	2	3	4	5
40. Take days off from work..............................	1	2	3	4	5

WORK ATTITUDES TOTALS (ITEMS 31 TO 40)= ___ +   ___ +   ___ +   ___ +___ =   ___

41. Feel this is generally not a good place to work............	1	2	3	4	5
42. Feel agency is overrun with problems........................	1	2	3	4	5
43. Coworkers make me angry...	1	2	3	4	5
44. Feel paperwork is excessive......................................	1	2	3	4	5
45. Feel there is no support group at the office................	1	2	3	4	5
46. Hate going to work..	1	2	3	4	5
47. Do not have privacy at my office...............................	1	2	3	4	5
48.Take brief daily breaks from work.............................	1	2	3	4	5
49. I have a feeling of dislike for my coworkers...............	1	2	3	4	5
50. Working conditions in our agency are generally poor....	1	2	3	4	5

WORK SETTING TOTALS (ITEMS 41 TO 50)= ___+   ___ +   ___ +   ___ +___ = ___

GRAND TOTAL FOR EACH CATEGORY= _____

Scoring   Procedure

In each section total the numbers for the five columns. Enter each total in the blank at the end of that section. Then add the numbers across and enter the total after the equal sign. This is the score for that individual section of the scale. Then add the score for each section and enter the number in the blank that says "grand total for each category." Then enter each sore on the set of stress thermometers on the following page. The grand total for each category should be entered on the thermometer labeled combine stress score.

STRESS SCALE SCORE SUMMARY SHEET

Scoring Instructions

Enter your score for each section of the Stress Scale on the appropriate "stress thermometer" printed below. You will have a numerical visual measurement of your stress levels in the five areas, as well as an overall stress score.

| Symptoms | Unhealthy Activities | Practice Performance | Work Attitude | Work Setting |

Appendix 8

Supervision Questionnaire

SUPERVISION QUESTIONNAIRE

PLEASE FILL IN OR CHECK THE APPROPRIATE BLANK FOR EACH QUESTION.

1. Sex of Practitioner: (1) Male   (2) Female

2. Sex of Supervisor: (1) Male   (2) Female

3. Age of Practitioner:

4. Age of Supervisor:

ANSWER EACH OF THE FOLLOWING QUESTIONS BY CIRCLING THE RESPONSE CATEGORY BELOW EACH QUESTION THAT BEST *DESCRIBES* HOW YOU FEEL ABOUT THE QUESTION. THE CODES FOR THE RESPONSES ARE:

SD = STRONGLY DISAGREE
 D = DISAGREE
MD = MILDLY DISAGREE
MA = MILDLY AGREE
 A = AGREE
SA = STRONGLY AGREE

5. My supervisor lets me do the work the way I think best.

SD   D   MD   MA   A   SA

6. I feel my supervisor has contributed to my professional growth.

SD   D   MD   MA   A   SA

7. My supervisor respects me as a professional and treats me as such.

SD   D   MD   MA   A   SA

8. I think my supervisor is fair.

SD   D   MD   MA   A   SA

9. Overall, I am satisfied with my supervisory experience.

SD   D   MD   MA   A   SA

10. I usually come out of my supervisory conferences or groups feeling pretty good.

SD   D   MD   MA   A   SA

11. I do not look forward to my supervisory sessions and dread them before-hand.

SD   D   MD   MA   A   SA

12. My supervisor's written and oral evaluations of my performance are similar to my self-evaluations of my level of performance.

     SD   D   MD   MA   A   SA

13. My supervisor knows how to set priorities.

     SD   D   MD   MA   A   SA

14. My supervisor is good at organizing work.

     SD   D   MD   MA   A   SA

15. My supervisor knows how to teach techniques.

     SD   D   MD   MA   A   SA

16. My supervisor emphasizes the quantity of work while I am more interested in the quality of my work.

     SD   D   MD   MA   A   SA

17. My supervisor rules with an iron hand.

     SD   D   MD   MA   A   SA

18. My supervisor is slow to accept new ideas.

     SD   D   MD   MA   A   SA

19. My supervisor insists that everything be done his or her way.

     SD   D   MD   MA   A   SA

20. My supervisor likes to give directions.

     SD   D   MD   MA   A   SA

21. My supervisor has a "just pay attention and listen" attitude.

     SD   D   MD   MA   A   SA

22. My supervisor seems to know what he or she is talking about when it comes to dealing with case material.

     SD   D   MD   MA   A   SA

23. My supervisor has adequate knowledge to function as a good supervisor as far as his or her teaching role is concerned.

     SD   D   MD   MA   A   SA

24. My supervisor tends to talk mostly about theory and does not bother to deal with applying theory to the practice component of my cases.

     SD   D   MD   MA   A   SA

25. My supervisor tends to assume that I know a lot more than I really do and often talks "over my head."

        SD   D   MD   MA   A   SA

26. My supervisor tends to assume that I know a lot less than I feel within myself I know.

        SD   D   MD   MA   A   SA

27. My supervisor has helped me develop more self-awareness.

        SD   D   MD   MA   A   SA

28. My supervisor seems more interested in analyzing me than my cases.

        SD   D   MD   MA   A   SA

29. When one of my cases drops out of treatment, my supervisor is more interested in how I contributed to this than in what motivated the client.

        SD   D   MD   MA   A   SA

30. My supervisor has helped to improve my efficiency as a practitioner.

        SD   D   MD   MA   A   SA

31. My supervisor has improved my effectiveness as a practitioner.

        SD   D   MD   MA   A   SA

32. When I go home at the end of the day, and I have had supervision. I can feel pretty good about my day's efforts.

        SD   D   MD   MA   A   SA

33. In absolute terms my caseload is too small, and I wish I had more cases.

        SD   D   MD   MA   A   SA

34. In absolute terms, my caseload is too large.

        SD   D   MD   MA   A   SA

35. My supervisor is friendly and can be easily approached.

        SD   D   MD   MA   A   SA

36. My supervisor encourages me to talk openly and freely with him or her.

        SD   D   MD   MA   A   SA

37. My supervisor makes me feel at ease when talking with him or her.

        SD   D   MD   MA   A   SA

38. My supervisor expresses appreciation when I do a good job.

    SD   D   MD   MA   A   SA

39. My supervisor does not always make himself or herself clear.

    SD   D   MD   MA   A   SA

40. My values about what constitutes good treatment are much different from those of my supervisor.

    SD   D   MD   MA   A   SA

41. I often seek advice of my co-workers rather than take the matter up with my supervisor.

    SD   D   MD   MA   A   SA

42. If I can get around it, I avoid conferences with my supervisor.

    SD   D   MD   MA   A   SA

43. It does not pay to confront my supervisor with an issue.

    SD   D   MD   MA   A   SA

44. My supervisor is usually looking for some issue to discuss in our conferences, and the best policy is to reveal as little as possible.

    SD   D   MD   MA   A   SA

45. My supervisor seems more concerned that I deal with my cases according to the rules and regulations rather than being concerned that I do the utmost to aid my clients.

    SD   D   MD   MA   A   SA

46. My supervisory experience has been of limited value because of the agency confines.

    SD   D   MD   MA   A   SA

47. It is no use to try to do something creative or innovative in this agency because there is always someone ready to put you down.

    SD   D   MD   MA   A   SA

48. Usually I am way behind on my dictation and should take some time to get caught up.

    SD   D   MD   MA   A   SA

49. The administrators in this agency are only concerned with output and really show little concern for the welfare of the practitioners.

    SD   D   MD   MA   A   SA

50. This agency seems to be constantly in a state of crisis, and we simply seem to just go from one crisis to another.

      SD   D   MD   MA   A   SA

51. There are so many problems in this agency that I avoid them and devote my time to doing a good job with my clients.

      SD   D   MD   MA   A   SA

52. All in all this agency is a pretty good place to work.

      SD   D   MD   MA   A   SA

ANSWER EACH OF THE FOLLOWING QUESTIONS BY CIRCLING THE RESPONSE CATEGORY BELOW EACH QUESTION THAT *BEST DESCRIBES* HOW YOU FEEL ABOUT THE QUESTION.

53. How often do you become annoyed with your supervisor?

      Never   Infrequently   Sometimes   Frequently

54. How often do you become angry with your supervisor?

      Never   Infrequently   Sometimes   Frequently

55. How often do you confront your supervisor?

      Never   Infrequently   Sometimes   Frequently

56. My supervisor allows me to observe directly his or her own methods of working with cases through allowing me to sit in on some of his or her interviews.

      Never   Infrequently   Sometimes   Frequently

57. My supervisor sits in on some of my own interviews as a means of gathering data to help me develop my own professional skill.

      Never   Infrequently   Sometimes   Frequently

58. My supervisor uses audio tape recordings of interviews in our supervisory conferences or groups.

      Never   Infrequently   Sometimes   Frequently

59. My supervisor uses videotaped interviews as supervisory material in our conferences or groups.

      Never   Infrequently   Sometimes   Frequently

60. My supervisor requires me to process record case material for use in supervisory conferences or groups.

      Never   Infrequently   Sometimes   Frequently

IN PERCENT, ON THE AVERAGE THE PROPORTIONING OF TIME IN MY SUPERVISORY SESSIONS IS:

61. _____ % discussing supervisor's personal problems.
62. _____ % discussing supervisor's cases.
63. _____ % discussing my personal problems.
64. _____ % discussing administrative matters.
65. _____ % discussing case material.
66. _____ % discussing my growth & development of self-awareness.
67. _____ % discussing everyday small talk that is unrelated to my work.

_____ TOTAL = 100%

68. How often do you have conferences with your supervisor?

(1) Never (2) Monthly or Less (3) Biweekly (4) Weekly (5) Daily

69. Supervisory conferences are usually held:

(1) at my request   (2) at request of supervisor

70. If I had my choice, I would prefer:

(1) individual one-to-one supervision.
(2) group supervision.
(3) combination individual and group supervision.
(4) no supervision.

71. On the average I conduct _____ interviews each day.

72. On the average each interview lasts _____.

IN PERCENT, ON THE AVERAGE MY WORK LOAD IS PROPORTIONED:

73. _____ % doing therapy
74. _____ % dictation
75. _____ % staff meetings
76. _____ % community work
77. _____ % other

78. IN THE SPACE PROVIDED, CHECK THE MODEL OF SUPERVISION THAT *MOST* CLOSELY PARALLELS THE ONE USED IN YOUR SUPERVISION:

_____ 1. Emphasis in supervision is placed on the three-part process of **help, teaching, and administration. Clinicians are expected to de**velop self-awareness. Regularly scheduled individual conferences are used to manage the flow and content of work of supervisees.

_____ 2. Supervision is viewed as strictly an administrative and teaching process. The supervisor avoids psychologizing the worker. The structure of supervision is regularly scheduled conferences with a specific agenda.

_____ 3. Emphasis in supervision is placed on teaching, and administration latitude is provided for a variety of supervisory styles adapted to individual practitioner needs. Clinicians are allowed to choose among available experts for advice. Individual conferences are used sparingly. There is some use of group seminars.

_____ 4. Role of individual supervisor is played down. The specific work group, which is set up on specialized skills and/or services, is the main supervisory unit and has virtually replaced the individual conference for supervisory decision making and problem solving.

_____ 5. The individual supervisor supervises several practitioners in a group arrangement. The group works together to establish the direction and content of supervision. Learning experiences and provided mainly through members of the group sharing ideas, information and observations with one another.

_____ 6. Clinicians function completely independently and only answer to their own consciences. No direct control is exercised over the clinician who is treated as a mature, experienced professional without need of supervision.

79. All supervisors are required to exercise authority and control in supervision from time to time. This question deals with how you view the source of authority and control used by your supervisor. CHECK THE BLANK THAT *MOST CLOSELY PARALLELS* THE SOURCE OF AUTHORITY USED BY YOUR SUPERVISOR.

_____ 1. Administratively assigned and agency sanctioned authority over practitioners.

_____ 2. Authority rests in ability to require or expect practitioners to reveal much about themselves in the supervisory relationship.

_____ 3. In part, authority depends on the ability to have influence beyond the job situation through, for example, evaluations.

_____ 4. Authority derives from the role as mediator of the relationship between clinician and the agency.

_____ 5. Authority derives from the fact that the supervisor knows more about some things than the clinician does.

_____ 6. Authority grows out of the personality of the supervisor and his or her ability to achieve cooperation from practitioners through diplomacy and skill in handling.

80. Along with their other duties, supervisors are required to perform teaching functions. This question deals with the teaching models used in your supervision. IN THE BLANK PROVIDED, CHECK THE MODEL THAT MOST CLOSELY PARALLELS THE ONE USED BY YOUR SUPERVISOR.

_____ 1. Basically the Socratic method is used. That is. supervisees are skillfully asked leading questions until they identify and recognize the material sought. The supervisor talks very little. The practitioner does most of the talking.

_____ 2. The major thrust of teaching is to provide information that will help clinicians avoid making errors and emphasis is placed on what not to do so as to avoid grave situations. This method is used to foster as much as possible the growth and self-expression of the clinician. The main function of teaching is viewed as provision for self-expression and development of self-awareness of the clinician.

_____ 3. Teaching in supervision centers around whatever experiences that emerge from the client treatment demands and the development of the essential skills necessary to provide treatment. Emphasis is placed on the relationship between knowing, feeling and doing in practice.

PLEASE COMPLETE THE FOLLOWING SENTENCES:

81. The things I like most about my supervisor are:

82. The things I dislike about my supervisor are:

83. Rank your supervisor from 1 to 10 (1 = low, 10 = high) according to how good a supervisor you think he or she is.

84. Rank yourself from 1 to 10 (1 = low, 10 = high) in terms of how good a clinician you think you are.

85. Do you think supervision has helped you improve your effectiveness and efficiency as a clinician? (1) Yes   (2) No

86. What do you see as the chief value of supervision?

87. COMMENTS:

Appendix 9

Long Form Stress Questionnaire

LONG FORM STRESS QUESTIONNAIRE

1. Sex: (1) Female   (2) Male

2. Age:

3. Race: (1)White   (2) Black   (3) Mexican American   (4) Other

4. Marital Status: (1) Married   (2) Divorced   (3) Single
   (4)Widowed   (5) Other

5. Do you have any children? (1) No   (2) Yes

6. If you answered yes to #5, how many children did you have?

7. Did you have any social work experience prior to working in this setting?
   (1) Yes   (2) No

8. If you answered yes to #7, how many years work experience did you have?

9. Religious preference: (1) Protestant   (2) Catholic   (3) Jewish
   (4) None   (5) Other

10. How often do you attend religious services?
    (1) Weekly or more   (2) Monthly or less   (3) Several times a year
    (4) Rarely   (5) Never

11. What is the highest degree you hold?
    (1) High school graduate   (2) BA   (3) BSW   (4) MA   (5) MSW

12. How many of your co-workers do you feel close to?

13. Do you feel you have experienced "burnout" due to your job?
    (1) No   (2) Yes

14. How many years have you worked at your present setting?

15. What is your job title?

16. How many years have you served in your current position?

ANSWER EACH OF THE FOLLOWING QUESTIONS BY CIRCLING
THE RESPONSE CATEGORY BELOW EACH QUESTION THAT BEST
DESCRIBES HOW YOU FEEL ABOUT THE QUESTION.
THE CODES FOR THE RESPONSES ARE:

         SD = STRONGLY DISAGREE
          D = DISAGREE
         MD = MILDLY DISAGREE
         MA = MILDLY AGREE
          A = AGREE
         SA = STRONGLY AGREE

17. I look forward to going to work most of the time.

    SD   D   MD   MA   A   SA

18. I feel capable of helping clients with their problems.

    SD   D   MD   MA   A   SA

19. When I have not helped a client I feel I have failed as a practitioner.

    SD   D   MD   MA   A   SA

20. I am able to concentrate on and listen to what the client says.

    SD   D   MD   MA   A   SA

21. I feel relaxed and at ease with clients.

    SD   D   MD   MA   A   SA

22. I experience exhaustion at work.

    SD   D   MD   MA   A   SA

23. I experience fatigue at work.

    SD   D   MD   MA   A   SA

24. I am able to understand clients' anger.

    SD   D   MD   MA   A   SA

25. I am able to interpret clients' anger.

    SD   D   MD   MA   A   SA

26. I become easily irritated at work.

    SD   D   MD   MA   A   SA

27. I become easily agitated at work.

    SD   D   MD   MA   A   SA

28. I have trouble viewing clients as individuals with unique problems.

    SD   D   MD   MA   A   SA

29. I feel apprehensive about meeting new clients.

    SD   D   MD   MA   A   SA

30. I try to avoid co-workers whenever possible.

    SD   D   MD   MA   A   SA

31. I feel that clients have not created their own problems.

    SD   D   MD   MA   A   SA

32. I suffer from chronic headaches.

    SD   D   MD   MA   A   SA

33. I suffer from persistent colds.

    SD   D   MD   MA   A   SA

34. I have frequent gastrointestinal upsets.

    SD   D   MD   MA   A   SA

35. I usually sleep well.

    SD   D   MD   MA   A   SA

36. I feel overwhelmed by my job most of the time.

    SD   D   MD   MA   A   SA

37. I do not have enough training in helping skills.

    SD   D   MD   MA   A   SA

38. We lack enough funds to accomplish agency goals.

    SD   D   MD   MA   A   SA

39. Excessive paperwork keeps me from doing a good job in this agency.

    SD   D   MD   MA   A   SA

40. I am sometimes confused about whether I am supposed to help or control clients.

    SD   D   MD   MA   A   SA

41. I get almost all my emotional needs met through my work.

    SD   D   MD   MA   A   SA

42. It seems hopeless to try to change things in this agency.

    SD   D   MD   MA   A   SA

43. When I go home at the end of the day, I can feel pretty good about my days's efforts.

    SD   D   MD   MA   A   SA

44. There is so much paperwork in this agency that one feels like giving up on accomplishing much.

    SD   D   MD   MA   A   SA

45. I often feel unappreciated and used by clients.

    SD   D   MD   MA   A   SA

46. I am reluctant to tell others what kind of work I do.

    SD   D   MD   MA   A   SA

47. It is difficult for me to unwind at the end of a workday.

    SD   D   MD   MA   A   SA

48. This agency seems to be constantly in a state of crisis, and we simply seem to just go from one crisis to another.

    SD   D   MD   MA   A   SA

49. Thre are so many problems in this agency that I avoid them and devote my time to doing a good job with my clients.

    SD   D   MD   MA   A   SA

50. All in all, this agency is a pretty good place to work.

    SD   D   MD   MA   A   SA

51. I spend more time watching television than I used to.

    SD   D   MD   MA   A   SA

52. I miss work frequently.

    SD   D   MD   MA   A   SA

53. I smoke more now than I used to.

    SD   D   MD   MA   A   SA

54. I drink more now than I used to.

    SD   D   MD   MA   A   SA

55. My supervisor expresses appreciation when I do a good job.

    SD   D   MD   MA   A   SA

56. I use drugs more now than I used to.

    SD   D   MD   MA   A   SA

57. I work more hours a week than the regular working hours of the agency.

    SD   D   MD   MA   A   SA

ANSWER EACH OF THE FOLLOWING QUESTIONS BY CIRCLING THE RESPONSE CATEGORY BELOW EACH QUESTION THAT BEST DESCRIBES HOW YOU FEEL ABOUT THE QUESTION.

58. How often do you become angry with your co-workers?

    Never   Infrequently   Sometimes   Frequently

59. How often do you become angry with your clients?

    Never   Infrequently   Sometimes   Frequently

60. How often do you become angry with your supervisor?

    Never   Infrequently   Sometimes   Frequently

61. How often do you find yourself making negative comments about clients?

    Never   Infrequently   Sometimes   Frequently

62. How often do you spend hours after work with co-workers?

    Never   Infrequently   Sometimes   Frequently

63. How often do you feel depressed over something that happens to you at work?

    Never   Infrequently   Sometimes   Frequently

64. How often do you feel exhausted even when you get enough sleep?

    Never   Infrequently   Sometimes   Frequently

65. Do you feel you have gone through several cycles of burnout in your job?

    (1) Yes   (2) No

66. Do you have a professional support group available to help combat burn-out?

    (1) Yes   (2) No

67. Do you have a professional support group or person that helps you combat work problems?

    (1) Yes   (2) No

68. Do you feel you have developed any physical signs or symptoms associated with your work?

    (1) Yes   (2) No

69. Do you feel you have developed any psychological signs or symptoms associated with your work?

    (1) Yes   (2) No

70. If you answered yes to either of the two previous questions, please explain.

COMMENTS:

Index

Abell, Walter, 395
Academy of Certified Social
    Workers, 67
Accrediting. *See* Credentialing
Action techniques. *See* Role Play
Active style of supervision, 101-102
Activity vs. practice, 7
Administrative activities
    in clinical practice evaluation,
      221-222
    clinical practitioners in, 71
    cost of, 17-18
    credentials and examinations,
      267-269
    dealing with other administrators,
      269-270
    duty to warn, 262-264
    in geriatric and gerontology
      settings, 314-315
    legal issues, 261-262
    record keeping, 258-261
    styles
      benevolent, affable democrat
        (BAD), 270-273
      cool, aloof decider (CAD),
        275-277
      jovial, outgoing klutz (JOK),
        273-274
      sadistic, authoritarian divider
        (SAD), 279-280
      sophisticated, learned, informed
        commander (SLIC), 274-275
      worried, anxious determinist
        (WAD), 277-279
    violence and safety, 264-267
    women and, 372-373
Adolescents
    child guidance movement and, 59
    in group homes, 318-324

Advocacy role and values, 87-88
Age and authority, 165
Agencies. *See* Organizations
Aging. *See* Geriatrics and
    gerontology settings
AIDS, 76
Alcohol abuse in social workers,
    231
Ambush interaction, 128
American Board of Examiners
    in Clinical Social Work, 10
American Medical Association, 60
Analysis and redefinition
    in supervision, 16-17
Anger
    authority and, 320-321
    stress and, 241
Anxiety. *See* Stress
Argyris, Chris, 399
Ariete, Silvano, 391-392,395
Art as Experience by John Dewey,
    387-388
Art in social work practice, 54-55
    as defense, 390-391
    definition, 380-381
    elements of
      audience and critics, 389-390
      creation, 385-388
      discipline, 388-389
      rehearsal, 389
    patterns and, 391-392
    qualities of, 395-397
    science and, 383-385
    supervision and, 392-394
    theory and, 197
    tradition of, 381-383
*The Art of Helping People Out
    of Trouble* by Karl
    DeSchweinitz, 54

Assessment
  clinical, diagnosis and, 32-34
  of consultation, 360-361
  of cotherapist activity, 353-354
  in credentialing, 267-269
  educational
    assessment scale, 426-427
    NASW Code of Ethics
      knowledge survey, 446-448
    of supervisees, 132-135
  history, 48-49
  of learning in clinical practice, 74
    administrative, 221-222
    audiovisual techniques, in,
      286-287,302
    criticism, 210-213
    decreasing defensiveness,
      205-206
    errors in practice and, 208-210
    follow-up, 210
    note taking, 217-218
    record keeping, 218-221
    research in, 215-217
    self-assessment, 214-215
    simplifying, 206-208
    supervision research, 222-225
  in long-term care facilities
    (LTCF), 316
  of role play, 297-298
  self-assessment of client interview,
    450-452
  self-assessment for clinical
    supervisor, 424
  of supervision, 13
Assessment scale for becoming
    a clinical supervisor, 424
Audiovisual techniques
  audiotaping, 291-292
  audio/video separation, 292
  effectiveness and efficiency,
    301-302
  as entertainment, 285-286
  ergonomics, 376
  in family therapy supervision, 338
  in live supervision, 299-301,302
  as measurement, 286-287
  research studies of, 284-285
  videotaping of therapy, 287-291
Authority
  age and, 165
  autonomy and, 165-169
  in criminal justice settings,
    317-322
  of group home residents, 322
  interaction and, 159-161
  in organizations, 155-156
    sex bias and, 369-371
  structure and, 161-163
  struggle with, 154-155
  style of supervisor and, 163-164
  supervision and, 36,156-159
Autonomy
  authority and, 165-169
  in rural practice, 325-327

Bagg, Alan R., 292
Beginning professionals. *See also*
    Students
  in cotherapist activity, 351-352
  elderly stereotyping and, 311
  in group supervision, 171-172
  stress and, 253-254
  supervision of, 27-28
Behavior
  ethics and, 91
  in stress, 240-243
  theory and, 189-190
Benevolent, affable democrat
    (BAD) administrator style,
    270-273
Bill of Rights for supervisees,
    39-40
Bissell, LeClair, 231
Bowen, Murray
  cotherapist activity, 349
  family of origin material, 344-345
  family therapy, 336-337
  style of supervision, 103
Brackett, Jeffrey Richardson, 394
Briar, Scott, 158

BSW's
  demand for, 65
  in generalist practice, 325
"Buddy system" and safety, 266
"Bug-in-the-ear" device
  in live supervision, 299-301,302
  in family therapy, 338
Burnout. *See* Stress

Cabot, Richard
  science and art in social work
    practice, 392-393
  medical setting for social work,
    52-53,54
Career advancement and women,
  373
Career choice and stress,
  230-231,245
Case material
  supervision of, 13,135-138
  supervisor/supervisee interaction,
    160-161
Casework
  vs. clinical practice, 8-9
  vs. psychotherapy, 63-64
Charity Organization Societies, 47
Chescheir, Martha W., 190
Child guidance movement, 58-59
Child welfare workers and stress,
  232
Client/clinical practitioner
    relationship
  AIDS, 76
  audiovisual techniques in, 301
  colleagues' clients and, 441-442
  in cotherapist activity, 352,356
  duty to warn and, 262-264
  ethics of, 436,439-440
  importance of, 73
  in 1970s, 68
  primary vs. secondary, 329-330
  proximity issues, 75
  in rural practice settings, 329-330
  stress and, 240-241

  supervision of, 135-136
  style of supervisor and, 97-98
  techniques in, 142-143
  theory and, 192
  values and, 84-88
  violence and, 264-267
Clinical assessment and diagnosis,
  32-34
Clinical exposure index, 285
Clinical practice. *See also* Clinical
    practitioners; Supervisees
  activity vs. practice, 7
  art in
    as defense, 390-391
    definition, 380-381
    elements of, 385-390
    patterns and, 391-392
    qualities of, 395-397
    scientifically based practice
      and, 383-385
    tradition of, 381-383
  assessment of learning in
    administrative, 221-222
    criticism in, 210-213
    decreasing defensiveness,
      205-206
    errors in practice and, 208-210
    follow-up, 210
    note taking, 217-218
    record keeping, 218-221
    research in, 215-217
    self-assessment and, 214-215
    simplifying, 206-208
    supervision research, 222-225
  defined, 8-11
  ethics and need for supervision in,
    25
  in mental health, 20-21
  philosophy of, 178-180
  practice theory, 181
  resurgence of, 20
  science in, 392-394
  stress in, 24-25
  techniques, 177-178
  theory, 183-184

application of, 200-201
explosion and, 21
theory of, 180-181
training for, 23-24
values and, 84-85
Clinical practitioner/client
relationship. *See*
Client/clinical practitioner
relationship
Clinical practitioners. *See also*
Clinical practice;
Supervisees
conflict with agencies, 162-163
stress in, 230-232
in therapy, 334-335
Clinical social work. *See* Clinical
practice
Clinical supervision. *See* Supervision
Code of Ethics of National
Association of Social
Workers. *See* National
Association of Social
Workers Code of Ethics
Colleagues, ethical responsibilities
to, 440-441
Common Human Needs by Charlotte
Towle, 60-61
Communication
consultation and, 358
discussion in supervision, 15
in group homes, 319-320
Communication pattern
in benevolent, affable democrat
(BAD) administrator style,
270
in cool, aloof decider (CAD)
administrator style, 275-276
in jovial, outgoing klutz (JOK)
administrator style, 273
in sadistic, authoritarian divider
(SAD) administrator style,
279
in sophisticated, learned, informed
commander (SLIC)
administrator style, 274

in worried, anxious determinist
(WAD) administrator style,
277
Communications devices, 376
Community service, 443
Competence style of authority,
163-164
Concepts in theory
defined, 185
paired or dual, 187
Conduct and comportment as a social
worker, 437-439
Conductor therapist style, 101
Confidentiality
duty to warn and, 262-264
ethics, 440
future trends, 75
value conflicts and, 85-86
Conflict
clinical practitioner and agency,
162-163
in cotherapist activity, 350,356
of staff in group homes, 321-322
supervisor style and, 119
values and, 83-84
Congruence of perceptions
in supervision, 12
Consistency of supervision, 13
Consultation
resistance to, 361-362
in rural practice, 328
structure, 359-361
vs. supervision, 11,169,356-358
type and focus, 358-359
Contact in consultation, 360
Continuing education and need
for supervision, 22-23
Continuity of supervision,
139-140,210
Contract in consultation, 359
Contracting as supervision
technique, 145-146
Conventional roles vs. interpersonal,
313
Conyngton, Mary, 53

Cool, aloof decider (CAD)
administrator style, 275-277
Coping strategies in supervision, 24
Cost of supervision, 17-18,71-72
Cotherapist activity
client access in, 352
client perception, 356
conflict in, 350
decision guidelines, 353
dominant therapist, 351
effectiveness of, 349-350
evaluation of, 353-354
joint style, 355-356
theory and, 355
Council on Social Work Education
art in social work practice, 382
Curriculum Policy Statement, 23
geriatric and gerontology settings
and, 312
Creativity
art and, 380-381,386-388
theory and, 197
Credentialing
administration and, 267-269
changes and need for supervision,
21-22
history of, 67,70
organizations, 430-431
Criminal justice settings
authority of social worker in,
317-318
group homes, 318-324
Criticism in supervision, 210-213
Culture of organization
and consultation, 359
Curriculum Policy Statement
of Council on Social Work
Education, 23
Cyclical pattern of burnout,
233-234

Daley, Michael R., 243
Davies, Joann F., 329
Death and dying, 308-310

Debriefing
in medical settings, 307
in role play, 298
Decision making
in benevolent, affable democrat
(BAD) administrator style,
272
in cool, aloof decider (CAD)
administrator style, 276
in jovial, outgoing klutz (JOK)
administrator style, 273
in sadistic, authoritarian divider
(SAD) administrator style,
280
in sophisticated, learned, informed
commander (SLIC)
administrator style, 274
in worried, anxious determinist
(WAD) administrator style,
278
Deductive vs. inductive method, 191
Defensiveness in supervision,
decreasing, 205-206
Depression
in medical settings, 308
stress and, 241
DeSchweinitz, Karl, 54-55
Dewey, John, 387-388
Diagnosis
assessment of knowledge of, 427
clinical assessment and, 32-34
in family therapy, 340
of mental health, 73-74
technique in, 144-145
theory in, 189
records, 260
supervisees' knowledge of, 133
Diminished perceptions, 31
Discharge records, 260
Discussion in supervision, 15
Distress. *See* Stress
Documentation. *See* Record keeping
Drug-abuse counselors, 86,87
DSM III-R Diagnosis, 73-74
Dual concepts, 187

Durkheim, Emile, 405
Duty to warn, 262-264
Dynamic intellectualism, 183
Dynamics and process in family
    of origin material, 346
Dyrud, Jarl E., 383

Eclecticism, 183
Education
    in agencies vs. universities, 48
    audiovisual techniques, 287-291
    in clinical practice
        administrative, 221-222
        criticism, 210-213
        decreasing defensiveness,
          205-206
        errors in practice and, 208-210
        follow-up, 210
        keeping simple, 206-208
        note taking in, 217-218
        record keeping, 218-221
        research in, 215-217
        supervision research,
          222-225
    audiovisual techniques in,
      287-291
    continuing, 22-23
    encouragement techniques, 150
    ethical responsibility of, 443
    family of origin material in,
      342-344
    field instruction
        1930s, 57
        1950s, 61
        1960s, 64-65
        1970s, 66
    NASW Code of Ethics, 93
    reading in, 146-148
    role play and, 292-293
    stress and, 245,247,250
    of substance-abuse counselors, 86
    for supervisors, 25-26
    supervisors in, 3,7,14,32
    of theory, 181-182

of techniques
    mechanics, 140-141
    technical skill and perspective,
      138-139
Educational assessment, 74
    of beginning professionals, 27
    self-assessment, 214-215
    scale, 426-427
    of supervisees, 132-135
Elderly. *See* Geriatrics and
      gerontology settings
Enabling in family therapy, 341,343
Encountering in family therapy,
    341,343
Endress, Anna H., 154-155
Environment. *See* Setting
Ergonomics, 375-376
Error acceptance learning, 205-206
Errors in clinical practice, 208-209
Espoused theory, 399
Ethics
    assessment of awareness, 133,426
    future trends, 74-75
    knowledge of, 90-92
    NASW Code of Ethics, 88-90
    need for supervision and, 25
    supervisor evaluation of, 224
    violations, 92-93
Evaluation. *See* Assessment
Examinations, 267-269. *See also*
      Assessment
Exhaustion stage of stress, 238-239
Expectations
    in stress, 237-238,254
    of supervisees, 42
    of supervisor, 40-42

Facts in theory, 184-185
Faculty-based field instructors,
    65
Failure to warn, 262-264
Family
    in criminal justice setting, 318
    in medical settings, 308-309
    1920s' focus on, 54

Family of origin material
in supervision
case example, 345-346
effectiveness of, 342-344
as focus, 348-349
history of, 344-345
practice and, 347-348
process and dynamics, 346-347
Family Service Association
of America Directors, 66
Family Therapy in Clinical Practice
by Murray Bowen, 344-345
Family therapy and supervision
audiovisual devices, 338
feminist, 371-372
individual therapy vs. family
therapy, 335-337
interactional issues, 337-338
in 1970s, 69
SEES system, 341-342
theory
diagnosis and, 340
vs. technique, 339-340
Fees and ethics, 440
Feminist practice
administration and, 372-373
agency function and, 368-369
family therapy, 371-372
sex bias and, 369-371
supervision and, 366-367
theory, 364-366
Fiduciary regulation, 17-18,71-72
Field instruction
1930s, 57
1950s, 61
1960s, 64-65
1970s, 66
Fisch, Richard, 391
Flexner, Abraham, 50
Follow-up of supervision
in evaluation, 210
importance of, 139-140
Freud, Sigmund
art and science in social work
practice, 385,396

feminist theory and, 369
influence on supervision,
51-53
style of supervision, 103
treatment of Dora, 208-209
Freudenberger, Herbert J., 236
Frink, Horace, 51
Function of supervision, 11-13

Gardner, George, 60
Garrett, Annette, 61
Gays, 76,369
Gender and supervision
background, 363-364
career advancement, 373
career choice, 230-231
discrimination, 362-363
evolution, 364
in feminist practice
administration, 372-373
agency function, 368-369
family therapy, 371-372
issues of supervision,
366-367
theory, 364-366
sex bias and, 369-371
stress, 374-375
General adaptation syndrome (GAS),
236
Generalist practice in rural settings,
324-325
Genuineness of staff in group home,
323-324
Geriatrics and gerontology settings
long-term care facilities (LTCF)
regulations, 315-317
role of social worker in,
312-315
role support in, 317
problems of, 310-312
Gestalt therapy, 180
Goals and objectives in supervisee
assessment, 134
Greben, S. E., 397
Group homes, 318-324

Group supervision
  considerations, 169-171
  vs. individual, 64-65
  role of supervisor, 172-173
  supervisee experience and,
    171-172
Guidelines
  for administrative evaluation,
    222
  for audiovisual and action
  technique efficiency and
    effectiveness, 302
  in cotherapist activity, 353
  for criticism
    of clinical material, 210-211
    dealing with, 212-213
  on death and dying in medical
    settings, 309
  for duty to warn, 263
  for geriatric and gerontology
    setting role differentiation,
    313-314
  for group home staff and resident
    process, 318-319
  for leisure activity, 249-250
  for record keeping
    clinical practitioner's personal,
      220
    legal, 219-220
    supervisory, 220
    for self-assessment, 214-215
  for supervisors and supervisees, 34
  for techniques of supervision, 150
  for theory application, 200-201

Haley, Jay, 349,390
  style of supervision, 103
Hamilton, Gordon, 61,384
High tech/high touch formula,
  375
History of supervision
  early
    assessment, 48-49
    institutional, 48

    origin, 47-48
    sociology and, 49-50
  Freudian influence, 51-53
  1920s
    family focus, 54
    social work as art, 54-55
  1930s
    field instruction, 57
    rank-and-file movement, 56-57
    treatment services, 57
  1940s
    child guidance, 58-59
    therapeutic eclecticism, 58
  1950s
    field instruction, 61
    professional status, 62
    psychiatry and, 59-60
    social science focus, 60-61
    systems theory, 62
    theory integration, 61-62
  1960s
    change and unrest, 63-64
    demand for practitioners, 65
    experimentation, 64-65
  1970s
    disillusionment, 65
    family therapy movement, 69
    field instruction, 66
    practitioner/client relationship,
      68
    private practice, 67-68
    professional status, 67
    systems theory, 68-69
    technology and specialization,
      65-66
  1980s
    credentialing, 70
    theory stagnation, 69
  1990s, 70-76
    practice theory and, 46
    Richmond, Mary, and, 53
Hollis, Florence
  casework text, 63
  social work as art, 382,393
Homans' hypothesis, 86-87

Homophobia
  of clinical practitioners, 76
  sex bias and, 369
Horney, Karen, 55,187-188
Hospice settings, 309-310
*How to Help: A Manual of Practical
  Charity* by Mary Conyngton,
  53
Hutchinson, Dorothy, 55,68
Hypotheses in theory, 185-188

Ideology and theory, 180-181
"If-then" technique, 143
Imagination in supervision, 16
Impulsive problem-solvers, 99-100
Individual supervision vs. group,
  64-65
Individual therapy vs. family,
  336-337
Inductive vs. deductive method, 191
Initial treatment plan (ITP) records,
  260
Institutional supervision, 48
Intake records, 260
Integrity, 438,442-443
Interaction
  in client/clinical practitioner
    relationship
    stress and, 240-241
    style of, 99
  in family therapy, 338
  in supervisor/supervisee
    relationship
    authority and, 159-161
    benevolent, affable democrat
      (BAD) administrator style,
      270-272
    in cool, aloof decider (CAD)
      administrator style, 275-276
    in jovial, outgoing klutz (JOK)
      administrator style, 273
    in sadistic, authoritarian divider
      (SAD) administrator style,
      279

    satisfaction and, 30-31
    in sophisticated, learned,
      informed commander
      (SLIC) administrator style,
      274
    stress and, 240-241
    theory and, 198-199
    in worried, anxious determinist
      (WAD) administrator style,
      277-278
Interactional perspective of
  supervision, 13-14
Interactional reactions of supervisors
  and supervisees, 120-130
Interpersonal Process Recall (IPR),
  287
Interpersonal roles vs. conventional,
  313
Intervention. *See also* Therapy
  assessment of knowledge of, 427
  models, 166
  techniques of, 178
Isolation and stress, 250-253

Job satisfaction in social workers,
  231-232
Joint style in cotherapist activity,
  355-356
Jovial outgoing klutz (JOK)
  administrator style, 273-274
Judson, Horace Freeland, 393
Jung, Carl G., 396-397

Kadushin, Alfred, 285,329,
  363-364
Kant, Immanuel, 7
Kenworthy, Marion, 54,381
Kramer, Charles H., 342

Langs, Robert, 208-209
Latent supervision, 148-149
Learning. *See* Education

Learning structure in contracting, 146
Learning Through Supervision by Annette Garrett, 61
Lebeaux, C. N., 364
Lee, Porter, 54,381
Legal liabilities
  administration and, 261-264
  record keeping and, 219-220
  of supervisor, 224-225
Leisure activity and stress, 245,248-250
Levi-Strauss, Claude, 14
Licensing. *See also* Credentialing
  administration and, 267-269
  changes and need for supervision, 21-22
Linguistic analysis, 291-292
Listening in supervision, 15-16
Live supervision, 299-301,302
  in family therapy, 337-338
Long-term care facilities (LTCF)
  role of social workers in, 312-315
    regulations, 315-317
    role support, 317

Machines in clinical practice, 375-376
Malpractice. *See* Legal liabilities
Mediation in agency/clinical practitioner conflict, 162-163
Medical settings
  death and dying, 308-309
  history of social work in, 52-53
  hospice care, 309-310
  knowledge base, 306
  organizational structure, 306-307
  psychological reaction
    of practitioner, 307-308
  terminal illness, 307
Men. *See* Gender and supervision
Mental health
  clinical practice in, 20-21
  diagnosis in, 73-74

Mental Hygiene and Social Work by Porter Lee and Marion Kenworthy, 54
Methods, defined, 178
Meyer, Adolf, 51
Milford Conference, 55,381-382
Minahan, Anne, 382,393
Minuchin, Salvador, 340
Mistakes in clinical practice, 208-209
Modalities, defined, 178
MSW's
  and BSW professionals, 325
  demand for, 65
  learning needs, 32
  in 1960s, 65
  in private practice, 67
Munson, Carlton E., research studies
  audiovisual techniques, resistance to, 285
  autonomous professional, 167
  cotherapist activity, 349-350
  gender and stress, 374
  learning needs of MSW's, 32
  research studies, 4-5
  self-analysis, 28
  students and stress, 232
  supervisees' expectations, 42
  supervision
    guidelines, 34
    style and authority, 163-164
    styles, 101-102
    training, 23-24,25-26
  therapist as role model, 334
  therapy vs. supervision, 37
  women
    career advancement, 373
    practitioners and supervisors, 363

Naisbitt, John, 375
National Association of Social Workers (NASW)
  clinical practice definition, 9
  in geriatric and gerontology settings, 312

history, 63,67
membership, 3
National Association of Social
    Workers Code of Ethics
    document, 434-444
    knowledge of, 90-92
    knowledge survey, 446-448
    supervision and, 88-90
National Conference of Charities
    and Corrections, 50
National Registry of Health Care
    Providers in Clinical Social
    Work, 9
Nature of organization
    and consultation, 359
Need for supervision
    changes in professional standards,
        21-22
    continuing education, 22-23
    ethics in clinical practice, 25
    mental health and clinical practice,
        20-21
    resurgence in clinical practice,
        19-20
    stress in clinical practice,
        24-25
    theory explosion, 21
    training for clinical practice and,
        23-24
Needs of supervisees, 29-32
Nelson, Gary L., 284-285
Nightingale, Florence, 388
Ninety-day review records, 260
Note taking. *See also* Record
        keeping
    in clinical practice evaluation,
        217-218
    in practitioner style, 98-99

Objectives and goals in supervisee
        assessment, 134
Objective tests in learning
        assessment, 74
Observation in supervision, 15

Office arrangement and violence
    and safety, 265
Office pathology, 122-123
Office rationality, 122-123
One-way mirror in supervision
    in family therapy, 338
    in live supervision, 299-301,
        302
Organizational perspective
    of supervision, 13
Organizations
    authority and, 155-156
    conflict with clinical practitioner,
        162-163
    conformity in contracts, 146
    constraints of, 121-123
    consultants in, 356-362
    credentialing, accrediting,
        and service, 430-431
    culture, 359
    ethical responsibility of social
        worker to, 442
    feminist practice and, 368-369
    field instructors, 65
    in medical settings, 306-307
    nature, 359
    need for supervision and, 28
    record keeping, 258-259
    relationships in, 358
    supervisees knowledge of, 134
Oversimplification response,
        124-125
Overwhelming clinical evidence
    in supervisor/supervisee
        relationship, 123

Paired concepts, 187
Paradoxing techniques, 92
Parallel process in live supervision,
        299
Patient. *See* Client/clinical
        practitioner relationship
Pattern recognition in supervision,
        17
Patterns of treatment, 140

Perceived organizational constraints
in supervisor/supervisee
relationship, 121-123
Perception in supervision, 16
Perlman, Helen Harris, 61-62,382
Persistent diagnosis, 33,123-124
Personality perspective
of supervision, 13
Perspective learning, 138-139
Perspectives of supervision, 13-14
Philosopher/philosophical
abstraction in supervision,
106-108,209,252
Philosophy of practice
defined, 178-180,397-399
Physical symptoms of stress,
241-242
Pincus, Allen, 382,393
Planning
of audiovisual device use in live
supervision, 338
in consultation, 359-360
in role play, 294-296
in technician style of supervision,
113-114
Prediction in supervision, 17
Preparation for supervisors, 25-26
Primary relationships vs. secondary,
329-330
Privacy
in client/clinical practitioner
relationship
audiovisual techniques and, 301
ethics, 440
of students and family of origin
material, 342-344
Private practice, emergence in 1970s,
67-68
Privatization, 72-73
Problem solving
in benevolent, affable democrat
(BAD) administrator style,
272
in cool, aloof decider (CAD)
administrator style, 276

in jovial, outgoing klutz (JOK)
administrator style, 273
in sadistic, authoritarian divider
(SAD) administrator style,
279-280
in sophisticated, learned, informed
commander (SLIC)
administrator style, 274
styles of, 99-100
in worried, anxious determinist
(WAD) administrator style,
278
Process and dynamics of family
of origin material, 346
Professionalism and professional
standards
autonomy and, 167
changes and need for supervision,
21-22
effects of supervision on, 225
ethics and, 437-438,442-443
history of, 62,67,70
in private practice, 67-68
Program implementation
in consultation, 358
Progress notes, 260
Propriety as a social worker, 437
Proximity issues
future trends, 75
violence and safety and, 266-267
Pseudo criticism desire, 125-126
Psychiatry
child guidance movement and,
58-59
providing psychotherapy, 20
social work and, 59-60
Psychoanalysis
in clinical practice, 8,20
feminist theory and, 365-366,
369
research studies
effectiveness, 215-216
practitioner perception
of session, 206-208
social work and, 57

theory
    comprehensiveness of, 191
    organization function, 188-189
    verification of, 190-191
Psychosocial therapy, 63-64
Psychotherapy. *See* Psychoanalysis

Questioning as supervision
    technique, 144-155

Rabin, Herbert M., 349
Random activity, 7,399-400
Rank-and-file movement, 56-57
Reactive style of supervision,
    101-102
Reading in supervision, 15,146-148
Reasoned neutrality, 121
Record keeping. *See also* Note
    taking
  as administrative activity, 258-261
  assessment of knowledge of, 427
  in clinical practice evaluation,
    218-221
  in consultation, 360
  in cotherapist activity, 353-354
  fiduciary regulation and, 72
  in long-term care facilities
    (LTCF), 316-317
Recreation and stress, 245,248-250
Reflective problem-solvers, 99-100
Regularity of supervision, 12
Regulations
fiduciary, 72
  in long-term care facilities
    (LTCF), 315-317
Reiter, Laura, 230-231,374
Relationships. *See specific types*
Reporting. *See* Record keeping
Researcher/practitioner relationships,
    222-223
Research studies
  audiovisual techniques
    audio vs. video, 292

    negative effects, 290
    resistance of, 284-285
  background, studies A-I, 4-5
  career advancement for women,
    373
  case study presentation,
    160-161
  in clinical practice evaluation,
    215-217
  cotherapist activity, 349-350
  ethics and, 438-439
  family of origin material
    in training, 342-344
  NASW Code of Ethics knowledge,
    90-91
  in 1960s, 64-65
  practitioner perception of session,
    206-208
  practitioners in therapy, 334
  researcher/practitioner
    relationships, 222-223
  stress in social workers, 230-232
    beginning professionals,
      253,254
    expectations, 237-238
  styles
    authority, 163-164
    supervisor, 101-102
  values and ethics, 82-83
  women
    career choice, 374
    practitioners and supervisors,
      363
Resistance
  to consultation, 361-362
  family of origin material and,
    346-347
  to supervision, 205-206
Resistance stage of stress, 238
Restraint of clients, 267
Reynolds, Bertha Capen, 204,
    364
Richmond, Mary
  art in social work practice,
    381,392

influence on supervision, 53
    role of supervision, 50
Rogers, Carl, 216
Role models
    supervisor as, 247
    therapist as, 334-335
Role of social worker
    in long-term care facilities
            (LTCF), 313-315,317
    in medical settings, 309-310
Role play
    procedures
        debriefing, 298
        evaluation, 297-298
        monitoring, 296-297
        physical setting, 298
        planning, 293-296
    value of, 292-293, 302
Role play deviance, 297
Rosenblatt, Aaron, 222-223
Rural practice settings
    description of, 324-325
    need for supervision, 327-328
    self-reliance in, 325-327
    use of relationship, 329-330

Sadistic, authoritarian divider (SAD)
            administrator style, 279-280
Safety and violence, 264-267
Sanction style of authority, 163-164
Sartre, Jean-Paul, 388
Schon, Donald A., 399
Science in social work practice
    artistic elements and, 383-385
    supervision and, 392-394
    tradition of, 381-383
Secondary relationships vs. primary,
        329-330
SEES system for analyzing family
            therapy interactional
            sequences
    components, 341-342,343
    origin, 5
Self-analysis. See Self-awareness

Self-Analysis by Karen Horney, 55
Self-assessment
    becoming clinical supervisor, 424
    in clinical practice evaluation,
            214-215
    form for practitioners, 450-452
Self-awareness
    of staff in group home, 323-324
    stress and, 244
    in supervisor/supervisee
            relationship, 127-128
Self-monitoring in cotherapist
            activity, 353-354
Self-reliance in rural practice,
            325-327
Selye, Hans, 230,236,238-239
Service as primary obligation, 438
Setting
    of role play, 298
    of supervision
        characteristics, 306
        criminal justice, 317-324
        geriatrics and gerontology,
            310-317
        medical, 306-310
        rural practice, 324-330
    in work and stress, 245,246-247
Sex and supervision. See Gender
            and supervision
Sexual activity in clinical practice,
        25
Shifting the dysfunction in family
            therapy, 341,343
Siporin, Max, 383
Situational perspective
    of supervision, 13
Social Diagnosis by Mary
            Richmond, 53,392
"Social Ethic," 156
Social reform, 50
Social sciences and social work
    early history, 49-50
    1950s, 60-61
Social Service and the Art of Healing
            by Richard Cabot, 54

Social work practice. *See* Clinical practice

Society, ethical responsibility to, 443-444

Sociology and social work
history, 49-50,60-61
theory, 189-190

Sophisticated, learned, informed commander (SLIC) administrator style, 274-275

Specialization in 1960s and 1970s, 65-66

Spencer, Herbert, 230

Staff conference in supervision, 52,54

Stereotyping of the elderly, 311

Streepy, Joan, 231-232

Stress
beginning professional and, 253-254
contributing factors, 243-244
dealing with, 244-246
future trends, 75
gender and, 374-375
isolation and, 250-253
need for supervision and, 24-25
principles of
behavioral indicators, 240-243
expectation source, 237-238
general adaptation syndrome, 236
process of reactions, 238-240
recreation and, 248-250
research studies of, among clinical practitioners, 230-232
of staff in group homes, 322-323
students and, 232-233
supervision and, 233-234, 246-247
of supervisors, 234-235
support in, 235-236

Stress scale
long form questionnaire, 468-472
short form, 454-456

Stress Without Distress by Hans Selye, 230

Structure
authority and, 161-163
of consultation, 359-361
in contracting, 146
of supervision, 12
of treatment, 177

Students. *See also* Beginning professionals
audiovisual techniques and, 290-291
in cotherapist activity, 352
family of origin material in training, 342-344
role play and, 293-296
stress and, 232-233

Studies. *See* Research studies

Studies A-I, 4-5

Sturdivant, S., 364-365

Style of family in family therapy, 341,343

Style of practice. *See also* Style of supervision
in cotherapist activity, 352,355-356
espoused theory in, 399
philosophy of practice in, 397-399
philosophy of life in, 397
random activity in, 399-400
technique in, 399
theory in use, 399
understanding of treatment process in, 399

Style of supervision, 6,18-19. *See also* Style of practice
administrator
benevolent, affable democrat (BAD), 270-273
cool, aloof decider (CAD), 275-277
jovial, outgoing klutz (JOK), 273-274

sadistic, authoritarian divider
(SAD), 279-280
sophisticated, learned, informed
commander (SLIC), 274-275
worried, anxious determinist
(WAD), 277-279
applying, 103-105
authority and, 163-164
as concept, 99-103
defined, 96-97
evaluation of clinical practice and,
209
observing, 97-98
as resource, 98-99
stress and, 252
substyles
philosopher/philosophical
abstraction, 106-108
technician/technical strategy,
111-114
theoretical orientation, 114
theoretician/theoretical
arguments, 108-111
Substance abuse in social workers,
231
Substance-abuse counselors, 86,87
Supervisees. *See also* Clinical
practice; Clinical
practitioners
Bill of Rights, 39-40
characteristics, 26-28
criticism of, 212-213
educational assessment of,
132-135
expectations, 42
NASW Code of Ethics and, 89
need of, 29-32
self-assessment, 214-215
supervisor styles, reaction to
ambush interaction, 128
expectations, 118-120
interactional reactions,
120-121
oversimplification response,
124-125

overwhelming clinical evidence,
123
perceived organizational
constraints, 121-123
persistent diagnosis, 123-124
pseudo criticism desire, 125-126
reasoned neutrality, 121
self-analysis, 127-128
theoretical speculation, 126-127
Supervision
administrative activities
credentials and examinations,
267-269
dealing with other
administrators, 269-270
duty to warn, 262-264
legal issues, 261-262
record keeping, 258-261
styles, 270-280
violence and safety, 264-267
art and science in social work
practice, 392-394
assessment of learning in clinical
practice
administrative, 221-222
criticism, 210-213
decreasing defensiveness,
205-206
follow-up, 210
note taking, 217-218
practice errors, 208-210
record keeping, 218-221
research in, 215-217,222-225
self-assessment, 214-215
simplification, 206-208
assessment scale for becoming
supervisor, 424
audiovisual techniques in, 284-292
authority and, 36,156-159
age, 165
autonomy, 165-169
in group model, 169-173
vs. independence, 154-155
interaction, 159-161
in organizations, 155-156

structure, 161-163
style, 163-164
beginning professionals, 27-28
characteristics, 35,38-39
consequences of, 37-38
cost, 17-18
defined, 10-11
in education, 3,7
expectations of, 40-42
five basic actions, 15-16
function, 11-13
guidelines, 34
history
    early, 47-50
    Freudian influence, 51-53
    1920s, 54-55
    1930s, 56-57
    1940s, 58-59
    1950s, 59-63
    1960s, 63-65
    1970s, 65-69
    1980s, 69-70
    1990s, 70-77
    practice theory and, 46
    Richmond, Mary, and, 53
live, 299-301,302
need for, 19-25
organizational obstacles, 28
perspectives, 13-14
practice research and, 222-225
preparation for, 25-26
role play
    procedures, 293-298
    value of, 292-293,302
settings
    criminal justice, 317-324
    geriatrics and gerontology,
        310-317
    medical, 306-310
    rural practice, 324-330
situations
    consultation, 356-362
    cotherapist activity,
        349-356
    ergonomics, 375-376

family of origin material in,
    342-349
family therapy, 335-342
gender and, 362-375
practitioners in therapy, 334-335
stress
    in beginning professional,
        253-254
    in clinical practitioners,
        230-232
    contributing factors, 243-244
    dealing with, 244-246
    general principles, 236-243
    isolation and, 250-253
    recreation and, 248-250
    students and, 232-233
    of supervisors, 234-235
    supervisors in, 233-234
    supervisor training, 250
    support in, 235-236
styles, 6,18-19
    applying, 103-105
    as concept, 100-103
    defined, 96-97
    observing, 97-98
    as resource, 98-99
    substyles, 105-114
    theoretical orientation and, 114
supervisees
    assessment and diagnosis, 32-34
    expectations, 118-120
    interactional reactions, 120-129
    needs of, 29-32
support for, 37
technique
    case material and, 135-138
    continuity and, 139-140
    contracting, 145-146
    educational assessment,
        132-135
    guidelines, 150
    knowledge level and, 138-139
    latent supervision and, 148-149
    mechanics of, 140-141
    overcoming difficulty, 141-143

questioning as, 144-145
reading as, 146-148
supervisor resistance and,
    149-150
treatment patterns, 140
theory in, 176-177
    abandonment of, 194-197
    application, 197-198
    components of, 190
    creativity and, 197
    elements of, 184-188
    functions of, 188-190
    guidelines for application,
        200-201
    interaction and, 198-199
    practice and, 183-184
    speculation, 192-193
    teaching, 181-182
    technique and, 193-194
    timing, 193
thought process, 16-17
vs. treatment skills, 36-37
values and ethics
    concepts of, 83-85
    knowledge of, 85-88
    NASW Code of Ethics,
        88-92
    research studies, 82-83
    violations, 92-93
Supervision questionnaire,
    458-465
Supervisor response strategy
in benevolent, affable democrat
    (BAD) administrator style,
    272-273
in cool, aloof decider (CAD)
    administrator style, 276-277
in jovial, outgoing klutz (JOK)
    administrator style, 273-274
in sadistic, authoritarian divider
    (SAD) administrator style,
    280
in sophisticated, learned, informed
    commander (SLIC)
    administrator style, 275
in worried, anxious determinist
    (WAD) administrator style,
    278-279
Supervisory intervention models,
    166
Support for supervisors, 37
Support role
    vs. nonsupport in supervisors, 29
    in supervision, 235-236,317
Systems theory, 62,68-69

Taft, Jessie, 58
Tarasoff rule, 262-264
Team functioning in medical
    settings, 310
Technical skill learning, 138-139
Technician/technical strategy in
    supervision,111-114,209,
    252
Technique, defined, 177-178
Technique in supervision
    case material and, 135-138
    continuity and, 139-140
    contracting, 145-146
    difficulties in, 141-143
    educational assessment and,
        131-135
    in family therapy, 339-340
    guidelines, 150
    knowledge level and, 138-139
    latent supervision and, 148-149
    mechanics of, 140-141
    in practice style, 399
    questioning in, 144-145
    reading as, 146-148
    supervisor resistance and,
        149-150
    theory and, 193-194
    vs. treatment, 36-37
    treatment patterns in, 140
Television. *See* Audiovisual
    techniques
Terminal illness, 307
Termination records, 260
The Family, 52,54

Theoretical speculation
   in supervisor/supervisee
     relationship, 126-127
Theoretician/theoretical arguments
   in supervision, 108-111
Theory
  abandonment, 194-197
  application, 197-198,200-201
  assessment of knowledge of, 426
  beginning professionals'
    knowledge of, 27
  clinical practice and, 183-184
  components, 190-192
  in cotherapist activity, 355
  creativity and, 197
  elements
    concepts, 185
    facts, 184-185
    hypotheses, 185-188
  ethics of, 92
  explosion and need
    for supervision, 21
  in family therapy
    diagnosis and, 340
    technique and, 339-340
  in feminist practice, 364-366
  functions
    explanation, 189-190
    organization, 188-189
    prediction, 190
  history of supervision and
    1930s, 46
    1950s, 61-62
    1960s, 63-64
    1970s, 68-69
    1980s, 69
  organizational, 28
  philosophy of practice and, 399
  speculation, 192
  supervisees' knowledge of, 133
  in supervision, 114,176-177
  supervision interaction and,
    198-199
  teaching of, 181-182
  technique and, 193-194

terminology clarification
  clinical practice, 181
  ideology and, 180-181
  methods, 178
  modalities, 178
  philosophy of practice, 178-180
  techniques, 177-178
  timing, 193
Therapeutic eclecticism, 58
Therapists as role models, 334-335
Therapy
  patterns, 140
  process, 260
  in practice style, 399
  vs. supervision, 36-37
Thistle, Pamela, 344
Thomas, Lewis, 394
Thought process in supervision,
    16-17
Timing and theory, 193
Timing element in contracting, 146
Towle, Charlotte, 60-61,62
Traditional supervisors vs. clinical
    supervisors, 37-38
Training. *See* Education
Treatment. *See* Therapy
Tuskegee Study, 224

Ullmann, Liv, 390

Values
  assessment of supervisees, 134
  concepts and behavior, 83-85
  knowledge and, 85-88
  in philosophy of practice, 179
  research studies of, 82-83
Videotapes. *See* Audiovisual
    techniques
Violence and safety, 264-267

Warning devices and safety, 266
Weisman, Avery, 309
Whitaker, Carl, 103,351

Whyte, William, 156
Wilensky, H. L., 364
Wolman, Benjamin B., 234-235,253
Women. *See* Gender and supervision

Worried, anxious determinist (WAD)
 administrator style, 277-279
Writing. *See* Note taking; Record
 keeping